THE COMPLETE EATER'S DIGEST AND NUTRITION SCOREBOARD

The Complete Eater's Digest and Nutrition Scoreboard

MICHAEL F. JACOBSON

ANCHOR PRESS/DOUBLEDAY
GARDEN CITY, NEW YORK
1985

Library of Congress Cataloging in Publication Data
Jacobson, Michael F.
The complete eater's digest.
Bibliography: p. 371
Includes index.
1. Food additives. 2. Food—Composition. I. Title.
TX553.A3J22   1985   641.1   82-45857
ISBN: 0-385-18245-7

Nutrition Scoreboard copyright © 1974, 1975 by Michael F. Jacobson
Eater's Digest copyright © 1972, 1976 by Michael F. Jacobson
New material in *The Complete Eater's Digest and Nutrition Scoreboard* copyright 1985
by Michael F. Jacobson

All Rights Reserved
Printed in the United States of America
First Edition

Preface

Food. It's such a simple four-letter word. Not very emotional. Food is something that we all grew up with. Ate it several times a day. But we never gave much thought to it . . . and sometimes still don't.

I remember when I was little that soda pop was the beverage we drank at dinner, if we didn't drink milk. And picnics meant hot dogs and hamburgers. Ball games at Wrigley Field meant peanuts and hot dogs. All summer long we played baseball in Hollywood Park and had a lunch and snacks at McDonald's —this was 1957 and it was probably one of the first—across the street. A friend behind the counter would give us four free hamburgers and fries for every one we paid for. Food was something that you ate to stop hunger.

Thinking back upon it, there wasn't much variety, either. I didn't dig my teeth into a stuffed lobster or steamed artichoke until my twenties. Food was hamburgers and french fries, hamburgers and mashed potatoes, frankfurters and macaroni, and some broccoli, carrots, and homegrown corn in the summer. On school days I would treat myself to some Fritos at lunch and to a couple of Hostess Twinkies after I got home. It certainly wasn't the best diet one could eat, but it certainly wasn't the worst, either. It was just what everyone ate. And anyone who ate anything different was a nut. I remember snickering at one crazy guy who used *honey,* instead of sugar, on his cornflakes; little did I realize then . . .

Somehow food didn't have much to do with health. Recently, I saw an old home movie, vintage 1959, showing our whole family at one of our Sunday backyard picnics. All the aunts and uncles as well as my brother and sisters and cousins were there. The uncles were making big, fat hamburgers on the outdoor grill. Everyone was smiling in the film. But, sadly, three of the four uncles are now dead, having had their coronaries at about the actuarially expected times. No one ever associated the hamburgers with the heart attacks. You just die "when your number is up."

I never did learn anything about nutrition in college or graduate school, though I could have recited metabolic cycles—how cells turn food into energy

—forward and backward. When I was an undergraduate at the University of Chicago, I lived, barely, for the better part of a semester on canned spaghetti and meatballs. One summer though, around 1964, I must have run into some early food freaks, because I became a vegetarian for several days. Unfortunately, I didn't get the right instructions. I thought vegetarians ate only vegetables, so it was a pound of broccoli one day, a pound of brussels sprouts the next, and so on. I never did hear about grains and beans, so that first brush with better nutrition was a short one.

In graduate school, while studying microbiology at M.I.T., diet was still not anything that I, or anyone I knew, cared about. Even though my lab was only one flight of stairs from the nutrition department, any inklings about nutrition eluded me totally. For snacks it was a Fresca out of the vending machine on the seventh floor. For lunch, it was a homemade bologna sandwich on white bread and some gloppy packaged pastry out of the machines in the basement, just a floor below the aforementioned nutrition department.

My ignorance of nutrition, my total obliviousness to something that could impact decisively on my health, was typical of virtually all Americans (except the few that we might have made fun of). We never thought about what we ate. Or why we ate it. Or who was persuading us to eat it. Or why our choices were limited. Or why our health departments were doing nothing to educate us. All we knew was that "Americans had the safest food supply in the world" and that per capita "Americans spent less on food than any other nation" and that "American supermarkets offered a wider choice of foods than you could get anywhere else in the world." And that was that.

I first got involved with food, in a professional way, when I went to Washington in 1970 to work with consumer activist Ralph Nader. James Turner, an attorney working with Nader, had just finished writing *Chemical Feast,* a book about the ineffectiveness of the Food and Drug Administration (FDA). This was just after the banning of the artificial sweetener cyclamate. Nader and Turner thought that it would be appropriate for me, having scientific training, to write a book about a large group of chemicals that FDA regulates. That I knew nothing about and had no previous interest in food additives, let alone that I had never even thought of writing a book, did not seem to bother my Washington guides. In the subsequent several years, I wrote two books, one about food additives, *Eater's Digest,* the other about nutrition, *Nutrition Scoreboard,* and have learned far more about these subjects than I had dreamt existed.

The present book is a total revision of those two books and a story of some of the things I have learned about chemicals in food, nutrition and health, why we eat what we do, the food industry, and how the government works. So after too many years, I at last learned that diet has an enormous effect on health. I was amazed to discover that the typical American diet contributes to many of the most common health problems, ranging from tooth decay and constipation to heart disease and stroke. While food additives introduce some of the problems, the foods themselves, laden with fat and salt, are responsible for the bulk of the problems. I hope that the *Complete Eater's Digest and Nutrition Scoreboard* convinces the reader that food can do a lot more than just slake hunger . . . and inspires every reader to make some dietary changes for the better.

Acknowledgments

It is a pleasure to thank publicly some of the many people who offered assistance and advice and helped educate me about nutrition and food additives in the past decade.

Jan Zimmerman, with help from the University of Maryland computer department, helped develop the formula for rating the nutritional value of foods. The present formula was built upon my original work with Jim Silverman, who, with his trusty slide rule, helped me develop the formula used in the first edition of *Nutrition Scoreboard*.

Bonnie Liebman is our resident nutrition expert at the Center for Science in the Public Interest. She has been a great help in explaining diet-related health problems, especially those related to excesses of fat, cholesterol, sodium, and sugar, and deficiencies of dietary fiber. Her many articles in *Nutrition Action* on fish, salt, cancer, dietary fiber, alcohol, "health foods," and other topics, as well as her thoughtful comments on this manuscript, were uniquely helpful. She was responsible for compiling most of the information in the charts on the fat, sodium, and sugar content of foods.

To Karen Jeffrey, a word of thanks for her help in gathering information about certain food additives. And another thank you to the scientists and secretaries in FDA's Division of Food and Color Additives for guiding me to the files on various additives. Ogden Johnson, nutritionist at Hershey Foods, provided useful comments on how industry is using numerous additives.

Many staff members of CSPI and other public interest groups over the years have also contributed in one way or another to this work. Ralph Nader provided me with my first postgraduate course in consumer advocacy. Patti Hausman, Greg Moyer, Frensch Niegermeier, Bill Schultz, Bruce Silverglade, and Bambi Batts-Young have all helped, either with specific suggestions and criticisms or by having written extremely informative books and petitions. D'Anne DuBois, my skilled and loyal assistant, Barbara Franklin, Jim Gollin, and Brian Corbin helped with background research or typing.

Contents

PREFACE	v
ACKNOWLEDGMENTS	viii
PART ONE: *Nutrition Scoreboard*	1
I. *The American Way of Eating*	3
II. *Rating the Nutritional Value of Foods*	31

      Protein
      Carbohydrate
      Fat
      Cholesterol
      Salt/Sodium
      Vitamins and Minerals
          Vitamin A
          Riboflavin (Vitamin B_2)
          Niacin (Vitamin B_3)
          Vitamin C
          Iron
          Calcium
          Calories

III. *Beyond the Nutrition Scoreboard Formula*	104

      Food Additives
      Trace Minerals
      Organically Grown Food
      Alcohol
      Food for Babies

IV. *The Nutritional Ratings of Common Foods*	113

      Beans, Nuts, and Seeds
      Grain Foods: Bread, Rice, and Pasta

       Meat, Poultry, Eggs, and Fish
       Dairy Foods
       Nondairy Beverages
       Vegetables
       Fruits
       Breakfast Cereals
       Desserts
       Snacks
       Condiments

NOTES   159

APPENDIX I. *The Nutrition Scoreboard Formula*   163

APPENDIX II. *1983 Advertising Budgets of Major Food Companies*   167

APPENDIX III. *Job Changes Between Government and Industry*   168

SELECTED BIBLIOGRAPHY   172

PART TWO: *Eater's Digest*   173

   V. *An Overview of Food Additives*   175
      Introduction
      Why Are Additives Used
      The Scope of This Book
      Safety: The Number One Priority
      How Are Food Additives Tested?
      Is the Government Guarding Your Health?
      Notes

   VI. *A Close-up Look at Food Additives*   209
      acesulfame-K
      acetic acid
      acetone peroxide
      adipic acid
      agar
      alginates
      alpha tocopherol
      aluminum compounds
      ammoniated glycyrrhizin
      ammonium compounds
      amylases
      arabinogalactan
      artificial coloring
          Blue 1

      Blue 2
      Citrus Red 2
      Green 3
      Orange B
      Red 3
      Red 40
      Yellow 5
      Yellow 6
artificial flavoring
ascorbic acid
ascorbyl palmitate
aspartame
azodicarbonamide
benzoyl peroxide
beta-carotene and Vitamin A
brominated vegetable oil
butylated hydroxyanisole (BHA)
butylated hydroxytoluene (BHT)
caffeine
calcium compounds
calcium and sodium propionate
calcium and sodium stearoyl lactylates and sodium stearoyl fumarate
caramel
carbon dioxide (carbonated water)
carboxymethylcellulose (CMC, cellulose gum), cellulose, and related compounds
carnauba wax
carrageenan
casein
chewing gum base
chlorine
chlorine dioxide
cinnamaldehyde
citric acid
corn syrup, high fructose corn syrup
cysteine
dextrin
dextrose (glucose, corn sugar)
dimethylpolysiloxane (methyl silicone, methyl polysilicone)
dioctyl sodium sulfosuccinate (DSS)
disodium guanylate (GMP), disodium inosinate (IMP)
EDTA (ethylenediamine tetraacetic acid)

ergosterol
ferrous gluconate
fructose
fumaric acid
furcelleran
gelatin
gluconic acid
glycerin (glycerol)
glycine (aminoacetic acid)
guar gum
gum arabic (acacia gum, gum senegal)
gum ghatti
gum guaiac
helium
hesperidin
hydrolyzed vegetable protein (HVP)
hydroxylated lecithin
invert sugar
iron compounds (ferric ammonium citrate, ferric phosphate, ferric pyrophosphate, ferric sodium pyrophosphate, ferrous citrate, ferrous lactate, ferrous sulfate, reduced iron)
karaya gum
lactic acid
lactose
lecithin
locust bean gum (carob seed gum, St. John's bread)
magnesium compounds (magnesium carbonate, magnesium chloride, magnesium hydroxide, magnesium phosphate, magnesium stearate, magnesium sulfate, and other magnesium-containing salts)
malic acid
maltol, ethyl maltol
manganese
mannitol
meat tenderizer
mono- and diglycerides and related substances
monosodium glutamate (MSG)
niacin
nitrous oxide
pantothenic acid (and sodium pantothenate)
papain
parabens

pectin (and sodium pectinate)
phosphoric acid
polydextrose
polysorbate 60, 65, 80
potassium compounds (potassium bicarbonate, potassium hydroxide, potassium phosphate, potassium sulfate, and other potassium salts)
potassium bromate, calcium bromate
potassium chloride
potassium iodide, cuprous iodide, potassium or calcium iodate
propyl gallate
propylene glycol, propylene glycol mono- and diesters
propylene glycol alginate
pyridoxine (or pyridoxine hydrochloride)
quillaia
quinine
riboflavin (or riboflavin-5 phosphate)
saccharin
silicates, silicon dioxide
smoke flavoring
sodium compounds
sodium benzoate
sodium erythorbate, erythorbic acid, sodium isoascorbate
sodium nitrate, sodium nitrite
sorbic acid, potassium sorbate
sorbitan monostearate
sorbitol
stannous chloride
starch
starch, modified
stearic acid, calcium stearate, stearyl citrate
succistearin
sucrose
sucrose polyester (SPE)
sulfiting agents—sulfur dioxide, potassium metabisulfite, sodium bisulfite, sodium metabisulfite, sodium sulfite
tannin, tannic acid
tartaric acid, potassium acid tartrate, sodium potassium tartrate, sodium tartrate
TBHQ (tertiary butylhydroquinone)
textured vegetable protein (TVP), isolated soy protein
thiamin mononitrate, thiamin hydrochloride

titanium dioxide
tragacanth gum
vanillin, ethyl vanillin, vanilla
vegetable oil
vitamin A (palmitate)
vitamin D (D_2)
xanthan gum
xylitol
yellow prussiate of soda

VII. *Food Additive Cemetery* — 352
cyclamate
diethyl pyrocarbonate
Red 2 (amaranth)
Red 4 (ponceau SX)
Violet 1

GLOSSARY — 360

BIBLIOGRAPHY — 371

INDEX — 376

ABOUT THE AUTHOR — 391

1
Nutrition Scoreboard

Some All-Star Foods

Food	Serving Size	Nutritional Score
wheat germ	1/2 cup	120
black beans	1/2 cup, cooked	93
spinach	2 cups, raw	93
sweet potato	1 medium, baked	82
tuna, water-packed	3 ounces	75
watermelon	10" × 1" slice	68
yogurt, lowfat, plain	8 ounces	64
whole wheat bread	2 slices	55

Some Junkyard Foods

Food	Serving Size	Nutritional Score
butter	1 pat	−13
American cheese	2 ounces	−18
hot dog	1 (1.6 ounces)	−20
chocolate éclair	1	−30
Hostess Twinkies	1 package	−34
Spam	3 ounces	−35
soda pop	12 ounces	−55

—avoid fat, cholesterol, salt, sugar—

I

The American Way of Eating

People who eat brown rice and whole wheat bread are sometimes called food faddists, while others who gobble Twinkies and Sugar Frosted Flakes are considered normal, red-blooded Americans. At a time when nutritionists and dentists decry diets high in fat and sugar, Betty Crocker and Sara Lee continue to be two of America's favorite cooks. While the most healthful meals are brimming over with green vegetables, whole grains, and fresh fruits, the big advertising budgets are pushing beer, soda pop, and fast-food hamburgers. Alice would feel quite at home in the wonderland of manufactured foods, food advertising, and corporate cooks.

Food is a fascinating subject. By examining our food supply from different perspectives, we can learn about economics, human behavior, politics, nutrition, farming, ecology, and toxicology. A comprehensive treatise on food would be monumental and would certainly tax to the breaking point the patience and intelligence of any mortal writer. For the present then, let us focus on two of the most interesting aspects of food: nutrition and its effect on health, and the factors that influence our eating habits.

Malnutrition means not eating the right balance of foods. In the United States we have three broad classes of malnutrition. The first is hunger. This is the most brutal form of poor nutrition. Secondly, some people have generally good diets, but, because of their food choices or special needs, are deficient in one or more particular nutrients. Finally, the most widespread form of malnutrition and the one we will be focusing on is *over*nutrition . . . too much of the wrong foods. This is a most deadly form of poor nutrition but, fortunately, one that anyone can defeat—inexpensively and deliciously.

America's war against hunger started in the 1960s and expanded greatly in the 1970s, when congressional hearings and the news media publicized the shocking extent of hunger. The United States now has numerous federal programs, including subsidized school breakfasts and lunches, special aid for pregnant or nursing women, elderly feeding programs, and food stamps to help ward off hunger. By 1980, 11.9 million children received free or reduced-price school lunches, 1.9 million mothers and babies benefited from the highly efficient and successful WIC (women/infants/children) program, and 19.2 million people received food stamps. This multifaceted program was so successful that hunger was virtually eradicated in the United States. But then came Ronald Reagan.

After moving into the Oval Office in 1981, President Reagan started making good on his campaign promises to reduce federal spending on domestic programs. He put a meat ax to the food programs, and once again hunger reared its ugly head. In 1981, funding for the school lunch program was cut by about one third. Less than half the number of people eligible for the food stamp and elderly nutrition programs were participating, partly due to lack of funding. Lack of funding also kept over 6 million low-income women and children—70 percent of those eligible—out of the WIC program. The President's official commission on hunger said that the number of hungry people could not be estimated with any accuracy (and presidential adviser Ed Meese said that people choose to be poor). But other surveys confirmed what common sense would suggest: when you reduce federal food programs, you end up with more hungry people. The privately funded Physician Task Force on Hunger in America estimated in 1985 that "up to 20 million citizens may be hungry at least some period of time each month" and relatively vulnerable to illness.

While governmental food assistance programs are not the final or most desirable answer for millions of poor people, they have been lifesaving for many. Hunger—and the need for government assistance programs—won't ever be eliminated completely, until poverty is wiped out.

The second kind of malnutrition relates not to hunger, but to specific nutrient deficiencies due to an ill-chosen diet. Women frequently have diets low in iron and calcium. Among some ethnic groups and in some regions of the country, diets may be deficient in vitamin A or other nutrients. Sometimes these specific deficiencies can be corrected by a well-designed program of nutrition education or, in the short term, by vitamin/mineral pills.

The U.S. Department of Agriculture (USDA) conducts surveys about every ten years to analyze the nutritional status of the population. The most recent survey (April 1977–March 1978) included about 34,000 individuals in 15,000 households. Americans were in great shape as far as protein, vitamin C, riboflavin (vitamin B_2), and niacin (vitamin B_3) were concerned. Almost every population/age group also consumed adequate amounts of phosphorus, vitamin A, thiamin (vitamin B_1), and vitamin B_{12}. Of the nutrients examined, the major problems were calcium, iron, magnesium, and vitamin B_6. Women, as well as older men and teenaged boys, tended to consume too little calcium, which is vital in maintaining strong teeth and bones. Inadequate iron was a problem for toddlers and women between twelve and fifty years of age. And all groups over two years of age had less than the Recommended Dietary Allowance for magnesium and vitamin B_6. Many people also consume too little zinc, selenium, folacin (a B vitamin), but intakes of these nutrients were not determined in the USDA study. Intake of some nutrients, such as iron for babies and vitamin C for the general population, increased significantly since 1965 due to the fortification of specific foods.

Although poor nutrition has traditionally been thought of in terms of vitamin, mineral, and protein deficiencies, millions of Americans suffer another kind of malnutrition: too rich a diet—too many calories, too much fat, too much salt (sodium), too much cholesterol, too much alcohol. It is somewhat ironic that after centuries of worrying about starvation, much of humankind finally overcame deprivation only to suffer the ravages of food excesses. This third form of malnutrition is by far the greatest nutritional problem in the United States, Canada, and most other technologically advanced nations. Millions of people are suffering incalculable pain, paying enormous medical costs, or dying prematurely, because of maladies ranging from tooth decay, constipation, and obesity to diabetes, stroke, heart disease, and cancer. These chronic, degenerative diseases are epidemic and account for about half of all deaths. Most people assume that these serious health problems are a natural and inescapable part of life. Wrong! These health problems are virtually unknown in some cultures. In short, these should be considered *unnecessary diseases*. We will discuss many of these diseases in greater detail later.

The unnecessary diseases take a toll that can only be called awesome. Consider the following statistics on various diseases caused by diet (sometimes in combination with other factors):

- 59,400 deaths from colon cancer in 1984 and 90,000 new cases[1] (high-fat diets, lack of dietary fiber)
- 37,300 deaths from breast cancer in 1984 and 115,000 new cases[2] (high-fat diets)
- 545,000 deaths from coronary heart disease in 1984 and 1,250,000 heart attacks[3] (too much fat and cholesterol)
- 60 million people have high blood pressure[4] (too much sodium and fat)
- 156,000 stroke deaths in 1983 and 550,000 cerebral hemorrhages[5] (too much sodium and fat)
- adult-onset diabetes accounts for 135,000 deaths (mostly heart attacks) each year[6] (too much fat, too little dietary fiber)
- 5,000 cases of blindness from adult-onset diabetes each year[7] (too much fat and sugar)

- the average seventeen year old in 1979–80 had eleven decayed, missing, or filled teeth; Americans spend billions each year repairing rotten teeth[8] (too much sugar)
- Americans spend about $400 million each year on laxatives to alleviate constipation[9] (too little fiber)
- approximately 14 percent of adult men and 24 percent of adult women are 20 percent or more above their desirable weight; one third of adults are 10 percent or more overweight[10] (too many calories, too little exercise).

The unnecessary diseases develop slowly and quietly—not like measles or the flu—and reflect the gradual disintegration of bodily organs and processes. They may begin in childhood, but not be evident until middle or old age. It is much harder to be concerned about an unseen enemy that will not reveal itself for twenty or thirty years than about an acute infectious disease—yet the two may be equally deadly. That the diseases are caused by eating tempting foods makes it all the harder to fend them off. Understanding the long-term ill effects of the average American diet is the first step you can take toward better health.

If health considerations are not impressive enough to cause most people to change their diets, rising food prices may be. The diet that is best for our health can also be relatively inexpensive. Meat is the most expensive item in most of our food budgets and a major source of fat and cholesterol. Coca-Cola costs more than milk, but has no real nutritional value—just lots of sugar and a dose of caffeine. Beans, lentils, brown rice, and potatoes are dirt cheap compared with the meat or cheese for which they can substitute. I estimate that people concerned about nutrition spend about one third less money on their food bills than those people whose shopping carts are overflowing with soda pop and hot dogs.

When calculating the true cost of food, we should really include the long-term health consequences of a bad diet. A good part of the many billions of dollars we spend every year in treating diabetes, diverticulosis (an intestinal problem), constipation, and heart disease more properly belongs in the food budget than in the health budget. For our nation as a whole, the direct (doctor and hospital bills, medicines, etc.) and indirect costs (time lost from work) related to heart disease come to about $65 billion a year. Alcohol-related problems translate into $120 billion costs. Cancer, stroke, dental caries, and diabetes add additional billions. How wonderful it would be if these vast sums could be devoted to more socially productive purposes than repairing clogged arteries, buying pills, and financing doctors' vacations.

In June 1974, the Senate Select Committee on Nutrition and Human Needs sponsored a three-day National Nutrition Policy Study that brought together many of the nation's leading nutritionists, food industry executives, economists, and public interest advocates. The panel on Nutrition and Health focused its attention on heart disease, obesity, diabetes, and similar health problems. The panel said that, "a few simple changes in the American diet and habits of life could greatly reduce the number of people who acquire these diseases and may die from them." In its report, the panel strongly recommended that Americans switch to a diet low in calories, saturated fat, sugar, cholesterol, and salt:

> The "alternative diet" is designed to prevent disease and, at the same time, is nutritionally adequate. Because it is largely but not completely derived from legumes [pod vegetables: beans, peas, peanuts, etc.], grains, vegetable and fruit products, it is less expensive to produce in terms of resources than the present American diet based much more on food products derived from animals.

It is ironic that the richest people in the history of the world should have such widespread diet-related diseases, while certain far more primitive populations have well-balanced diets and enjoy excellent health. An article in *Science* magazine described the !Kung* people, who have lived as hunters and gatherers in the Kalahari Desert of southern Africa for at least 11,000 years. Their diet consists of nuts, vegetables, and lean meat and lacks milk and grains. Researchers found very few cases of either nutritional deficiencies or excesses, with degenerative diseases being equally rare.[11]

The standard American diet offers much more variety than the !Kung enjoy, but we are paying the price. Our diet, loaded with fat, salt, and sugar, and containing little dietary fiber (roughage) is a novel experience for the human metabolic pathways, which during tens of thousands of years of evolution became accustomed to a diet more like the !Kung's.

But there have been holdouts—even in the United States. Some individuals and groups have avoided meat and much of the fare so widely advertised on television and sold in supermarkets, restaurants, and vending machines. Adherents to the Seventh-Day Adventist (SDA) faith provide an example and can serve as a basis of comparison for the rest of the population. SDAers eat little meat and consume somewhat less fat than the average American. Their diet is high in grains, fruits, and vegetables, and therefore relatively high in dietary fiber. Strict adherents are vegetarians, nonsmokers, and nondrinkers. With this kind of lifestyle, it is no accident that Seventh-Day Adventists are remarkably healthy. According to one study, their death rate is 35 percent lower than the general population's. They suffer 30 percent fewer deaths due to heart disease, 25 percent fewer deaths due to cancer, and 80 percent less cirrhosis of the liver. The risk of death due to mouth and lung cancer is half as great among Seventh-Day Adventists as the rest of the population.[12] The remarkable contrast between SDAers and the general population would have been even greater

---

* The "!" represents a clicking sound.

if only strict adherents to the Seventh-Day Adventist way of life had been included in the study.

The sound nutritional advice offered by the panel on Nutrition and Health got only a line or two in the newspapers back in June 1974, and did not cause many people to eat any differently, but it marked the beginning of a path that was to lead to major changes in America's nutrition policy and eating habits. Opposing the dietary changes, though, were industries whose profits depended upon the sale of foods that promoted illness, not health.

Eating the kind of diet that optimizes health should be a national priority. For many years, though, advice about eating was left almost exclusively to the food industry, and, boy, did they do a number on us! The ad budgets of big food companies are absolutely astonishing (see Appendix II). Hershey Foods Corp. spent $68 million on advertising in 1983. Campbell Soup Co. spent $126 million. Coca-Cola spent $282 million, a figure that McDonald's Corp. exceeded by $29 million. General Foods, which makes Jell-O, Cool Whip, Maxwell House Coffee, Oscar Mayer hot dogs, and other nutritional nothings, spent $386 million on radio, TV, newspaper, magazine, and billboard advertising. The top twenty food advertisers spent $4.4 billion on advertising. And this is only part of the picture. The companies generally spend about as much on other promotions: leaflets, brochures, "educational" movies, coupon discounts, shelf-markers in supermarkets, and trade shows. Though no one has calculated the total amount spent on food advertising and promotion a year, I would estimate that the grand total is about $15 billion.

Have you noticed that heavily processed, nonnutritious foods are advertised much more heavily than whole wheat bread, broccoli, and bananas? The reason for this gets to the heart of the problems with our food supply. If you grew broccoli, put your name on it, and started advertising it, some shoppers might go to the supermarket and look for your brand, because of its "delicate freshness," "rich, deep, farm-fresh color," or other advertised quality. However, right next to Jean Green's broccoli they might see other bunches of broccoli that looked exactly the same, but were a few cents cheaper, because their grower did not advertise. The chances are they would figure that the cheaper stuff was just the same as your broccoli and buy the former. So you ran the ads, but your competitor got the sales. Next time, though, you got smart. You froze the broccoli and smothered it in some gloppy sauce. Then you went out to advertise your product, and shoppers discovered that yours was the only frozen broccoli in Chef Jean's secret sauce. They were sold by the ad and then bought your brand, because there was no choice. Eventually, another company mimicked your product, so you had to develop a newer version, perhaps frozen broccoli with three different packets of sauce mixes, so the consumer could demonstrate his or her own culinary skill while making broccoli. The next twist would probably be an "all natural" frozen broccoli, with a special "no preservative added" sauce and a premium "natural" price! "Product differentiation" is the name of the game and the reason why most advertising is for heavily processed foods.

It is true that ads for potatoes or oranges do show up occasionally on TV. These are sponsored by state commissions (Washington apples, Idaho potatoes, Texas grapefruits, etc.). These campaigns are all too rare and quiet. People in the produce industry tell me that most growers are barely surviving and are reluctant to ante up the funds.

So what if companies advertise their junk on TV, you might say. Parents and teachers can teach kids what to eat and what to avoid. If you ever took a close look in the classroom, you'd find that many of the companies are actually feeding teachers and students pretty unpalatable fare in the form of charts, leaflets, filmstrips, movies, and ads and planted articles in classroom magazines. From McDonald's to the Pickle Packers International, Inc. to the National Macaroni Institute, the information comes pouring forth, each industry shouting the glories of its products. Some of the information is accurate, interesting, and responsible, some is subtly deceptive, and some is downright laughable. Many teachers, unfortunately, rely extensively on this, the most easily available and least expensive, information to supplement standard texts.

The National Soft Drink Association (NSDA), which represents the makers of billions of dollars worth of soda pop, will supply any teacher with plenty of pro-soda pop propaganda. NSDA has lovely pamphlets that are free to teachers. Students learn that their bodies need "lots of water every day" and that "soft drinks are about 90 percent purified water. And their good taste provides a pleasant alternative to water and juices." The association's pamphlet writer even managed to find a way to compare soda pop favorably to a peach: "The peach may give you certain vitamins that the soft drink does not, just as the soft drink gives you more liquid than the peach does." I'm glad someone out there is concerned about liquid deficiencies.

The makers of potato chips have the Potato Chip Information Bureau. The Bureau hired several professors and food writers to sing the praises of the greasy chips in its "Potato Chip Information Booklet." Ronald Deutsch, for instance, asks, "Do potato chips really have a useful role in nutrition?" and answers, not surprisingly considering who is paying him, "Of course." He contends that "The chip is simply a cooked slice of potato and the potato is one of the world's staple foods." Only fifteen questions later does he come to the issue of fat and salt. He defends these on the grounds that a bag of chips provides only a modest portion of one's fat intake. Students whose education is based on this propaganda could not be expected to know that the unprocessed potato is one of the most nutritious foods around. If you compare the price of a pound of potatoes to a pound of potato chips, you will understand instantly why chips are more heavily advertised than plain potatoes.

The sugar industry has received its share of lumps from nutritionists, so it, too, has revved up its pamphlet machine. This industry's educational arm is The Sugar Association, which asserts, "A primary objective of The Sugar Association is to convey the scientific facts concerning sugar and health to the consumer." So, get ready for the facts. The Sugar Association tells students that sugar "serves as a ready source of energy, particularly vital to children . . . the importance of sugar in providing an inexpensive, readily available source of calories cannot be underestimated." The Association says, "If one could eliminate sugar from the diet, or even cut it down, it would be most difficult to find substitute sources of calories." Somehow, I think that people who cut back on soda pop, cupcakes, and candy bars would eventually discover milk, bread, fruit, and other sources of calories.

The National Dairy Council, which has local offices scattered throughout the country, has for many years been teachers' major source of nutrition education materials. At least the dairy industry provides some healthful foods, like skim milk and low-fat cottage cheese, so it is conceivable that this information would be reasonably objective. Many of the council's materials provide straightforward facts about calories, vitamins, and minerals. But the dairy industry's Achilles heel is butterfat, and seldom is heard a discouraging word about the dairy (and other) foods that promote the nation's number one killer, coronary heart disease. The Dairy Council is in the position of having to defend and promote all dairy foods, including butter, ice cream, sour cream, and hard cheeses, all of which are high in fat. Dairy foods provide more than one fourth of our intake of saturated fat, the type of fat associated with the development of heart disease. Skim milk is seldom praised as being superior to whole milk.

One Dairy Council pamphlet, "A Girl, Her Figure, and You," advised that angel food cake and ice cream, or balls of cream cheese softened with cream or fruit juice rolled in chopped peanuts and served with fruit, are low-calorie desserts. The pamphlet, which was published until 1981, also contains the handy advice that "ice cream cones are good choices for snacks, desserts, and party time." A more recent and slicker pamphlet, "YOU, A Guide to Food, Exercise & Nutrition," notes that fat is "a terrific energy source" and "carries vitamins A, D, E, and K in the body," but never mentions ugly words like saturated fat and heart disease. The version of this pamphlet for girls manages to squeeze a cup of whole milk and a tablespoon of sour cream into a weight-loss menu plan.

In the classroom, children hear what society says about nutrition; in the school cafeteria, children eat foods that show what society really thinks about nutrition. School cafeterias have been a battleground for advocates and opponents of good nutrition in the past decade. In communities where parents or school food service directors care about nutrition, the students can eat mighty well. New York City recently had a dynamic food service director, Elizabeth Cagan, who did the undoable. She banished artificially colored and flavored foods and foods treated with BHA and BHT preservatives. She introduced whole grain breads, beans, and tofu (bean curd). In Fulton County, Georgia (suburban Atlanta), Sara Sloan instituted the nationally acclaimed Nutra-Lunch program. She treats the students as if they were her own children and provides natural, generally nutritious meals, often featuring salad bars. Examples like these refute those who say that kids will only eat meals like those served in fast-food restaurants. In most communities, though, school fare consists of bland, frozen dinners or overcooked canned foods, which reflect the school's concern about costs, nutrition, and the students.

While some nutrition advocates were promoting good foods in schools, others were focusing their efforts on the general public or people with diet-related diseases. One of the most effective popularizers of improved nutrition was Nathan Pritikin, who developed a rational plan unencumbered by food industry influences or tradition-bound thinking. While his physicians observed with skepticism, Pritikin changed his diet to almost pure vegetarian and started exercising. Within a few short years, his blood cholesterol level plummeted from around 300 down to 100.

The Pritikin Diet is a logical extension of laboratory, clinical, and epidemiological evidence that underscores the value of eating fruits, vegetables, whole grains, and low-fat animal foods, and minimizing the intake of fat, cholesterol, sodium, and refined sugars. The average American diet receives about 40 percent of its calories from fat; Pritikin recommends 8 to 10 percent. He is similarly strict on cholesterol and sodium. Though the diet is considered unrealistically and unnecessarily stringent by some critics, it is similar to the near-vegetarian diets enjoyed by millions of Asians and Africans.

Pritikin, who had no patience for filling out government grant applications and no access to the old-boy network, opened a diet-exercise center in 1976, which soon became self-sufficient. Most of the people who spent two to four weeks in Southern California relearning their eating and exercise habits became rejuvenated. They saw their cholesterol levels and blood pressures drop, lost weight, and found they could run for miles rather than walk for yards. Clients soon became disciples, and Pritikin support groups sprung up around the country. Pritikin wrote "how-to" books and cookbooks that made his theory and his program available to millions of people for a few dollars, instead of the several thousand it costs to stay at the Pritikin Research Center.

The medical establishment gave a cold shoulder to Pritikin's approach to improved health through nutrition and exercise. He was not a member of their club. Some of Pritikin's critics said that Pritikin was going in the right direction, but went overboard. While the scientific establishment resisted giving Pritikin any credit, many physicians, who were more interested in saving their patients' lives than in waiting around for the elusive definitive studies, endorsed the extremely low-fat, low sugar, low sodium diet and saw their patients undergo recoveries that would be considered miraculous were not the underlying scientific reasons known. Pritikin's groundbreaking efforts put effective pressure on the medical community to rely less on twenty-thousand-dollar-coronary bypass operations and more on brown rice and broccoli. Furthermore, unlike most self-styled book-writing diet experts, whose tracts are based on theory and anecdote, Pritikin put his diet into action and then kept careful records to document its effectiveness.[13]

While Pritikin was popularizing a rigorous, but optimal, diet, scientists continued with their research. Study after study confirmed the relationship between high fat intake and heart disease; high sodium intake and high blood pressure; low fiber, low carbohydrate diets and diabetes; and inadequate fiber intake and intestinal problems. The government sponsored several exciting, little experiments, where researchers sought to modify the lifestyle of entire communities and provide models for broader nutrition projects. The increasingly informative research on diet and health would soon form the foundation for improved governmental policies, which could promote changes in eating habits.

National nutrition policies, reflecting compromises between the public's health and commercial interests, change more slowly than one would like, but they have undergone a remarkable transformation in the past few years. The changes started with the 1974 National Nutrition Policy Study mentioned earlier. This was followed up in 1977 by the Senate Committee on Nutrition and Human Needs' groundbreaking report entitled "Dietary Goals for the United States." Though this document reflected the thinking of only one Senate committee, it was the first official enunciation of the need for a new national diet. The report went beyond vague generalities and called for a 25 percent reduction in fat intake, a 50 to 85 percent reduction in sodium intake, and a 40 percent reduction in refined sugar. The Senate report recommended that we eat twice as much starchy food, like potatoes and whole grain bread. That was splash number one.

The dietary goals report was released to the public just as Jimmy Carter was being inaugurated as President. Carter appointed new leadership to the Department of Agriculture, the primary agency for nutrition education. The Secretary of Agriculture, Bob Bergland, called on Harvard nutrition professor D. Mark Hegsted to be the department's top nutritionist. Hegsted had also been the main resource for the Senate committee's "Dietary Goals" report. And over in the Department of Health and Human Services, new appointees included Secretary Joseph Califano and Surgeon General Julius Richmond, both of whom saw the value in preventing disease, not just curing it.

Splash number two came from USDA. Assistant Secretary Carol Foreman fought for a law that banned certain junk foods from school cafeterias, a regulation that required low-fat or skim milk to be available in every school lunchroom, and a twenty-five-million-dollar Nutrition Education and Training program (NET) that enabled local school systems to produce innovative nutrition education materials and develop better school food programs. Efforts like these set a whole new tone for nutrition education. Gone were the days of "all food is good food."

The next major step forward was "Healthy People," the Surgeon General's 1979 report on disease prevention. This report endorsed diets higher in dietary fiber and lower in fat, sodium, sugar, and cholesterol. It also endorsed breast feeding. This report was the first expression of a new national nutrition policy. Coming from the office of the Surgeon General, the policy was infused with credibility and authority. (This is not to say that, behind the scenes, scientists at the research arm of the Department of Health and Human Services, the National Institutes of Health, were not quibbling and calling for more research before advising people to change their eating habits.)

The biggest splash of all came in February 1980, when the Department of Agriculture together with the Department of Health and Human Services issued a twenty-page pamphlet entitled "Nutrition and Your Health: Dietary Guidelines for Americans." This pamphlet dropped the Basic Four food groups and condensed nutrition advice into seven simple guidelines:

- eat a variety of foods
- maintain ideal weight
- avoid too much fat, saturated fat, and cholesterol
- eat foods with adequate starch and fiber
- avoid too much sugar
- avoid too much sodium
- if you drink alcohol, do so in moderation

The two government departments then took the message to the people. Nutritionists introduced the guidelines to professional organizations, textbook publishers, and newspaper and magazine food editors. Over six million copies of the dietary guidelines pamphlet were given out for free. Almost overnight the conventional wisdom about nutrition had changed. The focus on fat, sugar, whole grains, starchy foods, salt, and alcohol replaced the former emphasis on vitamin, mineral, and protein deficiencies. The huge thirty-year gap between scientific knowledge and public policies had been narrowed greatly. Hallelujah!

The changes in national nutrition policies did not come without great controversy and resistance, especially from the cholesterol lobby—the meat, dairy, and egg industries. Trade associations, like the American Meat Institute, American Egg Board, and National Pork Producers Council, tried to bully the politicians around. In 1977, farm-state senators on the Select Committee on

Nutrition and Human Needs were criticized severely, but to their credit they did not make significant changes in the "dietary goals." Their only noteworthy concession was changing "eat less meat" to "eat lean meat," hardly a terrible change. Some of the senators paid a heavy price at election time, and one of the reasons why George McGovern lost his Senate seat in 1980 was the wrath of South Dakota cattle ranchers.

In their efforts to fend off the nutrition reformers, food companies had a severe handicap: they had little credibility with the public. After all, who would believe that the sugar industry could be totally objective in talking about tooth decay and obesity? In the 1960s and 1970s, the food, chemical, and other industries got more sophisticated about public relations. They realized that anyone with the title of "professor" had instant credibility. Many professors realized the same thing . . . and quietly developed close and financially rewarding ties with industry.

Whenever a controversy erupts about a dietary component or environmental pollutant, a myriad of voices offers advice from every point of the spectrum: "Too much fat is dangerous." "We need more research, before people should be advised to change their eating habits." "Diets low in fat may be dangerous, due to vitamin and mineral deficiencies." For the average eater, who just wants a simple answer, the cacophony can be terribly confusing.

Once upon a time, the different actors in the drama were clearly identifiable: there were consumer advocates and environmentalists who often broke the bad news, government officials whose role it was to say that more information was needed, and industry representatives who offered boilerplate reassurances of safety. Now, with many professors renting out their credibility, the dramatis personae have become much more difficult to decipher. Like Shakespearean characters who wear disguises over disguises, the "experts" are not always who they appear at first blush to be.

Industry's defensive strategy includes such elements as:

- *preventive public relations and advertising campaigns* to assure the public that chemicals, various foods, and oft-criticized industries were all working for the public good. The beef, pork, coffee, sugar, and dairy industries have all mounted major ad campaigns to counter criticisms of their products and revive flagging sales.

- *greater involvement in congressional and presidential elections through campaign contributions* (political action committees). After a President and legislators sympathetic with industry were elected in 1980, companies worked closely with the new officials to weaken government regulations, laws, and entire agencies.

- *dominating reputable organizations,* such as the Food and Nutrition Board of the National Academy of Sciences–National Research Council.

- *sponsoring its own "scientific" or "consumer" organizations,* such as the Council on Agricultural Science and Technology and the American Council on Science and Health. Industry was aided here by its skein of consultants, grant recipients, and other politically conservative friends in the academic community.

While industry has every right to mount this multifaceted response, all too often the client agencies pretend to be something other than what they are. Groups describe themselves as "consumer health" or "independent scientific" organizations, even though they are directed largely by industrial consultants and financed in large part by food, chemical, oil, timber, steel, and other vested interests. At press conferences, scientists flaunt their university affiliations, but fail to disclose their connections (research grants, consulting arrangements, corporate directorships) with industries whose profits depend on the food or chemical that the scientist is defending. In a 1976 study entitled "Feeding at the Company Trough," Congressman Benjamin Rosenthal and the Center for Science in the Public Interest disclosed numerous instances in which outspoken nutritionists and food scientists had close ties with food and chemical companies.

While it is important to know about possible financial and other interests that might bias a professor (or anyone else), one should not assume that a grant or consulting fee will always determine someone's views. Usually, in fact, the grants confirm a professor's previously held positions rather than change his or her beliefs. Once the grants and consulting fees start flowing, though, it can be hard—financially and psychologically—for a professor to revise his or her views in ways that would adversely affect the parties who dispensed the grants.

Organizations To Watch Out For

- *Council on Agricultural Science and Technology:* Founded in 1972, CAST has issued numerous reports criticizing organic farming and defending pesticides, defending high-fat, nitrite-rich foods, and attacking the possible link between food additives and hyperactivity. However, CAST lost much of its credibility when its directors made a casting mistake on panels focusing on antibiotics in animal feed and on organic farming. Several scientists on the panels charged that CAST "has not acted in good faith with respect to its announced intention to prepare an unbiased report on antibiotics in animal feed . . ." and that the report on organic farming was "inherently biased" and "totally discredited." *Science* magazine and other mainstream journals publicized the phony "science," as well as CAST's financial dependency on major agribusiness and chemical companies.[14] Since then, CAST has issued relatively few reports.

- *American Council on Science and Health:* ACSH was founded in 1978 by Harvard School of Public Health nutrition professor—and consultant to the sugar, dairy, breakfast cereal, and other industries—Frederick Stare and his protégée Elizabeth Whelan. ACSH's main thrust is to defend the practices of the major food and chemical companies. Thus, ACSH defends saccharin, diets high in fat and salt, pesticides, caffeine, and even went so far as to have an article in its newsletter suggesting that small amounts of dioxin, a chemical that is toxic and is suspected of causing birth defects, are good for you. On the positive side, ACSH has been a vocal critic of cigarettes and health food quackery, such as "vitamin" B_{15}. ACSH's funders includes Coca-Cola, Stauffer Chemical, Dow Chemical of Canada, U.S. Steel, the U.S. Chamber of Commerce, Georgia-Pacific, the National Soft Drink Association, and dozens of other major corporations that use or produce substances ACSH defends.[15] In 1984, the Washington *Post* reported that an ACSH "friend of the court" brief defending formaldehyde and costing $47,966 was actually paid for by a major formaldehyde producer, Georgia-Pacific, and written by that company's law firm. This revelation further reduced ACSH's already meager credibility, especially among policy-makers in Washington.

- *International Life Sciences Institute (ILSI):* In 1978, shortly after controversies broke out over the safety of caffeine, representatives of the soft-drink, coffee, and other industries organized a new association that would sponsor research and defend the food industry. Currently, ILSI's membership roster reads like a who's who of the food and food-additive industries. The board of trustees includes representatives of Kellogg, Coca-Cola, and other companies, as well as several professors (who have received corporate grants and consulting fees), and two government officials. ILSI has a habit of holding conferences in Hawaii and other exotic places, with professors receiving expense-paid trips. I first encountered ILSI firsthand in 1982, when I attended its Washington press briefing on the effects of caffeine. Professors from Harvard Medical School and the University of Cincinnati proclaimed the safety of caffeine, without once alluding to the evidence indicating it poses a hazard to certain segments of the population. Even more shameful, neither the professors nor the moderator advised the press that ILSI was funded by industry and that the professors were serving as paid consultants.

- *Nutrition Foundation:* This organization was founded and directed by representatives of major food companies. In 1984 it merged with ILSI (see preceding entry). Much of NF's work was benign: it used food industry money to fund research projects and publish the monthly *Nutrition Reviews*. However, from time to time, the food industry used NF as an independent-sounding mouthpiece. NF criticized Food Day, a grass-roots educational project sponsored by Center for Science in the Public Interest in 1975–77. It also attacked the hypothesis that food additives could cause hyperactivity. In 1982, Dr. Albert Kolbye, a high-ranking FDA official, replaced William Darby as director of NF; Darby moved to the American Meat Institute.

- *Food and Nutrition Board:* For many years this committee of the prestigious National Research Council (itself affiliated with the National Academy of Sciences) did little but publish technical reports and devise "recommended dietary allowances" for nutrients. FNB was never an avant-garde organization, but in the mid-1970s food company employees and consultants dominated the group.

    In 1980 FNB published a hastily conceived, poorly researched report, "Toward Healthful Diets," that disputed links between high-fat diets and heart disease. (The report did acknowledge a link between sodium and hypertension, but its reasoning was just as flawed as elsewhere in the report.) The report got tremendous publicity, because most of its advice was opposite to that being given by the American Heart Association, National Cancer Institute, Surgeon General, and other normally reliable agencies. FNB members basked in the bright sunlight of publicity—for one day. The day after the report was published reporters realized they had been deceived: rather than being an organization of objective, independent experts, the FNB largely comprised of people who consulted for the meat, dairy, and egg industries and who had long been known as passionate defenders of the status quo. The shoddy report proved a great embarrassment to the National Academy of Sciences. The NAS–NRC's new leadership has been revamping the FNB so a similar problem would not occur again.

- *Calorie Control Council:* No, this is not another weight watchers group; it is the trade association of companies that make and use artificial sweeteners. It led the lobbying campaign to exempt saccharin from the law prohibiting cancer-causing chemicals. In 1979, the CCC distributed a pamphlet defending saccharin after a National Academy of Sciences (NAS) review panel had concluded that saccharin promoted cancer. The CCC took the panel's comments out of context to make it look like there was official controversy about saccharin's ability to promote cancer. One member of the NAS committee called the CCC's pamphlet "a complete distortion" and "a total misrepresentation." After that criticism, the CCC revised the pamphlet, deleting all references to the National Academy of Sciences report.

The food industry's efforts to turn back the clock on nutrition received a major boost in 1980 when Ronald Reagan was elected President. The Department of Agriculture, the lead agency for nutrition education, was basically given over to the meat industry. The Secretary of Agriculture, John R. Block, was a hog farmer. His top aide, Deputy Secretary Richard Lyng, had been president of the American Meat Institute for eight years. And one of the assistant secretaries, C. W. McMillan, had headed the National Cattlemen's Association. When Block testified at a Senate hearing on January 6, 1981, regarding his confirmation as Secretary, he dismissed nutrition education as a serious issue:

> I know that they are not the same, but hogs are just like people. You can provide protein and grain to a hog and he will balance his ration. He will eat about the right amount of protein to go along with the grain. He will not overeat on the protein or the grain. People are surely as smart as hogs. Really, I think people deserve that prerogative. I am not so sure that government needs to get so deeply into telling people what they should or should not eat.

Block and his aides swiftly dismantled the department's educational initiative. They either silenced or fired many of their nutritionists. They halted publication of a new pamphlet on nutrition education. The administration slashed the Nutrition Education and Training (NET) program budget by 80 percent and started charging exorbitant prices for previously free pamphlets, including the basic "Dietary Guidelines for Americans." And, perhaps most importantly, they responded to a congressional request by appointing a committee to review the dietary guidelines themselves.

The dietary guidelines review committee consisted of nine scientists, three of whom had been placed on the committee by the Department of Health and Human Services (DHHS). The six individuals chosen by USDA included at least five who consulted for the meat, dairy, egg, sugar, and processed foods industries. Several of these had been long-standing critics of the dietary guidelines. The chairman was Bernard Schweigert, former director of the American Meat Institute's research foundation. The committee was clearly formulated for one purpose only: gut the guidelines.

Several of the presumably distinguished members of the dietary guidelines review committee made revealing comments in the course of the early meetings. Frederick Stare (professor emeritus, Harvard School of Public Health) said, "It doesn't make a lot of difference if you have a lot of fat, a little fat, a lot of sugar, or a little sugar in the American diet." He also wanted to delete the recommendation to pregnant women that they abstain from alcohol. Robert Olson (University of Pittsburgh School of Medicine) said that the guideline "Avoid too much sugar" should be eliminated because it "plays into the hands of food faddists and other promoters of diets that are 'natural.'" Another member of the committee, Duke University professor Henry Kamin, said that a new guideline might read, "Please don't louse up your diet." Earlier he had suggested that all people needed to do was have foods of at least three different colors on their plates. Incredible as it sounds, these were the people formulating our national nutrition policy.

Fortunately, the three DHHS nominees believed strongly that the dietary guidelines should be maintained or even strengthened. These three were Sanford Miller, the director of FDA's Center for Applied Nutrition and Food Safety; Lester Salans, the director of the National Institute of Arthritis, Diabetes, and Digestive and Kidney Diseases; and Robert Levy, the former director of the National Heart, Lung, and Blood Institute. As this book was going to press, it appeared that the trio had staved off the carving knives and prevented any major dilutions of the already mild recommendations.

While Reagan's Department of Agriculture was foursquare against promoting good nutrition, the Department of Health and Human Services remained more supportive. FDA Commissioner Arthur Hull Hayes was an expert on high blood pressure. He knew full well the danger posed by diets high in sodium, most of which comes from salt (sodium chloride) in processed foods. Hayes, who served between 1981 and 1983, was a loyal Reaganite and opposed legislation that would have required processed foods to list sodium content on their labels. He also opposed mandatory reductions in the sodium content of foods. However, he used his office as a bully pulpit on the sodium issue. He urged consumers to ingest less salt and urged food processors to use less sodium in their products. He helped make sodium a page one issue. A number of companies began producing reduced-sodium foods and many began listing the sodium content on the label. FDA also issued a regulation in 1984 that requires companies using nutrition labeling (about 40 percent of packaged grocery products) to include sodium in the listing.

The other issue that moved forward concerned the relationship between diet and cancer. Between 1982 and 1984, the National Cancer Institute (NCI), a panel of the National Academy of Sciences–National Research Council, and the American Cancer Society all issued reports on the relationship between diet and cancer. The reports emphasized the apparent connection, which we will discuss in greater detail later, between high-fat, low-fiber diets and cancers of the breast, colon, and prostate. Together, these cancers kill about 110,000 Americans a year. In April 1985, the NCI began a public education campaign to alert people to this important reason for eating less fat and more fiber. NCI's free pamphlet "Diet, Nutrition and Cancer Prevention" is a must for every household (call 1-800-4-CANCER).

The Federal Trade Commission (FTC), along with the health agencies, plays a major role in determining what consumers hear about food and nutrition, because it regulates food advertising. Food producers, processors, and retailers spend billions of dollars a year on radio, television, and print advertising. Ads are the way that companies inform consumers of new products and remind us of the glories of old ones. In recent years, more and more companies and trade associations have been making health or nutrition claims in their ads. When the claims are honest, such ads not only sell a "better" product, but also have a more general educational effect. Not too long ago, companies never bragged about healthful ingredients. Now, innumerable ads emphasize "no added salt," "half the fat," "made with 100% whole wheat," and "contains no caffeine."

In the late 1970s, the FTC recognized that claims in many food ads were either confusing to consumers or outright dishonest and began to develop some ground rules for making claims in food advertising. For instance, when should a company be allowed to claim that its product is more nutritious than a competitor's? What does the word "natural" mean? Should ads bragging that a food gives "energy" be required to disclose that energy is a euphemism for *calories?* Some FTC staff members even urged that all ads include some rudimentary nutrition information.

The FTC staff's get-tough approach quickly ran into major opposition. The first problem developed when the FTC jolted food companies and broadcasters by a formal proposal to ban advertising on children's television shows. The FTC said such ads, being aimed at youngsters, were inherently unfair. The threatened food and broadcasting industries, along with other corporate allies, pressured Congress to order the FTC to halt the children's television proceeding. The second problem developed when President Reagan took office and appointed an economist, James C. Miller, to head the FTC. Miller believed fervently that the "free market" (a concept that exists primarily in academic textbooks) generally protects the consumer and that federal regulatory agencies were far too intrusive and generally unnecessary. Chairman Miller eliminated the FTC's division of food and drug advertising, then scuttled the nascent advertising guidelines, saying that the FTC should take a case-by-case approach.

Food processors quickly threw down the gauntlet to the FTC's case-by-case approach by coming out with a flock of questionable ads:

- The National Coffee Association, seeing coffee sales sliding sharply, mounted a major ad campaign around the slogan "coffee lets you calm yourself down and picks you up." Needless to say, caffeine-rich coffee has never calmed anyone down.

- Campbell Soup Company advertised that "soup is good food" and provided "health insurance" even though most of its soups are excessively high in sodium. For people with high blood pressure, such soups are anything but "good food."

- Del Monte's ad campaign held that canned vegetables are "as nutritious as fresh cooked." Most canned vegetables, however, contain much more sodium than fresh vegetables unless a consumer salts them heavily. Some of the water-soluble vitamins are also lost in the canning process and storage.

- Coca-Cola, PepsiCo, and Diet-Rite all advertised early in 1984 that their diet sodas were sweetened with NutraSweet, keeping secret the fact that the sodas also contained the cancer-promoting sweetener saccharin.

- Hillshire Farms and Bob Evans Farms' ads bragged that their sausages were made with lean meat. About 80 percent of the calories in their sausages come from fat. The Beef Industry Council waged a national campaign to persuade consumers that "beef gives strength" rather than being a major source of saturated fat.

- Ralston-Purina's Donkey Kong Junior "cereal" ads said, "It tastes like fruit and it's lots of fun. It's wild with fruit flavor." No fruit in this product, though; just artificial flavoring.

The FTC snoozed through all these advertising campaigns. Only after groups like Action for Children's Television and Center for Science in the Public Interest filed formal, legal petitions did senior FTC officials even look at the ads. And then, after months of delays, the FTC rejected virtually all of the criticisms. Meanwhile, though, the Better Business Bureau forced the coffee association and Del Monte to change or discontinue their ads, and the New York State Attorney General forced the cola companies, Campbell, and the beef industry, to change their ads. Practically the only food ads that the federal watchdog cracked down on were ones sponsored by health food companies, rather than those run by major national companies. With the FTC doing almost nothing, and companies making all kinds of subtly deceptive health claims, the average consumer surely has a tougher time making sensible, informed decisions at the grocery store.

What with all the conflicting voices screaming for the consumer's attention, the food label is one of our quiet allies. The most basic information about a food is the list of ingredients of which it is made. Most foods, except alcoholic beverages and those served at restaurants and cafeterias, bear a list of ingredients. The ingredients are listed in order of predominance: the major ingredient is listed first, the one used in smallest amount is listed last. From this listing you can often figure out approximately how much of several ingredients are present. For instance, if a breakfast cereal lists "wheat, corn, sugar . . .", you know that more wheat is present than corn or sugar and that sugar cannot constitute more than one third of the product. When an ingredient listing contains ten or twenty different ingredients, the product contains only small amounts of the last ingredients, especially if they are vitamins, minerals, flavorings, or preservatives. Of course, even "small" amounts of salt, which promotes hypertension, and unsafe additives may be too much.

Not every ingredient needs to be listed by name on products, and some ingredients do not have to be listed at all:

- artificial colors need not be listed on butter, cheese, or ice cream, thanks to an exemption won in 1938 by the dairy industry.

- artificial colors (except for the allergy-causing dye Yellow No. 5) and flavors do not have to be listed specifically. Foods often contain tiny amounts of ten or twenty different flavorings; listing each one would probably only cause confusion and distract attention from the major ingredients. However, only two or three artificial colorings are usually used to provide the desired hue to processed foods; it would be simple to list such colorings parenthetically: "artificial coloring (Yellow No. 6, Blue No. 1)." The European Economic Community requires specific listing of colorings.

- vegetable oils and sugars may be listed in the form "may contain soybean oil, lard, or palm oil." Such labeling is annoying to those who want to know exactly what a food contains. A Moslem or Jew might want to avoid a product if it contains lard, but would buy it if it has soybean oil. Similarly, a consumer trying to avoid saturated fats would avoid the product if it contained lard or palm oil, but not if it contained soy oil. Flawed as it is, the current labeling is actually an improvement over what was required in the early 1970s, when labels could simply list "shortening." A manufacturer that uses either/or labeling actually penalizes itself, because consumers may decline to buy a food even though it does not contain the undesired ingredient. (In 1985 FDA proposed that this vague form of labeling be extended to emulsifiers and thickening agents.)

Occasionally, an ingredient label can play tricks on you. For instance, the label on a box of "honey wheat thins" might list "flour, dextrose, corn syrup, honey, BHT." Flour is the major ingredient. However, the next three ingredients are different types of sugar. Together the sugars could comprise 75 percent, by weight, of the product, with honey providing just a small fraction of that.

Listing the actual percentage of each significant ingredient—say, those comprising 5 percent or more of the product—would answer a lot of questions about products. The "honey wheat thins" label might read "flour (60%), dextrose (20%), corn syrup (15%), honey, BHT." The consumer would know that sugars constituted about one third of the product and that only trivial amounts of honey were used.

The forty-billion-dollar-a-year fast-food industry has escaped ingredient labeling completely. If there were ingredient labeling, McDonald's would have to disclose the presence of pulverized chicken skin in Chicken McNuggets, of beef tallow as the fat in which foods are fried, and of Yellow No. 5 dye in a dozen products. Burger King customers might be surprised to learn that the fried potatoes contain corn sugar and that the fish fillet contains milk solids.

Fast-food restaurants are more like decentralized food manufacturing facilities that sell direct to the consumer than like a traditional restaurant. The foods generally come in packages, the menus are limited, and the recipes are constant from day to day and coast to coast. People with allergies and those concerned about heart disease vitally need ingredient information, but most fast-food companies are totally secretive. To correct this situation, in June 1985, the New York State Consumer Protection Board, Food Allergy Committee of the American College of Allergists, and the Center for Science in the Public Interest petitioned FDA and USDA to require ingredient labeling of fast foods. Maybe one of these days we'll see a "shake" labeled with:

> Milk, sucrose, nonfat milk solids, corn syrup solids, cream, guar gum, sodium hexametaphosphate, carrageenan, salt, imitation vanilla powder, sodium alginate, cellulose gum, dextrose, Yellow dyes No. 5 and 6.

Consumer groups have long advocated percentage ingredient labeling, but the food industry has resisted. Companies claim that such labeling would be exorbitantly expensive and would prevent last-minute, cost-saving changes of ingredients. Instead of ordering industrywide percentage labeling, FDA has reserved this approach for foods that contain one particularly valuable and "characterizing" ingredient that may be diluted by other ingredients. The only two products that now bear percentage labeling are certain fruit drinks and seafood cocktails. In the first case, a small amount of fruit juice may be diluted with five or ten times the volume of water. In the latter case, one or two shrimp might be smothered in a cheap tomato sauce. Much greater use of percentage labeling would help consumers make more sensible marketplace decisions.

As important as it is to know what ingredients a food contains, for people concerned about nutrition the fat, sodium, vitamin, and mineral content is equally important. With clear labeling, a consumer could choose, or avoid, products that contain a certain balance of nutrients. The Food and Drug Administration adopted its basic nutrition labeling regulation in 1973. Currently, a manufacturer must use nutrition labeling, if the label makes a nutritional claim, such as "high in vitamin C" or "loaded with nutrients." Fortified foods or enriched baked goods must also bear nutrition labeling, because FDA considers the mention of vitamins or minerals in the ingredient listing to be a nutritional claim. Manufacturers may also use nutrition labeling voluntarily; many companies do, but many still do not.

The current form of nutrition labeling requires the following information:

- serving size
- servings per container
- calories
- protein
- carbohydrate
- fat
- sodium (voluntary until July 1986)
- vitamin A
- vitamin C
- thiamin
- riboflavin
- niacin
- calcium
- iron

The content of other vitamins and minerals, as well as cholesterol and specific kinds of fatty acids, may be listed at the manufacturer's discretion, unless, of course, the company brags "low cholesterol" on the package. Also, if a food contains negligible amounts of vitamins and minerals a company may simply declare, "contains less than 2 percent of the U.S. RDA of [list of nutrients]."

Nutrition labeling provides important clues about a food's nutritional worth. A consumer can use it to avoid foods with hidden fat . . . or to compare the protein content of two brands of the same food . . . or to tally up his or her calcium intake during the day, if enough foods were appropriately labeled.

As valuable as nutrition labeling is, it is not without defects. The most obvious problem is that only certain foods are labeled. While the grocery industry predicted in 1975 that 85 percent of companies would use nutrition labeling "in the near future," by 1985 less than half of packaged foods were actually labeled. But even if all foods were labeled, the information provided is not always what the consumer wants and needs. Many people want to know how much sugar is in a product. Sugar, however, is generally tossed in with carbohydrate, making it impossible to distinguish the refined sugar from the starch or fiber in a frozen pie or cake mix. Only the breakfast cereal industry has voluntarily provided sugar content on package labels. Cereal companies and others add vitamins and minerals to their products to improve their nutritional value. The nutrients used are the very ones used in nutrition labeling. Thus, the product looks very nutritious, even though it may still be high in sugar or fat.

A key problem with nutrition labeling is that it highlights certain vitamins and minerals. This has the effect of downplaying the significance of the fat, dietary fiber (rarely listed), sodium, cholesterol (rarely listed), and sugar content of a food. In the late 1970s the FDA, USDA, and FTC were considering ways in which to improve nutrition labeling, but the Reagan Administration scuttled the review.

Ideally, nutrition labeling would be mandatory for all packaged foods. A food's sugar content (whether naturally occurring or added) should be stated clearly and not combined with total carbohydrate. The fat, sodium, sugar, starch, dietary fiber and calorie contents should be highlighted. This could be done using graphic techniques, such as boldface or colors, and by making the vitamin and mineral listing optional. Few people are suffering from deficiencies of thiamin and riboflavin, yet companies spend millions of dollars a year analyzing and then listing the amounts of these vitamins present. Sensible changes in food labeling could be both cost-saving and life-saving.

To say that nutrition has been the focus of great public controversy and interest in the past decade would be an understatement. The media's coverage of nutrition reflected and encouraged interest in foods on the part of the general public. Whereas in 1970 only "kooks" were eating yogurt and whole wheat bread, in 1985 such foods are staples for a large segment of the population. The new interest in eating a more healthful diet was not lost on corporate marketing executives. They saw the health food industry enjoying explosive growth . . . and figured that they could get in on the action. Companies began producing and marketing a wide variety of improved foods: canned vegetables without the added salt, fruit canned in juice instead of heavy syrup, chicken hot dogs with one third less fat than those made of beef and/or pork, cereals without artificial coloring and flavoring, breads loaded with fiber (never mind, for the moment, that the added ingredient is sawdust), cola beverages

PROPOSED NUTRITION LABELING FORMAT

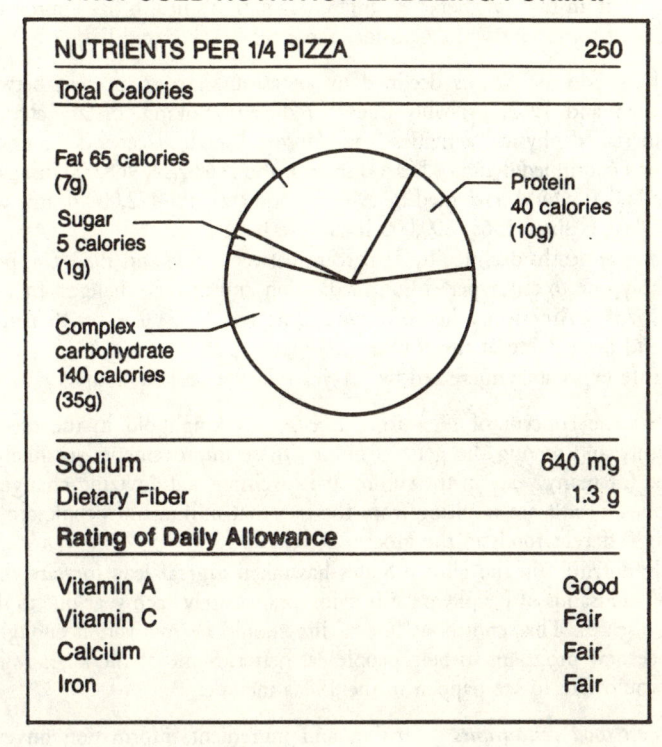

NUTRIENTS PER 1/4 PIZZA	250
Total Calories	

- Fat 65 calories (7g)
- Sugar 5 calories (1g)
- Complex carbohydrate 140 calories (35g)
- Protein 40 calories (10g)

Sodium	640 mg
Dietary Fiber	1.3 g

Rating of Daily Allowance

Vitamin A	Good
Vitamin C	Fair
Calcium	Fair
Iron	Fair

without caffeine, low-sodium salt substitutes, low-fat yogurt, and whole wheat bread are in every supermarket in the country. Oftentimes new products were boosted by multimillion dollar advertising campaigns.

Some of the biggest changes were occurring in the restaurant industry. Natural foods restaurants have been sprouting up all over (though many such restaurants specialize in high-fat, cholesterol-rich egg and cheese recipes). Many regular restaurants offer low-fat or skim milk and whole wheat bread (though sometimes it is caramel coloring, not whole wheat, that confers the dark color). Last but not least, fast-food restaurants have undergone a metamorphosis. They used to be hamburger joints. They served a small variety of foods, almost all of which were bad for your health. In the early eighties, fast-food chains began diversifying their menus, sometimes with nutritious foods. Wendy's and Burger King have salad bars that they promote with beautiful TV spots. Kentucky Fried Chicken offers corn on the cob. Several chains offer baked potatoes. Who would have ever predicted that hamburger joints would have piles of alfalfa sprouts at all-you-can-eat salad bars!

Stimulated, in part, by dietary changes, our nation's health has improved in a number of important ways. Consider these remarkable statistics:

- Heart disease deaths declined by an astounding 36 percent between 1968 and 1983, probably due to reduced smoking, dietary changes, increased physical activities, and improved medical care. If Americans had continued dying of heart disease at the 1968 rate, 968,000 instead of 546,000 would have died in 1983. In other words, 422,000 deaths were averted. Since 1968, 800,000 lives have been saved.[16]
- Stroke deaths declined by 51 percent between 1968 and 1983, this probably due to antihypertension medication and dietary changes. In 1983, 157,000 Americans died of stroke. This was 158,000 fewer than if we had been dying at the 1968 rate.[17]
- Life expectancy increased by 3.1 years in the decade of the 1970s.[18]

Now that the concept of *preventing disease* is taking hold in the medical community and among the general public, these improvements are likely to continue for many years in the future. It is exciting that amazing changes in the public's health are resulting from the fact that millions of people are just choosing different foods in the grocery store.

While nutrition in the United States has taken a great leap forward, hundreds of thousands of people are still dying prematurely each year due to diet-related diseases. That enormous loss of life should be motivation enough to introduce new programs to help people eat better. Some of the key advances that I would like to see happen in the 1980s include:

- *Fast-food restaurants:* nutrition and ingredient information on every wrapper; wider variety of foods, including fresh fruits, vegetables, and whole wheat hamburger buns; prepackaged nutritious meals designed for children.
- *Supermarkets:* more use of in-store posters, shelf-markers, newspaper advertisements, and house brands to help shoppers buy the most nutritious, least expensive foods possible; signs next to produce to indicate whether pesticides, waxes, and colorings have been used; greater availability of organically grown foods.
- *Growers and distributors:* much more advertising and point-of-purchase cooking information to promote the sale of fruits, vegetables, beans, grains, low-fat dairy foods, and other basic foodstuffs.
- *Food processors:* more grain foods made with whole grains or half whole grain and half refined grain; greatly reduced fat, sugar, and sodium content of foods; less reliance on artificial colors and flavors; clear ingredient and nutrition information.
- *FDA, USDA, and FTC:* improve the clarity of nutrition labeling, emphasizing fat, sugar, fiber, and sodium; require that all processed foods

list the calorie, sodium, fat, and sugar content; set gradually decreasing limits on the fat and sodium content of hot dogs, canned foods, and many other processed foods; ban deceptive labels and ads.
- *Industry, health organizations, and government agencies:* massive nutrition education campaigns, integrated with other health information and coupled with universal screening programs so that every citizen has a sense of his or her state of health.
- *Consumers:* more thoughtful buying decisions at grocery stores, restaurants, and vending machines; greater involvement in consumer advocacy groups that promote better local and national policies.

As bitter controversy gives way to broad consensus in the area of fat, sugar, and salt, new nutrition debates are centering around the use of "megadoses" of vitamins and minerals to prevent or treat diseases. Two-time Nobel laureate Linus Pauling has been vocal about the value of preventing colds and treating certain cancers with huge doses of vitamin C. Others cite niacin (vitamin B_3) as a cure for some cases of schizophrenia. Thousands of women are taking vitamin B_6 supplements to alleviate PMS (premenstrual syndrome) and calcium supplements to help prevent osteoporosis. Research is suggesting that vitamin A may reduce the risk of several types of cancer. Some observers say that vitamin supplements can favorably affect people with behavioral problems. In these and other areas of biomedical research, the evidence is suggestive, but still fragmentary and inconclusive.

The "pioneers" of megavitamin therapy (or "orthomolecular medicine") say "give supplements a try; you have everything to gain and nothing to lose. Even large amounts of these substances are certainly safer than potent, synthetic prescription drugs." All too often, however, proponents of megavitamins cite studies that support their views without acknowledging other reports that refute some or all of the earlier evidence.

The "establishment" holds that "the vitamin-pushers are modern-day charlatans, getting rich by exploiting people's fears. They endanger lives, because individuals with serious diseases may take useless vitamin pills or other potions instead of seeking more traditional medical aid." The cynics in the establishment say that the widespread consumption of supplements has resulted in Americans having the most valuable urine in human history. Those who criticize the use of nutrition supplements demand perhaps an unattainable level of evidence supporting their efficacy and safety, oftentimes exaggerate the likelihood of harm that might result from taking large doses of vitamins or minerals, and ignore the possible benefits. They also, more naively, maintain that supplements are unnecessary, because "Americans are the best-fed people in the world," blithely ignoring the fact that large segments of the population do not consume anywhere near the recommended amounts of calcium, vitamin B$_6$, magnesium, and other nutrients.

Bigger and better studies will eventually clarify what appears now to be conflicting research. Until that distant day, though, what are people supposed to do? The top priority is to eat a diet that provides the recommended amounts of nutrients. Only real food provides a wide range of nutrients, including even some nutrients that may not have yet been discovered. Supplements include only those nutrients that were intentionally included. But fulfilling our nutrient requirement from real food may be easier said than done, especially because so many people lead sedentary lives that require relatively low caloric intakes. The less food one eats, the harder it is to get the required nutrients. We need to be switching to a "high nutrient density" diet, one with fewer calories, but more nutrients. Lots of vegetables, whole grains, and other nutrient-rich, low-calorie foods is the way to go.

The next step—whether or not to take supplements—is more controversial. Individuals going the supplement route have to figure out what dosages to take and because individual circumstances vary greatly, this is hardly the place for detailed advice. It certainly wouldn't hurt anyone to take, "just for insurance," a multivitamin/mineral supplement containing approximately 100 percent of the RDA of the various nutrients. Beyond this, growing bodies of research point to real benefits—and little risk—of larger amounts of certain vitamins or minerals:

- Women who suffer from PMS may enjoy tremendous relief from large doses of vitamin B$_6$; they should be aware that amounts above several hundred times the recommended level (the RDA is about 2 milligrams a day for adult women) have been found to cause serious side effects; less heroic doses (100–200 milligrams a day) have not caused problems.

- Women who do not consume much calcium (from dairy foods, fish bones, and certain vegetables) should take a calcium supplement to minimize bone loss.

- With growing evidence pointing to an increased cancer risk from inadequate consumption of vitamin A and selenium, one should consider taking these as well. Here, though, large amounts can be toxic, so one should not take more than two or three times the RDA of vitamin A (carotene, the plant form of the vitamin, is totally harmless) and one or two times the RDA of selenium. With these and certain other nutrients, the benefit/risk equation has "moderate likelihood of benefit" on one side and "tiny chance of risk" on the other. In such a situation, it makes sense to take the supplements without waiting for the level of proof that research scientists rightfully demand before coming to a final verdict.

We have focused primarily on the nutritional content and health effects of foods, but let's not forget that foods and meals have traditionally served important social and psychological roles in our lives. The lifestyle of Americans has changed dramatically in the last forty years and with it our eating habits. The pace of our lives has become increasingly frenetic. Many people don't even make time to treat themselves to a good breakfast, but settle for a cup of coffee, doughnut, and cigarette. More and more foods are of the instant variety—devoid of what country music singer Mary Kay Place called "vitamin L, the most important one of all"—what with toaster-tarts and drink mixes for breakfast, vending machine sandwiches and beverages for lunch, and frozen or fast-food dinners for supper. The availability of these convenience foods has aided and abetted the disappearance of the family meal, as has the increasing proportion of women who work. The exodus of young families to suburbia has stranded many elderly people who must now shift for themselves or rely on government programs for food and companionship.

Although new food additives are now tested for adverse physiological effects, new foods and dietary patterns are not being studied for adverse sociological and psychological effects. But they should be, because we are rapidly headed for an Orwellian Nutri-Pill, which will contain all of our known nutritional requirements. Breakfast cereals fortified with 100 percent of our daily requirement of ten or more nutrients, Space Stick candy bars, and Instant Breakfasts offer a glimpse of the future, and the food technologists are working feverishly in their laboratories developing "newer and better" concoctions. A vending machine dispensing Nutri-Pills may be the kitchen and dining room of tomorrow. We must stop and ask ourselves if we really prefer missing out on the social opportunities that a meal with family or friends offers. Foods also serve as a link between nature and people. The supermarket is already a far cry from a farm. Are we really ready to take the next step and dissociate nutrients completely from the animal or vegetable sources from which we have obtained them for hundreds of thousands of years? Is a rubber nipple and glass bottle an adequate substitute for the human breast and mother's warmth? Questions like these deserve careful study by sociologists and psychologists. While they study, however, the food industry will be churning out new foods and new "food concepts." Therefore, it is urgent that we consider the role of foods and eating in our own lives. Our diet is too important to be left to the food industry.

I have tried to emphasize the dietary changes most of us should concentrate on: eating more vegetable foods (fruits, vegetables, grains, beans, nuts), less fat-laden meats and dairy foods, and fewer sugary, salty, greasy snack foods. The principles of a good diet are really quite simple. One does not have to read a hundred books or make the study of foods the whole focus of one's life to understand these principles and translate them into meals. But considering how important good nutrition is for our health and considering that we eat a thousand meals and perhaps another thousand snacks a year, is it unreasonable to devote perhaps a day or two of one's life to studying nutrition in order to understand clearly a few lifesaving rules? Once we integrate these rules into our lives, we can stop worrying about the composition of our diet and spend more time on other matters.

I receive many letters from people who say that the *Nutrition Scoreboard* system has helped them and their family or friends eat better. Many want to know what they can do to help improve the nutritional quality of foods at the store and the eating habits of the public. I urge two things. First, they should spruce up their own habits, both for their own well-being and to set an example for others. Second, they should join the fight for better nutrition. The best way to go about this is to join or start a local or national citizens' action group. Define a specific problem about which you are concerned, and then go to work and try to solve it. Fight for better foods in your own or your child's school cafeteria; get your local TV and radio stations to run pro-nutrition spots; press your local health department to require that wherever foods are vended from machines, at least half the choices should be nourishing. If you are not a joiner, work alone. Write letters to the editor, write to your legislators, complain to your supermarket or cafeteria manager. Individuals and groups have had numerous successes in improving food locally and have contributed immeasurably to the effort to rewrite America's nutrition policies. Not only are these activities satisfying, they are also fun, especially when combined with lots of potluck dinners. And with the thought of a joyous meal on our mind, let's now rate the nutritional value of the foods on our plate.

II

Rating the Nutritional Value of Foods

There are two common ways of communicating information about the nutritive value of foods. One approach is to recite truthful generalities about foods, such as "we should eat a protein source at every meal," or "this or that food is rich in this or that vitamin." The Basic Four (protein foods, dairy products, grains, fruits and vegetables) approach to nutrition is in this vein—the good foods are given a pat on the back, while the bad foods are ignored. As government nutrition surveys (and sales figures for soda pop and snack foods) prove, this approach was hardly a complete success.

The second popular approach is almost diametrically opposed to the first. Where the first offers generalities, the second chokes in details. Some books have page after page of nutritional analyses of foods. The plethora of numbers is enough to scare off any but the most dedicated nutrition hounds. Listed in the tables are the actual quantities of fat, protein, vitamins, and minerals contained in foods. With all the numbers, it requires a great effort to determine what constitutes a serving, whether the indicated amount of a nutrient makes a significant contribution to the person's diet, and how one food compares to another. Expressing the data on a per-serving basis (rather than per-100 grams) and listing it as a percentage of the RDA helps some. But huge tables can be terribly confusing, and they are almost useless to most of us.

Nutrition Scoreboard takes a different approach. We rate various foods for you, using a formula that gives a food credit for its nutritious ingredients and deducts credit for substances that Americans generally eat too much of (see Appendix I). The substances that get positive credit are:

- protein
- naturally occurring carbohydrate (including starch, dietary fiber, glycogen [animal starch], and sugars)
- Vitamin A, B_2 (riboflavin), B_3 (niacin), C (ascorbic acid)
- iron, calcium
- polyunsaturated fat

The substances that most people eat too much of and for which we subtract points are:

- sugar, corn syrup, and honey
- saturated and monounsaturated fat
- high fat content
- cholesterol
- sodium

None of these ingredients is inherently bad, and moderate amounts do not pose a problem for most people. But the average, sedentary American consumes enough of these substances to increase the risk of developing obesity, tooth decay, stroke, heart disease, and possibly certain cancers.

One additional factor in the formula rewards foods that are rich in nutrients and low in calories . . . and penalizes foods that are relatively low in nutrients, but high in calories.

As an example of how the formula works in practice, the following table breaks down the ratings of a glass of whole milk and a piece of pound cake:

Whole Milk (8 oz.)

Nutrient	Points
Protein	11.8
Carbohydrate (milk sugar)	8.4
Fat	−24.0
saturated fat −16.6	
monounsaturated −2.4	
polyunsaturated 1.0	
total fat quantity −6.0	
Cholesterol	−1.8
Calcium	10.4
Iron	0.4
Sodium	−1.6
Vitamin A	1.2
Vitamin B_2	15.6
Vitamin B_3	0.4
Vitamin C	1.2
Nutrient-Calorie factor	6.0
TOTAL	27.8

Pound Cake (1 med. slice)

Nutrient	Points
Protein	1.8
Carbohydrate	1.6
starch 11.2	
added sugar −9.6	
Fat	−16.0
saturated fat −7.6	
monounsaturated −4.0	
polyunsaturated 1.6	
total fat quantity −6.0	
Cholesterol	−3.0
Calcium	0.2
Iron	0.8
Sodium	−0.4
Vitamin A	0.4
Vitamin B_2	1.2
Vitamin B_3	0.2
Vitamin C	0.0
Nutrient-Calorie factor	−4.4
TOTAL	−17.5

Like any other system, our food rating system is not perfect. For instance, a food's rating does not indicate which nutrients contribute how many points. Thus, two foods with similar ratings—buttermilk (+46) and orange juice (+47)—could have totally different nutrient contents. Milk contains generous amounts of protein, calcium, riboflavin, and vitamin A, while orange juice contains a large amount of vitamin C and small amounts of several other nutrients. You could drink orange juice until you turned blue in the face, but you would die of malnutrition unless you obtained protein, calcium, and riboflavin from milk or other foods.

A few people may think that to have a nutritious, balanced diet all they have to do is consume the appropriate amounts of certain vitamins, minerals, and protein every day. They may pop a vitamin-mineral supplement to start the day and devour a large steak to satisfy their protein requirement at the end of the day. In between they might consume two cans of soda pop, four candy bars, several cups of coffee, a six-pack of beer, seven doughnuts, and a couple of imitation puddings. Obviously, this diet will look good if you just consider the vitamins, minerals, and protein. Equally obviously, it is a rotten diet. A slug of vitamins and minerals will not counterbalance the detrimental effects of the sugar, alcohol, and fat any more than painting the outside of a house improves an ugly interior. Our goal should be a diet composed of good foods, foods that will provide us with generous amounts of nutrients without the fat, cholesterol, sodium, and refined sugar. The makings of a good diet can be obtained from most grocery stores: fruits, vegetables, low-fat dairy products, beans, nuts, whole grains, lean meat and poultry, and fish. Let *Nutrition Scoreboard* be your guide to the best of these foods.

Protein

Protein, the stuff of which muscle, enzymes, hair, and cellular structures are made, is absolutely essential in a good diet. Fortunately, most North Americans are blessed with diets that provide more than enough protein. The average young man in his twenties gets twice the recommended dietary allowance of protein. That excess drops gradually as men get older, but even those over sixty-five get 30 percent more protein than they need. Similarly, the average young woman consumes 50 percent more protein than she needs, while women over sixty-five still get 20 percent more.[19]

Despite the rarity of protein deficiencies, food companies know that "protein" is a magical "buy" word and use it in their advertising as much as possible.

- Golden Griddle pancake syrup: "That's right, your kids get 40 percent more protein from a 'Golden Griddle' breakfast."
- Skippy peanut butter: "Salami's nutritious and so is ham and tuna salad. But ounce per ounce, Skippy has more protein than those."
- National Pork Producers Council: "The new pork is much leaner than ever—higher in protein, too."

Never mind that pancake syrup has essentially no protein and that peanut butter and pork are both usually high in fat.

Proteins are molecules. They are made up of amino acids linked end to end in long chains, much like cars in a long freight train. There are twenty different amino acids (analogous to twenty different kinds of freight cars), and the number of each variety and the specific order in which they are linked is characteristic of each protein. The body can produce some, but not all, of the amino acids. The "essential amino acids"—those which the body cannot produce—must be obtained from foods. These are isoleucine, leucine, lysine, methionine, phenylalanine, threonine, tryptophan, and valine.

The value of the protein content of a food depends on how much of the eight essential amino acids it contains. The best quality protein provides the best balance of all eight amino acids. Egg, milk, cheese, soy, fish, and meat all have excellent-quality protein. The protein in beans, peas, and most other vegetables is generally of lower quality, because it contains relatively little of certain of the essential amino acids. The lowest-quality, almost worthless, protein is gelatin. A person whose diet includes mainly poor-quality protein foods must consume more protein than one whose diet is rich in eggs, dairy products, meat, fish, and soy.

Proteins with different amino acid compositions complement one another if eaten within a period of several hours. That is, an essential amino acid that is in short supply in one food may be supplied to the body by another food. This concept is explained lucidly in Frances Moore Lappé's exquisite book *Diet for a Small Planet*. Thus, a mixture of different foods in the diet will result in an amino acid mixture that is more balanced than that of any of the component foods. Some people go to great lengths to eat meals with complementary proteins. Except for pure vegetarians (vegans) who eat no milk, meat, or eggs or for those few individuals whose diets are based on a narrow range of foods, it's not worth worrying about protein complementarity in a nation in which most people consume 150 percent or more of the recommended protein intake.

If anything, Americans ought to worry about ingesting too much rather than too little protein. In a 1980 speech to the American Meat Institute, the U.S. Department of Agriculture's top nutritionist, Dr. Mark Hegsted, warned of problems associated with both protein and meat. For one thing, there is good evidence that diets high in protein promote osteoporosis, the disease process that results in gradual bone loss, particularly in older women. Traditionally, scientists had thought that bone loss was due solely to inadequate calcium in the diet. However, osteoporosis is a problem even among Scandinavian women who consume high levels of calcium. By contrast, populations that consume less calcium than we do, but also consume much less protein, are not afflicted with osteoporosis.[20] High protein diets increase the rate at which the body excretes calcium.

One obvious problem with many protein-rich foods is that they are often also high in fat. It is amusing to see the meat industry tout hot dogs as high protein foods when, in fact, they usually contain more than twice as much fat as protein. A hamburger sandwich at a Roy Rogers restaurant provides 20 percent more fat than protein; cheddar cheese contains about one third more fat than protein; and whole milk contains equal amounts of both protein and fat. If we carelessly choose high-protein foods, we will probably choose a high-fat diet and increase our risk of heart disease.

The points for protein that some foods receive are listed in the Protein Scoreboard.

Protein Scoreboard

Food Name	Serving Size	PROTEIN SCORE	Percent U.S. RDA
Lobster meat, cooked	3 oz.	20.0	60
Chicken, skinless, baked	3 oz.	20.0	60
Turkey, roasted	3 oz.	20.0	60
Flounder, baked	3 oz.	19.2	58
Round steak	3 oz.	18.9	57
Cod, broiled	3 oz.	18.0	54
Tuna fish, in water	3 oz.	17.5	53
Pork chop, baked, lean	3 oz.	16.9	51
Leg of lamb	3 oz.	16.9	51
Sirloin steak, choice	3 oz.	16.7	50
Beef liver	3 oz.	16.6	50
Ham, baked	3 oz.	16.6	50
Shrimp	3 oz.	15.3	46
Hamburger, 25 percent fat, regular	3 oz.	14.0	42
Cottage cheese, 1 percent fat	1/2 cup	10.4	31
Yogurt, low-fat, plain	1 cup/8 oz.	8.8	26
Black beans	1/2 cup	5.6	17
Chick-peas, cooked	1/2 cup	5.1	15
Low-fat milk, 2 percent	1 cup	6.0	18

Carbohydrate

Carbohydrate is probably the most misunderstood component of our food. Carbohydrates are vilified, shunned, and feared by millions of eaters. Many people consider starchy foods a one-way ticket to obesity and that white sugar is another name for poison. As we shall see, these views are way off the mark.

The category "carbohydrate" includes a wide range of substances. The common feature is that they consist primarily of carbon, hydrogen, and oxygen atoms. The hydrogen and oxygen atoms are in a ratio of two to one, just as in water. Hence the name *carbo-* (from carbon) *hydrate* (from water).

Most people in the world today and for millennia in the past ate diets that consisted largely of foods rich in one important carbohydrate—starch. These foods, such as potatoes, rice, cassava, and wheat, also usually contain (or contain*ed*) another important carbohydrate—dietary fiber. Fiber includes a variety of compounds that are largely indigestible. The collective name for starch and fiber is complex carbohydrate.

A third kind of carbohydrate that occurs in natural foods, primarily fruit and dairy products, is sugars. These are small molecules and are called simple carbohydrates. Finally, sugars that are purified and isolated from other natural substances constitute a fourth kind of carbohydrate in our diet. These so-called "refined" sugars now comprise a major part of the diet for millions of people and are added to thousands of manufactured foods. To understand better the effects that carbohydrates are having on our health, let us examine in greater detail each of the four basic types.

STARCH

Believe it or not, even though starch has become almost a dirty word in some quarters, we should be eating *more* starchy foods. Many foods high in starch, such as potatoes, whole wheat bread, dried beans, corn, and peas, are excellent low-fat sources of vitamins, minerals, and protein. Bread and potatoes used to be the backbone of our diet, but they have gradually been replaced by foods high in refined sugar and fat.

Back around 1910, Americans ate about one third more carbohydrate than we do now. And of that carbohydrate, two thirds was complex carbohydrate (mainly starch) and only one third was sugar (both natural and refined). Now we eat more sugar than starch, and most of the sugar is refined.

The typical diet is excessively high in fat and refined sugar. To help bring that diet into better balance, we need to replace a lot of the fat and sugar with something else, namely starchy foods. In 1977 the Senate Select Committee on Nutrition and Human Needs recommended that we increase our intake of starch and natural sugars from 28 percent to 48 percent of our calories. In 1980 the U.S. Department of Agriculture and the Department of Health and Human Services urged people to "eat foods with adequate starch and fiber" and to "select foods which are good sources of fiber and starch, such as whole grain breads and cereals, fruits and vegetables, beans, peas, and nuts." The only nonplant food that contains any starch is liver, which contains a small amount of animal starch, or glycogen.

Though starchy foods have not had a great reputation, the most important dietary change most people could make is to eat more starchy foods and fewer fatty and sugary foods.

DIETARY FIBER

The second type of carbohydrate considered in the Nutrition Scoreboard formula is dietary fiber. Dietary fiber is a complex mixture of substances that the body digests poorly or not at all. While some types of fiber make it through the body undigested, other types are broken down by bacteria in the large intestine. The methane and carbon dioxide that those bacteria produce may cause gas or bloating. Fiber used to be dismissed as "mere roughage" until its important properties were discovered—or remembered—in the late nineteen sixties.[21] The dietary fiber contents of a variety of common foods are listed in the following table.

Dietary Fiber Content of Common Foods

No recommended daily allowance has been set for dietary fiber, but a reasonable target to shoot for would be 25 to 35 grams per day.

Food	Serving Size	Fiber (grams)
100% Bran	1/3 cup (1 oz.)	8.5*
All-Bran	1 oz.	7.9*
Whole wheat bread	2 slices	5.4*
Rye bread	2 slices	5.4*
Peas	1/2 cup, cooked	5.2*
Apple	1 large	4.9*
Kidney beans	1/2 cup, cooked	4.5*
Parsnips	1/2 cup, cooked	4.4*
Bran Chex	1 oz.	4.4*
40% Bran Flakes	1 oz.	3.9*
Orange	1	3.8
Baked potato	1 medium	3.8
Spinach, corn	1/2 cup, cooked	3.2*
Raisin Bran	1 oz.	3.0*
Carrot	1 raw	3.0
Broccoli	1/2 cup, cooked	2.9
Shredded Wheat	1 oz.	2.6*
Pear	1 small	2.5
Zucchini	1/2 cup, cooked	2.5
Green pepper	1 raw	2.4*
Rye wafers	3	2.3*
Tomatoes	1 small, raw	2.0
Popcorn, plain	2 cups	1.9
Brussels sprouts	1/2 cup, cooked	1.8
White bread	2 slices	1.6
Strawberries	1/2 cup	1.6
Green beans	1/2 cup, cooked	1.6
Rutabaga	1/2 cup, cooked	1.6
Kale	1/2 cup, cooked	1.4
Graham crackers	2	1.4
Turnips	1/2 cup, cooked	1.3
Brown rice	1/2 cup, cooked	1.3

Peaches, plums	1 medium	1.3
Asparagus, eggplant	1/2 cup, cooked	1.2
Spaghetti	1/2 cup, cooked	0.8
Iceberg lettuce	1/2 cup, raw	0.5

* A single serving of these foods contains at least 2 grams of insoluble fiber, the type of fiber that increases stool bulk and is most likely to protect against cancer.

Dietary fiber can be divided into two types: those that dissolve in hot water and those that don't. The insoluble fibers, including cellulose, hemicellulose, and lignin, come from the walls of plant cells, and are found in whole grains, beans, vegetables, and other plant products. Wheat bran is by far the richest source of insoluble fiber. This valuable bran is lost when whole wheat flour is refined to produce white flour.

The soluble forms of dietary fiber include gums, pectins, and mucilages. Beans, fruits, and oat bran are good sources of soluble fibers, though most plant foods contain both types of fiber. Animal foods never contain fiber.

Denis P. Burkitt, an eminent British surgeon, deserves the greatest credit for studying and then publicizing the importance of eating adequate amounts of fiber. Burkitt worked for many years in rural African hospitals and became familiar with the health conditions of people whose diets were rich in dietary fiber. He noted that despite a heavy patient roster, there were almost no cases of varicose veins, obesity, bowel cancer, appendicitis, constipation, or diverticular disease of the colon (a sometimes painful ailment that is common in the West).[22] To verify his own observations, he analyzed the experiences of two dozen East African mission hospitals.[23] He also visited remote, rural hospitals to determine how many cases they recorded of each type of common "Western" disease. Finally, he conducted simple studies of the intestinal action of rural Africans, urban Africans, and Europeans living in Africa. Of these three groups, rural Africans consume the most fiber and Europeans the least. His findings led him to conclude that some of the most common diseases of people who live on Western refined diets rarely afflict people who eat diets high in fiber and starch and low in sugar and fat.

The beneficial effect of fiber on constipation is something that has been long known but largely forgotten. Americans spend over four hundred million dollars a year on laxatives, an expense that would be largely unnecessary if the sufferers ate foods higher in fiber. TV programs are punctuated frequently by commercials for laxatives, but only rarely for the fruits, vegetables, and grains that would prevent constipation.

Persons on low-fiber Western diets have relatively small, hard, and infrequent stools. Such stools permit the colon to segment, which results in high pressures in the area of segmentation. The abnormally high pressure is believed to cause outpouchings of the intestinal wall.[24] This sometimes painful condition is called diverticulosis. Its more serious form is called diverticulitis. Thousands of Americans develop this serious disease every year. Many gastroenterologists are now recommending that patients who suffer from diverticulosis or constipation be treated with a high-fiber (the insoluble type found in wheat bran) diet to soften the stool.[25] Adequate fiber produces a large, soft stool that can be moved without increased pressure.

A diet high in fiber can probably help prevent obesity. Vegetables, fruits, beans, and other high-fiber foods are not only comparatively low in calories, but their bulk gives a feeling of fullness that may translate into pushing oneself away from the table. In one recent study, researchers at the University of Alabama found that people eating a high-fiber diet spent one third more time eating, but consumed only half as many calories as people on a low-fiber diet.[26]

Dr. James Anderson, professor of medicine and clinical nutrition at the University of Kentucky, has shown that high-fiber, high-carbohydrate, low-fat diets can benefit diabetics. Diabetics who eat this diet can greatly reduce or even eliminate their use of insulin or other drugs. Most of Anderson's patients' weights, blood cholesterol levels, and blood sugar levels decline. Anderson usually combines a high-fiber diet with an exercise program.[27]

To continue singing the glories of fiber, there are studies indicating that fiber-rich foods reduce the risk of heart disease. The soluble types of fiber appear to decrease "bad" low-density lipoprotein (LDL) cholesterol and increase the "good" high-density lipoprotein (HDL) cholesterol.[28] As a part of their heart-protecting benefit, note that foods high in fiber are also low in fat and cholesterol, unless the chef piles on a lot of cheese or butter.

A number of researchers, including Burkitt, have suggested that consuming too little dietary fiber can increase the risk of colon cancer, which kills 51,000 Americans a year.[29] Burkitt and his British colleagues theorized that diets rich in whole grains, beans, and vegetables might protect against cancer by speeding waste through the intestinal tract. They also thought that large, fiber- and water-filled stools would dilute the concentration of any cancer-causing chemicals that might be present.

While there are still more questions than answers, both the fat and fiber content of a diet appear to play significant roles in colon cancer. According to Drs. Bandaru Reddy and Ernst Wynder of the American Health Foundation, high-fat diets stimulate the production of bile acids. Populations that eat high-fat diets tend to have high levels of bile acids in their stools and also have high rates of colon cancer. Reddy and Wynder discovered that while Finns and New Yorkers both eat about the same amount of fat, the Finns have only one half the cancer rate of New Yorkers. But the Finns consumed much higher levels of dietary fiber and excreted three times the stool volume as did New Yorkers. The researchers theorized that the large, watery stools diluted the concentration of bile acids, which might cause cancer by irritating the intestinal wall.

The Japanese, on the other hand, eat the same amount of fiber as Americans and have similar size stools. Yet they have only one fourth our rate of colon cancer. Presumably that is because they eat very little fat. The comparison of Americans and Japanese suggests that fat intake is a more powerful determinant of colon cancer than fiber.

Though the exact benefits of dietary fiber are still a bit fuzzy, both the American Cancer Society and the U.S. Department of Health and Human Services have urged Americans to increase their intake of fiber. Even if fiber-rich foods play less of a role in preventing cancer than is now thought, such foods are still nutritionally valuable for numerous other reasons.

The only negative thing to say about fiber is that both the insoluble and soluble forms can bind minerals, such as calcium, magnesium, iron, and zinc. These bound nutrients are unavailable to the body. Considering that vegetarians generally have at least as much iron in their blood as the rest of the population, it seems unlikely that people who up their fiber intake need to worry about developing mineral deficiencies. Many researchers believe that the nutrient losses due to fiber would be insignificant in well-nourished individuals, and they note that after several months on a high-fiber diet the body adapts and extracts the minerals from foods more efficiently. This concern does serve as a warning not to go overboard in adding huge amounts of bran to your diet. Rather, double or triple your fiber intake by eating a different mix of foods.[30]

NATURAL SUGARS

Many fruits and some vegetables are sweet because of their natural sugar content. These sugars include sucrose (table sugar), glucose (same as dextrose or corn sugar), fructose, and several others. Dairy products contain the sugar lactose. When we got sugar only from natural sources it did not pose much of a problem, because it was present in bulky foods and was usually associated with a variety of nutrients. It is difficult to get excessive amounts of sugar from natural foods. For example, an orange contains only about one third as much sugar as a can of orange soda.

Regardless of their source, sugars can promote tooth decay. For this reason, even though naturally occurring sugars are components of nutritious foods, they are given less credit in our rating system than starch and fiber, but more credit than refined sugars.

REFINED SUGARS[31]

Children have probably always had a sweet tooth. Thousands of years ago, the sweet tooth could only be satisfied with honey, fresh fruit, or dried fruit.

Refined sugar was occasionally available, but only as a real luxury. Today, our sweet tooth can be satisfied by either inexpensive pure sugar or any of the thousands of cakes, candies, ice creams, soft drinks, and other manufactured products that line grocery store shelves.

Sugar use reflects availability and price. As inventors developed ways of producing sugar more efficiently, people ate more and more of it. In the 1820s Americans consumed only about 10 pounds per year, while in the 1870s we ate 40 pounds per year.* By 1910 that was up to 87 pounds. Now, the average person consumes about 125 pounds per year. Of that, 75 pounds comes from sugar cane and sugar beets, 48 pounds from corn (dextrose and corn syrup), plus another pound or two from honey. We eat about twice as many pounds of refined sugar as sugar from fruit and dairy products. Weight-conscious people should be aware that 125 pounds of sugar provides 227,000 calories.

We have included honey in the refined sugar category, because it is basically a thick solution of sugar-water. Despite what some "health food" books claim, honey contains virtually no vitamins or minerals. It often makes foods sticky, causing them to be particularly conducive to tooth decay. Some people believe that honey causes a smaller rise in blood sugar than does table sugar. In fact, on a scale of 1 to 100, with 100 representing the food that sends blood sugar soaring the highest, honey rates a disturbing 87. Table sugar rates 59.

The few good things that can be said about honey are that (a) it is sweeter than sugar, so slightly less can be used; (b) its image of healthfulness may encourage people to eat truly healthful foods; (c) it is a better bread-spread than high-fat butter; (d) it adds moisture to baked goods so you can use a little less fat; and (e) it is so expensive that we tend to use it sparingly.

A major—and underappreciated—problem with sugar relates to the sheer quantity we consume. Refined sugar comprises 10 to 20 percent of American diets. That means that people must obtain 100 percent of their nutrients from only 80 to 90 percent of their food. That feat is getting harder and harder to accomplish as we eat fewer and fewer calories, reflecting our sedentary lifestyle.[32]

Subtle effects due to sugar's diluting the nutritional quality of the diet would be virtually impossible to discern. For instance, might the reduced vitamin intakes make some children more susceptible to disease-causing germs? . . . or cause decreased attention span in 2 percent of the population? . . . or increase slightly the risk of cancer? Such uncertainties may never be answered . . . and we may have to rely on common sense to tell us that replacing 125 pounds per year of healthful foods with 125 pounds of refined sugar just does not make sense.

---

* Government statistics on the use of sugar and other commodities actually measure availability at the wholesale level, rather than how much is actually eaten. Wastage occurs in warehouses, stores, and homes, so these "consumption" figures overestimate true consumption. Nevertheless, they are the best figures available and are consistent from year to year.

Aside from diluting the nutritional quality of the diet, the one major effect that has been positively linked to sugar is tooth decay, or dental caries. Dr. Abraham Nizel, associate professor of Oral Health Services at Tufts University, told a congressional committee in March 1973, that:

> Over the last ten years, my students and I have done thousands of diet evaluations on patients with rampant caries at Tufts University School of Dental Medicine. We never found a single patient whose caries problem could not, in part, be traced to the patient's inordinate consumption of sugar. Every package of sugar-sweetened Life Savers, cough drops, breath mints, candies, chewing gum and soft drinks should be labeled with a statement warning that excessive frequent daily use of these products can produce significant amounts of dental plaque and dental decay.[33]

Sugar is most conducive to tooth decay when it is eaten in a solid or sticky form. A candy bar is much worse for the teeth than is soda pop, though the latter, too, promotes tooth decay. Also, between-meal sugar promotes tooth decay more than sugar eaten during a meal, because it is more likely to stick in the cracks and crevices of teeth. (Sugar itself does not cause decay; bacteria in the mouth digest the sugar and produce acid—it is this acid that eats away the teeth.)

The National Institute of Dental Research (NIDR) does not have any firm figure on the cost of dental caries. However, judging from decade-old figures presented at a congressional hearing, Americans probably now spend upward of six billion dollars a year repairing rotten teeth.

As rampant as tooth decay is, the tide of the battle against decay has turned. A study done in 1979–80 found that children between the ages of 5 and 17 had about one third fewer decayed, missing, or filled teeth than did children in a similar (but not identical) survey conducted between 1971 and 1973.[34] The decline in tooth decay represents a major triumph in the annals of public health. Still, about 25 percent of children had unfilled cavities.[35] In 1985 the Centers for Disease Control reported that 51 percent of nine-year-old children had no cavities compared to only 29 percent in the early 1970s.

While reduced sugar consumption by some children may have contributed to this remarkable decline in decayed teeth, the greatest credit belongs to fluoride. Fluoride strengthens the tooth's enamel and impairs the ability of decay-causing bacteria to convert sugars to acids.[36] In communities with water supplies that are naturally high in fluoride, decay rates are relatively low. This observation led public health officials and dental experts to advocate the addition of fluoride to water supplies that contained less than about 1 ppm fluoride. The majority of the U.S. population now drinks fluoridated water. (Too much fluoride, be it from water, dentifrices, or other sources can discolor teeth and should be avoided.)

Sugar is a tasty, concentrated source of calories and probably promotes obesity. Almost every nutritionist makes that charge, yet few studies have been done to prove it. One recent, but hardly definitive, British study found that "when sucrose is included in the diet in realistic amounts most individuals do not compensate for the increased energy [caloric] intake by eating less food, and most gain weight."[37]

Dr. John Yudkin of London University and author of the book *Sweet and Dangerous* has argued that sugar is the major cause of heart disease.[38] He cites studies that correlated the level of sugar consumption with the rate of heart disease in different populations. In general, populations that eat a lot of sugar have a high incidence of heart disease. These studies alone, however, are not persuasive, because sugar and fat consumption often increase in tandem, and there is overwhelming evidence that a high-fat diet is a major cause of heart disease.

The latest arguments about sugar center on the possibility that it affects behavior. Some people contend that high-sugar diets even cause criminal behavior, and several judges and probation officers specify low-sugar diets as a condition of probation. Some doctors believe, based on their observations of patients, that diets high in sugar cause hyperactivity in children. FDA's Dr. Thomas Sobotka, an expert in neurobehavioral toxicology, thinks the possible link should "definitely be investigated." He added that "Clinical observations, though not scientifically sound, do indicate something may be there. We're going to have to start looking at nutrition and brain function in general, and sugar is a good place to start . . ."[39]

The studies have begun to trickle in, and it is obvious that the sugar-behavior story is a complex one. University of Illinois psychiatrist Mortimer D. Gross had one patient, a 5-year-old boy, whose mother said he was sensitive to sugar. Gross gave the child a drink containing 5 teaspoons of sucrose, and within ten minutes the boy became "easily frustrated, hyperactive, and difficult to control."[40] The mother, too, was sensitive to sucrose. Other sugars did not affect either person. Gross then tested 50 other hyperkinetic patients. Not a single one reacted to sucrose, suggesting that the sensitivity is rare.

Dr. C. Keith Connors, at Children's Hospital in Washington, D.C., specializes in the effect of diet on behavior.[41] In one study involving severely disturbed children, two sugars (sucrose and fructose) "produced significant increases in directly observed activity level . . ." In a second study, children did not perform as well after eating a high-carbohydrate breakfast as after a high-protein breakfast. Sucrose, added to the high-carbohydrate meal, heightened the detrimental effect. Meanwhile, Connors and Dr. Judith Rapoport at the National Institute of Mental Health found that in certain situations sucrose slightly *reduces* motor activity and can even have a beneficial effect on behavior.[42]

One conclusion to draw from these studies is that sugar is best consumed in small quantities and together with a balanced meal. Least desirable is eating large amounts of sugar together with other carbohydrates—a cupcake and soda-pop snack, for instance.

Biochemists are beginning to understand just how diet might affect behavior. It appears that sugar and other carbohydrates, as well as amino acids, affect neurotransmitter levels in the brain. Neurotransmitters are the chemicals that enable brain cells to communicate with one another. High blood sugar levels, which are most readily caused by eating sugary or starchy foods in the absence of protein foods, may raise levels of serotonin, one of the neurotransmitters. In a test setting, effects can be seen. In one study, babies given a sugar solution containing a stiff dose of the amino acid tryptophan, which the body converts to serotonin, fell asleep significantly faster than babies not given the chemical.[43] More research is needed to determine to what extent behavioral effects occur in the real world.

The eye of the storm about sugar's behavioral effects centers on a condition known as hypoglycemia, the fancy name for low blood sugar. Health food stores are filled with books describing how low blood sugar causes irritability, fatigue, depression, confusion, anxiety, shakiness, headaches, schizophrenia, alcoholism, drug addiction, crime, and divorce. Millions of people claim to suffer from hypoglycemia, but most doctors doubt the disease even exists, except in individuals who have cancer of the pancreas or other unusual medical conditions.

Hypoglycemic attacks are said to occur a couple of hours after eating high-sugar foods. At first, blood sugar levels rise rapidly. Then the pancreas releases a spurt of insulin, enabling cells in the body to take in the sugar and causing blood sugar levels to fall rapidly to below-normal levels. It is then, say the sufferers, that hypoglycemia strikes. Respond the doubters: "All the symptoms are psychosomatic."

To correlate blood sugar levels with moods and behavior, physicians feed patients two or three ounces of glucose and then monitor both blood sugar and behavior for several hours. This is called a glucose tolerance test, or GTT. Thousands of GTTs have been done, but only a handful have correlated blood sugar and mood. In the few studies that did attempt to correlate blood sugar and mood, only occasionally did depression or other mood changes coincide with low sugar levels.[44] One study found that individuals whose blood glucose fell to a relatively low level performed slightly less well than other people on a test designed to reflect mental acuity.[45] Other studies, though, including one done at the Mayo Clinic, have not found a relationship between blood sugar levels and symptoms.[46] In a study done at the University of Alabama, two people who complained of adverse symptoms during a GTT were retested with saccharin in place of sugar. Even though saccharin has no effect on blood sugar, one of the patients again claimed to have symptoms. It is such findings that suggest that many cases of hypoglycemia are psychosomatic.

The glucose tolerance test certainly does not mimic the way most people eat. When the Mayo and Alabama researchers tested their subjects after eating a meal, rather than just sugar, many fewer subjects experienced symptoms. Yet, a child who drinks a bottle or two of soda pop on an empty stomach is doing the equivalent of a glucose tolerance test and might very well experience problems. People who feel weak, cold, shaky, sleepy, or depressed after eating carbohydrates should make a special effort to eat real meals, with their mix of carbohydrate, protein, and fat.

It is quite possible that a sugar-rich diet might affect behavior by mechanisms having nothing to do with blood sugar levels. In other words, the problems experienced by millions of "hypoglycemics" might be real, but the cause may pertain to neurotransmitter or hormone levels, not blood sugar.

Despite sugar's adverse health effects, our taste buds just love sugar, and the food industry has done everything possible to capitalize on this weakness. Companies sweeten foods that are not naturally sweet (like breakfast cereals), tempt children by describing in TV commercials how sweet and delicious their products are, and make sweet foods available wherever we turn. Many infants and toddlers start life with presweetened desserts and then quickly graduate to cupcakes and soda pop. In the face of all this encouragement to eat sugary products, an occasional warning from a dentist, teacher, or parent is doomed to failure.

Bonnie Liebman, nutrition director at the Center for Science in the Public Interest, and I have compiled a listing of the sugar content of many foods. I would like to have provided a more complete listing, but most food companies keep the sugar content of their products a deep, dark secret.

Sugar Content of Foods

Food (Serving size)	Percent of Total Calories from added sugar	Teaspoons of added sugar
BEVERAGES		
Liqueurs, cordials *(0.7 oz.)*	33	1.5
Brandy, cognac *(1 oz.)*	41	1.7
Carnation Chocolate Instant Slender *(1 packet)*	33	2.3
Dessert wine *(3.5 oz.)*	35	3.0
Carnation Chocolate Instant Breakfast *(1 packet)*	37	3.0
Birds Eye Orange Plus *(6 oz.)*	50	3.3
Gatorade *(8 oz.)*	100	3.5

RATING THE NUTRITIONAL VALUE OF FOODS

Food (Serving size)	Percent of Total Calories from added sugar	Teaspoons of added sugar
Nestea Light *(8 oz.)*	100	3.7
PDQ chocolate flavor *(3–4 tsp.)*	91	3.8
Ovaltine Malt Flavor *(4–5 tsp.)*	77	4.3
Nestle Chocolate Quik *(2–3 heaping tsp.)*	80	4.5
Capri Sun (all flavors) *(6.8 oz.)*	90	5.5
Nestea Iced Tea, sugar *(8 oz.)*	97	5.7
Nestle Hot Cocoa Mix *(1 oz.)*	84	5.8
Country Time Lemonade Flavor, concentrate *(8 oz.)*	100	6.0
Kool-Aid, sweetened *(8 oz.)*	100	6.0
Carnation Chocolate Slender *(10 oz.)*	45	6.3
Cranberry Juice Cocktail *(8 oz.)*	73	6.4
Hawaiian Punch *(8 oz.)*	100	6.5
Ssips, orange *(8.5 oz.)*	89	7.3
Hi-C Grape *(8 oz.)*	97	7.3
Tang *(8 oz.)*	100	7.6
Canada Dry ginger ale *(12 oz.)*	95	8.0
Canada Dry tonic water *(12 oz.)*	98	8.4
Sprite *(12 oz.)*	100	9.0
Coca-Cola *(12 oz.)*	100	9.8
Teem *(12 oz.)*	100	9.3
Pepsi Cola *(12 oz.)*	100	10.0
On Tap root beer *(12 oz.)*	100	10.3
Mountain Dew *(12 oz.)*	100	11.0
Patio orange soda *(12 oz.)*	100	11.8
Shasta orange soda *(12 oz.)*	100	11.8

BREAKFAST CEREALS

See p. 149

CAKES

Coffee cake, yeast *(2.3 oz.)*	6	1.3
Cupcake, no icing *(2½" dia.)*	28	1.5
Coffee cake, crumb *(2.3 oz.)*	16	3.2
Cupcake, w/icing *(2½" dia.)*	40	3.2
Applesauce cake, no icing *(2.3 oz.)*	31	3.8

Food (Serving size)	Percent of Total Calories from added sugar	Teaspoons of added sugar
Gingerbread, no icing (2.3 oz.)	31	4.1
Twinkies (1)	47	4.8
Yellow cake, no icing (2.3 oz.)	38	4.9
Pound cake, no icing (2.3 oz.)	29	5.0
Marble cake, no icing (2.3 oz.)	36	5.0
Chocolate cake, no icing (2.3 oz.)	39	5.3
Chocolate pudding cake (2.3 oz.)	42	5.6
Upside down cake (3.2 oz.)	39	5.9
Sponge cake, no icing (2.3 oz.)	51	6.3
Cinnamon coffee cake (2.3 oz.)	44	6.4
Spice cake, no icing (2.3 oz.)	26	6.5
Angel food cake, no icing (2.3 oz.)	61	6.8
German chocolate cake, w/icing (3.2 oz.)	33	7.6
Sara Lee chocolate cake (3.2 oz.)	37	7.9
Strawberry shortcake, whipped cream (3.8 oz.)	57	8.4
Yellow cake, w/icing (3.2 oz.)	46	9.0
Marble cake, w/icing (3.2 oz.)	50	9.8
Black forest cake, w/icing (3.2 oz.)	53	10.0
Sponge cake, w/icing (3.2 oz.)	59	10.7

CANDY

Certs (1)	100	0.5
Wrigley's gum, all flavors (1)	92	0.6
Pine Bros. cough drops (1)	98	0.6
Beech Nut chewing gum (1)	98	0.6
Lifesavers (1)	100	0.6
Fruit Stripe chewing gum (1)	100	0.6
Beech Nut cough drops (1)	100	0.6
Salt water taffy (1)	88	1.0
Starburst Fruit Chews (1)	88	1.0
Replay chewing gum (1)	99	1.1

RATING THE NUTRITIONAL VALUE OF FOODS

Food (Serving size)	Percent of Total Calories from added sugar	Teaspoons of added sugar
Raisinets *(1 oz.)*	16	1.2
Hubba Bubba bubble gum *(1)*	100	1.5
Now and Later *(1 square)*	100	1.5
Chuckles *(1)*	100	1.6
Bubble Yum bubble gum *(1)*	100	1.8
Betty Crocker Cherry Fruit Bar *(1)*	31	1.8
Peanut M & M's *(14)*	34	3.0
Whoppers *(1 oz.)*	34	3.1
Chunky *(4 squares)*	34	3.1
Plain M & M's *(31)*	40	3.5
Royals Mint Chocolates *(1 oz.)*	43	3.8
Reese's Peanut Butter Cup *(1.6 oz.)*	28	4.8
Cotton candy *(1 cone)*	100	5.2
Marshmallows *(4 large)*	100	5.3
Good & Plenty *(1 oz.)*	100	6.2
Dots *(1 oz.)*	100	6.2
Jelly beans *(10)*	100	6.6

CANDY BARS

Food (Serving size)	Percent of Total Calories from added sugar	Teaspoons of added sugar
Quaker Honey & Oat Granola Bar *(1 oz.)*	20	1.5
Chocolate Slender Bar *(1 oz.)*	25	2.2
Twix Peanut Butter *(1 oz.)*	29	2.3
Summit Cookie Bar *(1 oz.)*	26	2.7
Mr. Goodbar *(1 oz.)*	28	2.7
Hershey's Milk Chocolate w/Almonds *(1 oz.)*	32	3.2
Nestle's Milk Chocolate w/Almonds *(1 oz.)*	34	3.2
Hershey's Krackel *(1 oz.)*	34	3.2
Nestle's Crunch *(1 oz.)*	34	3.2
$100,000 Bar *(1 oz.)*	35	3.2
Snickers *(1 oz.)*	38	3.3
Twix Caramel *(1 oz.)*	36	3.3
Nature Valley Granola Cluster *(1 oz.)*	50	3.3
Mars Bar *(1 oz.)*	38	3.4
Hershey's Milk Chocolate *(1 oz.)*	34	3.4
Nestle's Milk Chocolate *(1 oz.)*	39	3.6
Nestle's Choco-Lite *(1 oz.)*	39	3.6
Milky Way *(1 oz.)*	49	3.9

Food (Serving size)	Percent of Total Calories from added sugar	Teaspoons of added sugar
CONDIMENTS		
Whipped topping, pressure can (2 Tbs.)	24	0.4
French dressing (1 Tbs.)	9	0.4
Ketchup (1 Tbs.)	63	0.6
Table sugar (1 tsp.)	100	1.0
Relish (1 Tbs.)	62	1.0
Honey (1 tsp.)	100	1.4
Jellies, jams, marmalades (1/2 Tbs.)	88	1.5
Cranberry sauce (1 Tbs.)	96	1.5
Chocolate fudge topping (1 Tbs.)	54	2.1
Molasses, light (1 Tbs.)	100	3.2
Maple syrup (1 Tbs.)	100	3.3
Golden Griddle Syrup (1 Tbs.)	100	3.3
Karo Pancake & Waffle Syrup (1 Tbs.)	100	3.8
COOKIES*		
Graham crackers (2 large)	25	0.9
Keebler Pecan Sandies (2)	14	1.5
Oatmeal raisin cookies (2)	22	1.7
Granola cookies (2)	22	1.7
Peanut butter cookies (2)	21	1.8
Keebler Coconut Chocolate Drop (2)	19	2.0
Keebler Elfwich (2)	29	2.0
Sandwich cookies (3)	25	2.1
Brownies w/nuts (1 oz.)	28	2.3
Fig bars (2)	38	2.3
Applesauce cookies (2)	37	2.3
Almond cookies (2)	21	2.4
Keebler Pitter Patter (2)	22	2.5
Keebler Rich 'n Chips (2)	25	2.5
Butter cookies (6)	31	2.5
Ginger snaps (4)	39	2.8
Sugar cookies (2)	40	3.0

* Serving size for all cookies is about one ounce.

DAIRY PRODUCTS		
Vanilla ice milk (1/2 cup)	47	2.7
Chocolate milk, 2% fat (1 cup)	24	2.7
Dannon frozen yogurt, vanilla (1/2 cup)	50	2.8

RATING THE NUTRITIONAL VALUE OF FOODS

Food (Serving size)	Percent of Total Calories from added sugar	Teaspoons of added sugar
Blintz, cheese filling *(1)*	34	2.9
Vanilla ice cream *(1/2 cup)*	34	2.9
Dannon frozen yogurt, fruit *(1/2 cup)*	66	3.7
Ice cream sandwich *(3 oz.)*	26	3.8
Heinz Baby Food Custard Pudding *(7.8 oz.)*	37	3.9
Dannon lowfat yogurt, flavored *(1 cup)*	33	4.2
Ice cream soda *(10 oz.)*	47	6.0
Dannon lowfat yogurt, fruit *(1 cup)*	37	6.0
Ice cream sundae *(1/2 cup)*	46	9.5
Thick shake *(11 oz.)*	44	9.6

FRUITS & VEGETABLES

Food (Serving size)	Percent of Total Calories from added sugar	Teaspoons of added sugar
Cream-style corn, canned *(1/2 cup)*	23	1.5
Glazed carrots *(1/2 cup)*	42	2.0
Peaches, light syrup, canned *(1/2 cup)*	50	2.3
Pineapple, heavy syrup, canned *(1/2 cup)*	54	3.0
Sweet potato, syrup, canned *(1/2 cup)*	38	3.1
Pears, heavy syrup, canned *(1/2 cup)*	59	3.6
Beets, w/Harvard sauce *(1/2 cup)*	50	3.8
Peaches, heavy syrup, canned *(1/2 cup)*	64	4.0
Applesauce, sweetened *(1/2 cup)*	60	4.3

OTHER DESSERTS & SNACKS

Food (Serving size)	Percent of Total Calories from added sugar	Teaspoons of added sugar
Blueberry muffin *(1.6 oz.)*	12	1.1
Bran muffin *(1.6 oz.)*	17	1.2
Banana nut bread *(1.6 oz.)*	12	1.4
Danish pastry *(2.3 oz.)*	9	1.5
Jelly doughnut, yeast *(1.8 oz.)*	13	1.7
Glazed doughnut, cake *(1.5 oz.)*	18	1.8
Heinz Baby Food Dutch Apple Dessert *(4.5 oz.)*	35	2.2

Food (Serving size)	Percent of Total Calories from added sugar	Teaspoons of added sugar
Chocolate covered doughnut, cake (1.5 oz.)	22	2.3
Cream puff, no icing (4.6 oz.)	13	2.3
Apple strudel (1/5th)	16	2.7
Crepes, fruit filled (2)	28	2.7
Apple crisp (1/2 cup)	27	2.7
Eclair, w/icing (3.5 oz.)	18	2.8
Blueberry, Cherry Pop-tart (1.8 oz.)	25	3.3
Chocolate pudding (mix) (1/2 cup)	41	4.1
Jell-O (1/2 cup)	95	4.2
Cracker Jacks (1 oz.)	60	4.3
Hunt's Snack Pack, vanilla (1 can)	37	4.4
Popsicle (1)	100	4.5
Frosted Choc. Fudge Pop-tart (1.8 oz.)	36	4.5
Sherbet (1/2 cup)	80	6.7
Caramel apple (1)	58	7.6

MISCELLANEOUS FOODS

Skippy Peanut Butter (2 Tbs.)	11	1.3
Coconut, sweetened (1/4 cup)	30	1.6
Pork & beans (1/2 cup)	25	2.4
Beans & franks (3/4 cup)	19	3.3

PIES†

Sweet potato pie (4.6 oz.)	9	1.5
Mince pie (4.6 oz.)	14	2.6
Fried apple pie (2.6 oz.)	18	2.7
Banana custard pie (4.6 oz.)	20	3.3
Pumpkin pie (4.6 oz.)	21	3.6
Coconut custard pie (4.6 oz.)	20	4.0
Cherry pie (4.6 oz.)	21	4.4
Peach pie (4.6 oz.)	21	4.5
Apple pie (4.6 oz.)	22	4.9
Chocolate cream pie (4.6 oz.)	37	7.5
Lemon meringue pie (4.6 oz.)	38	7.8
Chocolate chiffon pie (4.6 oz.)	35	8.9
Lemon chiffon pie (4.6 oz.)	39	9.8
Pecan pie (4.6 oz.)	35	12.0

† A 4.6 oz. serving is 1/7 of a pie.

NATURAL SUGARS

Fruit and some milk products contain naturally occurring sugars. While they are chemically identical to refined sugars, the sugars in fruit and milk are always accompanied by vitamins, minerals, or fiber.

DAIRY PRODUCTS

Food	Teaspoons of natural sugar	Food	Teaspoons of natural sugar
Vanilla ice milk (1/2 cup)	1.0	Dannon lowfat yogurt, flavored (1 cup)	3.9
Vanilla ice cream (1/2 cup)	2.1	Dannon lowfat yogurt, plain (1 cup)	4.3
Dannon frozen yogurt, fruit (1/2 cup)	2.2	Dannon lowfat yogurt, fruit (1 cup)	6.3
Milk (1 cup)	3.0		

FRUIT

Food	Teaspoons of natural sugar	Food	Teaspoons of natural sugar
Strawberry (1/2 cup)	1.1	Orange (1)	2.9
Blueberry (1/2 cup)	1.4	Apple (1)	3.4
Plum (1)	1.7	Honeydew (1/10)	3.5
Grape (10)	1.8	Orange juice (6 oz.)	3.6
Grapefruit (1/2)	1.9	Pear (1)	4.0
Cherry, sweet (10)	2.0	Banana (1)	4.9
Peach (1)	2.0	Apple juice (6 oz.)	5.2
Apricot (3)	2.1	Watermelon (1/2 cup)	6.2
Cantaloupe (1/4)	2.2	Raisins (1/4 cup)	6.3
Pineapple (1 slice)	2.4	Prunes (10)	9.9
Tangerine (1)	2.9	Dried figs (5)	17.0

Fat

The number one nutritional problem in the United States, Canada, and Western Europe is that people eat too much fat.

If you wanted to make just one change in your diet, you should eat less fat.

Sugar, cholesterol, sodium, refined flour, food additives, and food contaminants have all been criticized, justifiably, for the harm they cause. However, diets high in fat cause more harm to our health than any of those other dietary demons.

High-fat diets promote diseases that account for about 800,000 deaths annually, or almost half of all deaths. For at least three decades, there has been ample evidence that a diet high in saturated fat promotes diseases of the heart. In the past several years, a consensus has developed that diets high in any kind of fat probably increase the risk of cancers of the breast, colon, and prostate.

On top of everything else, fat is the most concentrated source of calories. While one gram of protein or carbohydrate provides four calories of energy, and a gram of alcohol provides seven, one gram of fat provides nine calories of energy. No wonder that fatty foods are likely to promote obesity.

Despite the problems associated with it, fat is a necessary constituent of the diet. It provides and facilitates the absorption of fat-soluble vitamins (vitamins A, D, E, and K) and contains the essential nutrients linoleic acid, linolenic acid, and arachidonic acid. It also provides energy (calories) and flavor. A little bit of fat is fine; large amounts consumed over many years can be deadly.

Many common and traditional foods are rich sources of fat, so anyone who decides to switch to a low-fat diet may have to make some jarring adjustments (see the following table). Butter, margarine, mayonnaise, salad oils, and shortening provide about 10 percent of our fat. This is probably the easiest fat to avoid, because we can see it and we consciously use it. Harder to see and avoid is the fat in red meat, poultry, and fish, which account for over 40 percent of our fat intake. Some of this fat can be cut away, before or after cooking, but the rest of it is part and parcel of the food itself. The most invisible fat is that in dairy foods, where the butterfat is dispersed in milk, ice cream, and cheeses. There is no way to cut away the fat. We can only be alert to its insidious presence, choose low-fat varieties, and eat modest portions. Dairy foods provide about 15 to 20 percent of our fat. The remainder of the fat we consume comes from nuts, seeds, eggs, and other minor sources. Most fruits and garden vegetables are essentially fat-free.

Sources of Fat in the American Diet[47]

Food	Percent of Total Dietary Fat
Meat, poultry, fish	41
Milk, cheese, ice cream, etc.	17
Bread, cakes, cookies, other grains	15
Vegetables, fruits, legumes, nuts, seeds	12
Margarine, butter, shortening, oils	10
Eggs	4
Sugar, sweets	1
TOTAL	100

The average American obtains about 40 percent of his or her calories from fat. This represents an increase from 32 percent of calories in the early years of the century and is one of the most important dietary changes that has occurred. It resulted from an increase in meat consumption, as well as a much more hefty increase in vegetable oils (primarily from processed foods). In 1910, only 16 percent of Americans' dietary fat came from vegetable sources, compared to about 45 percent currently.

There is no "right" fat intake, though the less we consume the better. Considering that fat is in such a wide variety of foods, the strictest, balanced diet imaginable would provide about 10 percent of its calories in the form of fat. The American Heart Association, National Academy of Sciences Committee on Diet, Nutrition and Cancer, and the National Cancer Institute have recommended a very moderate target of 30 percent calories from fat. I urge health-conscious people to aim for a stiffer, but still readily attainable, goal of 20 to 25 percent fat calories. People suffering from heart disease would do well to be even stricter, aiming for 10 to 20 percent of calories from fat.

The percentage of your calories coming from fat is difficult to estimate. Ideally, you would keep a careful record of the kinds and quantities of food you ate over a several-day period. Then you would look up the calorie and fat contents in the appropriate tables. To make the task a little easier, we have provided a chart that gives average caloric intakes for different age and sex groups (see page 61). Once you have estimated your caloric intake, look on the chart and decide what percentage of fat you want to strive for. The chart indicates how many grams of fat per day you should eat. Next, using your diet record and the "Fat Content of Foods" listing, tally up the amount of fat in your daily diet and compare the total to your personal goal. There are numerous home computer programs that can take the drudgery out of these calculations.

Another route to a low-fat diet is to forget all the tables and simply be very aware when you eat foods that contain significant amounts of fat. Then make it a habit to avoid some of these foods, eat smaller portions of others, and buy reduced-fat varieties. Several painless ways of reducing your fat intake (and possibly your waistline) include:

- Drinking skim milk (0 percent fat) or 1 percent milk (whole milk contains about 3.3 percent butterfat).
- Eating beans, pasta, rice, potatoes, and other starchy foods; and low-fat cottage cheese, fish, and chicken (without the skin) instead of meat.
- Avoiding hot dogs, bologna, and other luncheon meats; fat provides about 80 percent of their calories.
- Cutting off as much excess fat as possible from meat, both before and after you cook it.
- Eating a different grade of meat. "Choice" and "prime" cuts are highest in fat; "good" grade is low in fat, cheaper, and perfectly acceptable in stews, soups, etc.
- Using less butter, margarine, or cream cheese on bread, or switching to honey, jam, yogurt, or apple butter, or eating the bread plain.
- Eating fresh fruit, low-fat frozen yogurt, or ice milk instead of doughnuts, pies, pastries, cakes, or ice cream for dessert or snacks.

- Poaching or steaming vegetables, fish, and other foods, instead of frying or sautéing them.

The kind of fat in your food is also important, because different fats have different effects on the body. Saturated fat raises blood cholesterol levels and increases the risk of coronary heart disease, stroke, and other arterial diseases. On the other hand, polyunsaturated fats tend to reduce blood cholesterol, though one gram of "poly" fat lowers cholesterol only half as much as a gram of saturated fat raises cholesterol. Several recent studies indicate that monounsaturated fats, which are especially abundant in avocado and olive oil, may also reduce blood cholesterol.[48]

The following table lists the amounts of the different types of fat in common foods. Note that foods with large amounts of saturated fat, like cheese and pork, contain some polyunsaturated fat, while foods we normally think of being polyunsaturated, like soybean oil, still contain some saturated fat. Note also that coconut oil, which is commonly used in imitation dairy products, is more highly saturated than butterfat or lard and tends to raise cholesterol levels.

Fatty Acids in Common Foods[49]

Item	Saturated (percent)	Monounsaturated (percent)	Polyunsaturated (percent)
Safflower oil	10	14	76
Sunflower oil	11	19	70
Soybean oil	14	24	62
Corn oil	14	29	57
Olive oil	15	73	12
Avocado	17	69	14
Margarine, tub-type (average)	19	35	46
Peanut oil	21	49	30
Margarine, stick-type (average)	21	50	29
Cottonseed oil	26	22	52
Salmon, chinook, canned	27	49	24
Chicken, with skin	31	44	25
Herring (Atlantic), fillet	35	39	26
Lard (pork, ham)	44	46	10
Tallow (beef)	51	44	5
Butterfat (milk)	66	30	4
Coconut oil	93	6	1

The key problem with saturated fat is that it promotes heart disease. Heart disease is without a doubt the number one killer in the United States and other

Western nations. Virtually all researchers and expert committees have concluded, after studying the great body of scientific research that is available, that eating too much saturated fat, as well as cholesterol, definitely contributes to heart disease in a large fraction of the population, particularly men and older women.

There are two basic links in the logic concerning fat and heart disease: (1) eating more saturated fat (and cholesterol) raises blood cholesterol levels, and (2) the higher one's blood cholesterol levels, the greater one's risk of heart disease. Numerous studies establish each of these crucial points, and one can reasonably infer that saturated fat increases the risk of heart disease. Experimentally, it is very difficult to establish that eating more saturated fat leads directly to a higher risk of heart disease, but, as we shall see later, several studies do provide direct evidence of this.

Cholesterol levels in blood are powerfully influenced by one's dietary intake of fat and, to a somewhat lesser extent, cholesterol. Carefully controlled studies have shown that saturated fats, such as coconut oil or butter, raise cholesterol levels dramatically.[50] Also, in similarly controlled studies, food cholesterol raised cholesterol levels in blood.

Many studies have shown that the higher the level of cholesterol in blood, the greater the risk of heart disease. The most extensive and well-known of these studies has been conducted in Framingham, Massachusetts, since 1950. It and other studies have shown that 35–44-year-old men whose cholesterol levels are 260 or above have five times the risk of coronary heart disease as men whose cholesterol levels are below 200.[51]

The critical, and most difficult, point to establish is that lowering blood cholesterol levels can actually reduce the risk of heart disease. In 1984 the National Heart, Lung and Blood Institute reported the results of a key, ten-year-long, $150 million study.[52] The study involved 3,806 men who had high cholesterol levels. All of the men were urged to adopt a cholesterol-lowering diet. In addition, half of the men took cholestyramine, a cholesterol-lowering drug, for seven to ten years, though some of the men were more religious about taking the somewhat unpleasant medicine than others. The other half of the men took a placebo, a powder that did nothing. Neither the patients nor the researchers knew who was taking what until after the study was over. The drug-takers quickly experienced sharp drops in their cholesterol levels. More importantly, those taking the drug enjoyed a 24 percent reduction in fatal heart attacks. The men who adhered to the drug regimen most rigidly had the greatest reductions in heart attack rates. The researchers concluded that, as a rule of thumb, each 1 percent decline in blood cholesterol led to a 2 percent decline in heart disease risk. Though this landmark study used a drug, rather than diet alone, heart disease researchers believe that the results are directly applicable to what would happen if people ate a cholesterol-lowering diet and did not take drugs. This study has made believers out of almost everyone, including major segments of the meat industry. The American Meat Institute, The National Cattlemen's Association, the National Pork Producers Council, National Meat Association, and the National Live Stock and Meat Board released a "statement of principles" that included the following:

> We believe that overwhelming scientific evidence points to a diet of moderation and variety. Individuals with specific health concerns that require dietary modification should be diagnosed and have diets prescribed by a physician. *We agree with the concept of the dietary guidelines recommending the avoidance of too much fat, sodium, and sugar.* [emphasis added]

One of the most exciting current areas of heart research concerns the different forms of blood cholesterol. The two basic forms, present in everyone's blood, are called high-density lipoprotein (HDL) and low-density lipoprotein (LDL). Researchers have discovered that the HDL form consists of cholesterol leaving the bloodstream, and actually reduces the risk of heart disease. The LDL form has the potential for sticking to arterial walls, causing heart disease.

Traditional cholesterol tests measured the total amount of HDL, LDL, and other forms of blood cholesterol. This measure is still an excellent indicator of overall risk of heart disease, even though it does not distinguish between beneficial and undesirable forms of cholesterol. The reason for this is that almost everyone has substantially more LDL than HDL, so total cholesterol generally reflects the amount of LDL. However, most medical laboratories can now provide separate measurements of total cholesterol and HDL-cholesterol. The ratio of the two is one of the best estimates of heart disease risk—the smaller the ratio of total to HDL, the better. For example, a person might have a total cholesterol level of 180 and an HDL count of 50. Both the ratio, 3.6, and the total cholesterol level indicate a relatively low risk of heart attack. According to Dr. William Castelli, director of the Framingham heart disease study, people with a ratio over 4.5 should go on a cholesterol-lowering diet.

A good health goal is to boost one's HDL level, and scientists have identified several factors that correlate with high HDL. The most obvious one, though out of anyone's control, is to be a young woman. High HDL levels in young women apparently contribute to their low rate of heart attack. More under our control is another important factor: exercise. Long distance runners and other athletes tend to have above average HDL levels. Studies of nonrunners who were induced to run regularly (about ten or more miles per week) demonstrated that running increases HDL-cholesterol.[53] Alcohol consumption also correlates with high HDL levels, though the latest research indicates that there are actually several different kinds of HDL and that alcohol lifts levels of a kind that does not reduce heart disease risk.[54]

Though the largest, best controlled, and most sophisticated studies have been conducted only recently, there has been evidence since the early years of this century that fat promotes heart disease. Back in 1908, a Russian scientist gave rabbits atherosclerosis by feeding them meat, milk, or eggs.[55] As the evidence piled up through the decades, one health agency after another began advising consumers to eat less fat. In 1961 the American Heart Association first spoke out. Then in 1968 the governments of Finland, Sweden and Norway, all nations having high heart disease rates, recommended diets low in fat and high in starchy foods. In 1972 the Inter-Society Commission on Heart Disease Resources, which had representatives from twenty-nine medical societies, recommended cholesterol-lowering diets. The Commission had calculated that if Americans' blood cholesterol levels were 10 percent lower, heart disease would drop by 24 percent. A 15 percent reduction would reduce heart disease by 35 percent.

It took the federal government a few years longer—because of pressure from the obvious agricultural interests—to formally advise the public to eat less fat and cholesterol, but the Surgeon General of the United States finally did so in July 1979:

> Americans would probably be healthier, as a whole if they consumed . . . less saturated fat and cholesterol.

Once the Surgeon General made it official, the Department of Agriculture and the Department of Health and Human Services mounted educational campaigns. The keystone of the effort was a pamphlet entitled "Nutrition and Your Health" that emphasized seven "dietary guidelines." The most important guideline advises "Avoid too much fat, saturated fat, and cholesterol."

Americans' eating habits have been changing in a direction consistent with the official recommendations. Our consumption of eggs—a major source of cholesterol—dropped from 403 per person in 1945 to 326 in 1962 to 263 in 1982. Many people are switching from beef, which is high in saturated fat, to chicken and fish, which are low in saturated fat. Margarine and salad oils, both low in saturated fats, have largely replaced butter and lard in American homes. Also, low-fat and skim milk are gradually replacing whole milk as the "standard" milk. Presumably, such remarkable dietary changes in the "right" direction would lead to reduced heart disease rates, and, indeed, Americans' heart disease rates have plummeted. Between 1968 and 1983, mortality due to heart disease decreased 36 percent. What with better medical care, more effective drugs, more people exercising, and fewer adult men smoking, it is impossible to apportion the credit accurately to diet and each other factor. But we should have a feeling of real satisfaction that our improved health habits are yielding major benefits.

If it weren't bad enough that diets high in saturated fat promote heart disease, several kinds of studies also indicate that diets high in any kind of fat promote several different cancers. In 1979 the National Cancer Institute first publicized the evidence that high-fat diets are a cancer risk. At Senate hearings, NCI director Dr. Arthur Upton testified that "animal studies as well as

> **COOKBOOKS FOR LOW-FAT EATING**
>
> **Recipes low in all fats**
>
> 1. *The Alternative Diet Book,* William Connor, Sonja Connor, Martha Fry, and Susan Warner. University of Iowa Publications (Iowa City), 1976.
> 2. *The Live Longer Now Cookbook,* Jon Leonard and Elaine Taylor. Grosset and Dunlap, New York, 1977.
> 3. *The Good Heart Cookbook,* Ellen Stern and Jonathan Michaels. Ticknor & Fields (New Haven), 1982.
> 4. *Deliciously Low,* Harriet Sobel-Roth. New American Library (New York), 1983.
> 5. *Don't Eat Your Heart Out Cookbook,* Joseph Piscatella. Workman (New York), 1982.
>
> **Recipes low in saturated fat and cholesterol**
>
> 1. *The American Heart Association Cookbook,* Ruthe Eshleman and Mary Winston. David McKay, Inc. (New York), 1973.
> 2. *The Jewish Low-Cholesterol Cookbook,* Roberta Leviton. Erikkson Press (Middlebury, VT), 1978. ($15.95 to Erikkson Press, Battell Building, Middlebury, VT 05753)
> 3. *Laurel's Kitchen,* Laurel Robertson. Nilgiri Press (Petaluma, CA), 1976.

studies of human populations suggest that a high-fat intake may be associated with an increased risk of cancer. Both saturated and unsaturated fats have been incriminated." The National Cancer Institute issued a series of dietary recommendations, including one that stated ". . . in view of the suggestive association between fat consumption and the risk of cancer, a high intake of fat should be avoided."[56]

To help clarify relationships between diet and cancer and reduce public confusion, the National Academy of Sciences appointed a top-level committee to review the literature. In 1982 the Committee on Diet, Nutrition, and Cancer issued a major report. The committee concluded that:

> of all the dietary components studied, the combined epidemiological and experimental evidence is most suggestive for a casual relationship between fat intake and

the occurrence of cancer. Both epidemiological studies and experiments in animals provide convincing evidence that increasing the intake of total fat increases the incidence of cancer at certain sites, particularly the breast and colon, and, conversely, that the risk is lower with lower intakes of fat.

The NAS committee recommended that:

> the consumption of both saturated and unsaturated fats be reduced in the average U.S. diet. An appropriate and practical target is to reduce the intake of fat from its present level (approximately 40%) to 30% of total calories in the diet. The scientific data do not provide a strong basis for establishing fat intake at precisely 30% of total calories. Indeed, the data could be used to justify an even greater reduction.

In 1984 the American Cancer Society joined the growing chorus by urging people "to cut down on total fat intake." Also in 1984 the National Cancer Institute started a public education campaign. One of its eight "cancer prevention tips" is to "Eat foods low in fat."

DETERMINING YOUR FAT INTAKE

The less fat in your diet the better. The minimum possible amount is about 10 percent of your total caloric intake. The average American diet has about 40 percent of its calories from fat. A reasonable target to shoot for, unless you are suffering from advanced heart disease, is 25 percent or less of your calories.

To determine how many total calories and how many calories from fat you should consume, use the following chart:

	Average Daily Caloric Intake	Maximum Advisable Calories from Fat	Maximum Advisable Grams of Fat
Children 6–11	2,000	500	56
Females			
12–17	1,800	450	50
18–44	1,600	400	44
45 and over	1,400	350	39
Males			
12–17	2,600	650	72
18–54	2,400	600	67
55 and over	2,000	500	56

Now that you have learned the maximum number of grams of fat you should consume in a day, use the following tables to calculate how much fat you actually consume.

Fat Content of Foods

Food/Producer	Serving Size	Fat (grams)*
BEVERAGES (Nondairy)		
Beer, Wine, Liquor	1 serving	0.0
Coffee, Tea	6 oz.	0.0
Fruit Juices & Fruit Drinks	6 oz.	0.0
Soft Drinks	12 oz.	0.0
Milk Chocolate Cocoa Mix (Swiss Miss)	6 oz.	2.0
CONDIMENTS & SAUCES		
Ketchup	1 Tbsp.	0.1
Tomato Sauce (Del Monte)	1/2 cup (4 oz.)	0.5
Mustard (French's)	2 Tbsp.	1.0[L]†
Cremora Non-Dairy Creamer (Borden)	1 tsp.	1.0
Half & Half (Land O' Lakes)	1 Tbsp.	1.6[S]
Beef Gravy (Franco-American)	2 oz.	2.0[S]
Homestyle Spaghetti Sauce (Ragu)	4 oz.	2.0[P]
Reduced Calorie French Dressing (Kraft)	1 Tbsp.	2.0[P]
French Onion Dip (Kraft)	2 Tbsp.	4.0[S]
Salad Dressing (Hellman's)	1 Tbsp.	5.0[P]
Whipping Cream (Land O' Lakes)	1 Tbsp.	5.0[S]
Spaghetti Sauce (Prego)	4 oz.	6.0[L]
French Dressing (Kraft)	1 Tbsp.	6.0
Sour Cream (Land O' Lakes)	3 Tbsp.	7.5[S]
Tartar Sauce (Hellman's)	1 Tbsp.	7.7[P]
Italian Dressing (Wishbone)	1 Tbsp.	8.0[P]
Mayonnaise (Hellman's)	1 Tbsp.	11.0[L]
CRACKERS & CHIPS		
Whole Wheat Matzo (Manischewitz)	1 (1 oz.)	0.0
Golden Rye Crisp Bread (Wasa)	2 1/2 (1.1 oz.)	0.0
Pretzels (Mister Salty)	5 (0.9 oz.)	1.0
Popcorn, plain	2 cups	2.0
Stoned Wheat Thins (Interbake)	4 (1 oz.)	2.0
Triscuits (Nabisco)	7 (1.1 oz.)	5.0

* 1 teaspoon contains about 4 grams of fat.
† S = Tends to raise blood cholesterol (saturated)
P = Tends to lower blood cholesterol (polyunsaturated)
L = Little effect on blood cholesterol
No mark indicates that data were not available.

Food/Producer	Serving Size	Fat (grams)*
Wheatsworth (Nabisco)	9 (1 oz.)	6.0
Doritos Tortilla Chips (Frito-Lay)	1 oz.	7.0
Ritz (Nabisco)	9 (1 oz.)	8.0
Fritos Corn Chips (Frito-Lay)	1 oz.	10.0
Potato Chips (Wise)	1 oz.	10.0
Toasty Peanut Butter Sandwich (Lance)	1 1/4 oz.	10.0
Popcorn, regular (Jiffy Pop)	2 cups	11.0

DAIRY PRODUCTS & EGGS

MILK

Skim Milk	8 oz.	0.0
Buttermilk	8 oz.	2.2[S]
Lowfat Milk, 1% fat	8 oz.	2.5[S]
Lowfat Milk, 2% fat	8 oz.	4.6[S]
Chocolate Milk, 2% fat	8 oz.	5.0[S]
Whole Milk, 3.3% fat	8 oz.	8.0[S]

CHEESES

Cottage Cheese, 2% fat (Breakstone)	1/2 cup	2.0[S]
Lite-Line Pasteurized Process Cheese Product (Borden)	1.5 oz.	2.0[S]
Low Skim Edam (Dorman)	1.5 oz.	4.5[S]
Cottage Cheese, 4% milkfat (Sealtest)	1/2 cup	5.0[S]
Mozzarella, part skim (Kraft)	1.5 oz.	7.5[S]
Farmer's Cheese (Sargento)	1.5 oz.	7.5[S]
Velveeta (Kraft)	1.5 oz.	9.0[S]
Ricotta, part skim	1/2 cup	9.7[S]
Swiss (Land O' Lakes)	1.5 oz.	11.6[S]
Cheddar (Kraft)	1.5 oz.	13.5[S]
Cream Cheese (Philadelphia)	1.5 oz.	15.0[S]

EGGS

Egg Beaters (Fleischmann's)	1/4 cup	0.0
Egg	1 large	5.5[S]

YOGURT

Fruit Lowfat Yogurt (Dannon)	1 cup (8 oz.)	3.0[S]
Plain Lowfat Yogurt (Dannon)	1 cup (8 oz.)	4.0[S]
Fruit Yogurt (Yoplait)	3/4 cup (6 oz.)	4.0[S]
Plain Yogurt (Columbo)	1 cup (8 oz.)	7.0[S]

FAST FOODS

Hamburger Sandwich (McDonald's)	1 (3.6 oz.)	9.7[S]
Taco (Jack-in-the-Box)	1 (2.9 oz.)	10.8
French Fries (Burger King)	1 (2.4 oz.)	11.0[S]

Food/Producer	Serving Size	Fat (grams)*
Vanilla Milkshake (Gino's)	1 (14 oz.)	12.1[S]
Apple Turnover (Hardees)	1 (3 oz.)	13.7[S]
Superstyle Cheese Pizza (Pizza Hut)	2 sl. (¼ pie)	14.0
Egg McMuffin (McDonald's)	1 (4.9 oz.)	14.7[S]
Cheeseburger Sandwich (Burger King)	1 (4.4 oz.)	17.0[S]
Chicken Thigh (Kentucky Fried Chicken)	1 (3.1 oz.)	17.5[L]
Roast Beef Sandwich (Roy Rogers)	1	18.7[S]
Hamburger Sandwich (Wendy's)	1 (7 oz.)	26.0[S]
Big Mac (McDonald's)	1 (7.2 oz.)	33.0[S]
T-Bone Steak Platter (Rustler)	1	53.0[S]
Triple Cheeseburger Sandwich (Wendy's)	1 (14 oz.)	68.0[S]

FATS & OILS

Margarine, Diet	1 pat (1 tsp.)	1.8[L]
Margarine, Whipped	1 pat (1 tsp.)	2.3[L]
Butter, Whipped	1 pat (1 tsp.)	2.3[S]
Margarine, Stick or Tub	1 pat (1 tsp.)	3.7[L]
Butter, Stick	1 pat (1 tsp.)	3.7[S]
Corn, Safflower, Sesame, Soy, Sunflower Oils	1 tsp.	4.4[P]
Olive, Peanut Oils	1 tsp.	4.4[L]
Coconut, Palm Oils, Lard	1 tsp.	4.4[S]

FISH

Cod, Turbot, Flounder, Sole, Haddock	4 oz.	1.0[P]
Light Tuna, water-packed (Chicken of the Sea)	3 oz.	1.1[L]
Halibut, Red Snapper	4 oz.	1.6[L]
Scallops, Crab	4 oz.	2.0[P]
Catfish	4 oz.	5.1[L]
Rainbow Trout	4 oz.	6.4[L]
Salmon, Sockeye, canned	3 oz.	9.5[P]
Light Tuna, oil-packed (Chicken of the Sea)	3 oz.	10.3[L]
Filet of Sole in Lemon Butter Sauce (Gorton's)	4 oz.	12.4
Mackerel, Atlantic	4 oz.	13.8[L]
Batter Fried Fish Sticks (Gorton's)	4 (4 oz.)	24.0
Family Fried Clams (Mrs. Paul's)	4 oz.	25.0[L]

RATING THE NUTRITIONAL VALUE OF FOODS

Food/Producer	Serving Size	Fat (grams)*
FRUITS & VEGETABLES		
Fruits, fresh, frozen, canned, dried	1 serving	0.0
Vegetables, fresh, frozen, canned	1 serving	0–1
Japanese Style Vegetables (Birds Eye)	3.3 oz.	6.0
Sweet Peas in Butter Sauce (Green Giant)	1 cup	6.0[S]
Coconut, shredded	1/4 cup	7.0[S]
Broccoli with Cheese Sauce (Birds Eye)	5 oz.	12.0[P]
Avocado	1/2	15.4[L]
GRAIN FOODS		
Rice, Barley, Bulgur, Bran, Pasta, Millet	1 cup	0–1
Egg Noodles (Mueller's)	1 cup	3.0[S]
BREADS & PANCAKES		
100% Stone Ground Whole Wheat Bread (Arnold/Orowheat)	2 sl. (1.6 oz.)	2.0
White Bread (Wonder)	2 sl. (2 oz.)	2.0
Jumbo Buttermilk Frozen Waffles (Aunt Jemima)	1 (1.3 oz.)	2.1
Complete Pancake Mix (Log Cabin)	3 (4") cakes	3.0
Taco Shells (Old El Paso)	2 (0.8 oz.)	4.8[P]
Homestyle Frozen Waffles (Eggo)	1 (1.4 oz.)	5.0
Croissants (Sara Lee)	1 (0.9 oz.)	6.0[S]
Easy Mix Cornbread (Aunt Jemima)	1/6 (1.7 oz.)	6.0
Bisquick (Betty Crocker)	1/2 cup (2 oz.)	8.0
Chicken Flavored Stuffing Mix (Stove Top)	1/2 cup, prepared	9.0
Buttermilk Pancake Mix (Hungry Jack)	3 (4") pancakes	12.0
CEREALS		
Cream of Wheat (Nabisco)	1 oz.	0.0
Corn Flakes (Kellogg)	1 1/4 cup (1 oz.)	0.0
Rice Krispies (Kellogg)	1 cup (1 oz.)	0.0
Raisin Bran (Post)	1/2 cup (1 oz.)	1.0
Oatmeal (Quaker)	2/3 cup (1 oz.)	2.0[L]
Wheat Germ (Krotochmor)	1/4 cup (1 oz.)	3.0[P]
100% Natural (Quaker)	1/4 cup (1 oz.)	6.0[S]

Food/Producer	Serving Size	Fat (grams)*
MEATS & POULTRY		
Turkey, light, w/o skin	4 oz.	3.6[L]
Turkey Roll, white (Land O' Lakes)	3 oz.	3.6[L]
Chicken, light, w/o skin	4 oz.	5.2[L]
Round Steak, lean	4 oz.	5.3[S]
Beef Liver	4 oz.	5.3[S]
Sirloin Steak, lean	4 oz.	8.0[S]
Turkey Franks (Louis Rich)	1 (1.6 oz.)	8.0[L]
Turkey, dark, w/o skin	4 oz.	8.1[L]
Bacon (Oscar Mayer)	3 sl. (0.6 oz.)	9.3[S]
Chicken, dark, w/o skin	4 oz.	11.0[L]
Chicken Franks (Weaver)	1 (1.6 oz.)	11.0[L]
Lamb, Rib Chops, lean	4 oz.	12.0[S]
Veal, Round Roast, lean	4 oz.	12.0[S]
Chicken, light, w/skin	4 oz.	12.1[L]
Beef Franks (Eckrich)	1 (1.6 oz.)	13.0[S]
Breakfast Links (Morning Star Farms)	3 (2.3 oz.)	13.5[L]
Bologna (Oscar Mayer)	2 sl. (1.6 oz.)	13.7[S]
Pork Chops, loin, lean	4 oz.	16.1[S]
Canned Ham (Swift Premium)	4 oz.	17.0[S]
Chicken, dark, w/skin	4 oz.	17.6[L]
Deviled Ham (Underwood)	1/2 can (2.3 oz.)	20.0[S]
Brown n' Serve Sausage (Swift)	3 (2.2 oz.)	21.0[S]
Ground Beef, lean	4 oz.	22.6[S]
Spam (Hormel)	3 oz.	23.0[S]
Sirloin Steak, untrimmed	4 oz.	26.0[S]
T-Bone Steak, untrimmed	4 oz.	49.3[S]
NUTS & BEANS		
Dried Beans, Lentils Split Peas	1 cup, cooked	0–1
Refried Beans (Old El Paso)	8 oz.	2.0[S]
Pork n' Beans (Campbell)	8 oz.	4.0[S]
Tofu	2.5" × 2.8" × 1"	5.0[P]
Red Kidney Beans, seasoned with pork (Luck's)	7.5 oz. (7/8 cup)	6.0[S]
Soynuts (Planters)	1 oz.	7.0[P]
Soybeans	1 cup	10.0[P]
Cashews	1 oz.	13.0[L]
Peanuts (Planters)	1 oz.	15.0[L]
Crunchy Peanut Butter (Peter Pan)	2 Tbsp.	16.0[L]
PREPARED DISHES		
Long Grain and Wild Rice (Minute Rice)	1/2 cup, prep.	4.0

Food/Producer	Serving Size	Fat (grams)*
Hungry Jack Mashed Potatoes (Pillsbury)	1/2 cup, prep.	7.0
Lasagna Dinner (Chef Boy-ar-dee)	1/4 pkg., prep.	9.0[S]
Noodles Romanoff (Betty Crocker)	1/4 pkg., prep.	12.0[S]
Macaroni & Cheese (Kraft)	3/4 cup, prep.	14.0[S]

CANNED

Food/Producer	Serving Size	Fat (grams)*
Spaghetti with Tomato Sauce and Cheese (Franco-American)	7.4 oz.	2.0[S]
Chicken Chow Mein (La Choy)	3/4 cup	3.0[L]
Beef Stew (Dinty Moore)	7.5 oz.	9.0[S]
Spaghetti & Meat Balls (Chef Boy-ar-dee)	7.5 oz.	11.0[S]
Chili with Beans (Hormel)	7.5 oz.	16.0[S]
Chili No Beans (Hormel)	7.5 oz.	28.0[S]

FROZEN

Food/Producer	Serving Size	Fat (grams)*
Filet of Fish Divan Dinner (Stouffer's Lean Cuisine)	12 3/8 oz.	3.0
Lasagna (Stouffer)	10.5 oz.	14.0[S]
Fried Chicken Breasts (Swanson)	1 (3.2 oz.)	16.0
Cheese Pizza (Celeste)	1/3 pie (6 oz.)	17.4
Pepperoni Party Pizza (Totino's)	1/2 pie (6 oz.)	22.0
Salisbury Steak Dinner (Banquet)	11 oz.	24.5[S]
Cheese Soufflé (Stouffer)	6 oz.	26.0
Hungry Man Veal Parmigiana Dinner (Swanson)	20.5 oz.	34.0
Hungry Man Turkey Pie (Swanson)	1 (16 oz.)	47.0
Steak House Beef Tenderloin Dinner (Morton)	9.5 oz.	64.0[S]

SOUPS

Food/Producer	Serving Size	Fat (grams)*
Tomato Cup-A-Soup (Lipton)	6 oz.	1.0
Minestrone (Progresso)	8 oz.	2.0[P]
Chunky Chicken (Campbell)	10 3/4 oz.	8.0[L]
Cream of Mushroom (Campbell)	10 oz., prep.	8.7

SWEETS & DESSERTS

CANDY

Food/Producer	Serving Size	Fat (grams)*
Chewing Gum, Hard Candy, Mints, Marshmallows	1 piece	0.0

Food/Producer	Serving Size	Fat (grams)*
Cinnamon Granola Bar (Nature Valley)	1 (0.8 oz.)	4.0[S]
M & M's, plain (M&M/Mars)	1 bag (1.7 oz.)	10.3[S]
Chocolate Figurines (Pillsbury)	2 (1.8 oz.)	10.3[S]
Baby Ruth (Nabisco Brands)	1 (1.8 oz.)	11.0[S]
Milk Chocolate Bar (Hershey)	1 (1.2 oz.)	11.0[S]
Peanut Butter Cups (Reese's)	2 (1.4 oz.)	12.1[S]
Breakfast Squares (General Mills)	2 (3 oz.)	17.0

FROZEN DESSERTS

Frozen Lowfat Yogurt (Dannon)	1 cup (8 oz.)	2.0[S]
Strawberry Ice Milk (Light 'n Lively)	3/4 cup (3.5 oz.)	3.0[S]
Orange Sherbet (Land O' Lakes)	3/4 cup (6 oz.)	3.1[S]
Vanilla Ice Cream (Breyers)	3/4 cup (3.8 oz.)	12.5[S]
Chocolate Ice Cream (Häagen-Dazs)	3/4 cup (6 oz.)	25.5[S]

PUDDINGS & GELATIN

Gelatin, all flavors (Jell-O)	1/2 cup, prep.	0.0
Vanilla Instant Pudding (Royal)	1/2 cup, prep.	5.0[S]
Chocolate Ready-to-Eat Pudding (Swiss Miss)	1/2 cup (4 oz.)	6.0

SWEET TOPPINGS

Jams, Jellies, Sugar, Honey, Syrup	1 Tbsp.	0.0
Chocolate Syrup (Hershey)	2 Tbsp. (1 oz.)	1.0[S]
Vanilla Rich n' Easy Frosting Mix (Pillsbury)	for 1/2 cake	5.0
Chocolate Ready to Spread Frosting (Betty Crocker)	for 1/2 cake	8.0

SWEET BAKED GOODS

MIXES

Blueberry Muffin Mix (Betty Crocker)	1/12 pkg.	4.0
Double Fudge Brownie Mix (Duncan Hines)	1 prep.	5.0
Devil's Food Cake Mix (Duncan Hines)	1/12 cake	6.0
Supermoist Carrot Cake Mix (Betty Crocker)	1/12 cake	12.0
Yellow Cake Mix (Pillsbury Plus)	1/12 cake	12.0

FROZEN

Pound Cake (Sara Lee)	1/15 (1.1 oz.)	7.4[S]

Food/Producer	Serving Size	Fat (grams)*
Chocolate Chip Cookies (Pillsbury)	3	8.0
Honey Buns (Morton)	1 (2.3 oz.)	11.0
Cinnamon Raisin Danish (Pillsbury)	2 (2.7 oz.)	11.0
Pecan Coffee Cake (Sara Lee)	1/4 (1.6 oz.)	11.5S
Cream Cheesecake (Sara Lee)	1/2 (3.3 oz.)	16.0S
Apple Pie (Mrs. Smith's)	1/8 (5.8 oz.)	17.0S
READY TO EAT		
Ginger Snaps (Nabisco)	4 (1 oz.)	3.0
Graham Crackers (Nabisco)	4 (1 oz.)	3.0
Chocolate Cupcakes (Hostess)	1 (1.8 oz.)	5.0
Cherry Pop Tart (Kellogg)	1 (1.8 oz.)	5.0S
Chips Ahoy Cookies (Nabisco)	3 (1.1 oz.)	7.0
Oreo Cookies (Nabisco)	3 (1.1 oz.)	7.0
Old Fashioned Donuts (Hostess)	1 (1.5 oz.)	10.0
Cheese Danish (TastyKake)	1 (2.3 oz.)	14.5
Peach Pie (Hostess)	1 (4.5 oz.)	20.0
Honey Bun (Hostess)	1 (4.8 oz.)	34.0

Cholesterol

"Is cholesterol really bad for you?" This is certainly one of the most asked health questions in the United States. Unfortunately for lovers of eggs, the answer for the past twenty-five years has been an unequivocal "yes."

The cholesterol issue is confusing, partly because the word cholesterol can apply to two different things: the cholesterol in food and the cholesterol in our bloodstream. The amount of cholesterol in one's blood is a key gauge of one's risk of heart attack.

Blood cholesterol levels are influenced by several factors. First, the human liver and intestine can produce cholesterol, usually about 500–1,000 milligrams a day. This insures that the body will always have adequate cholesterol for the production of sex hormones, transport of essential fatty acids, and formation of the insulation around nerves.

Another important determinant of blood cholesterol levels, as we have seen, is the amount and kind of fat in the diet. Other factors, such as eating certain kinds of dietary fiber and engaging in frequent aerobic exercise, also affect cholesterol levels somewhat.

Finally, cholesterol in food significantly affects blood cholesterol levels. The average male consumes about 400 milligrams of dietary cholesterol per day, and the average female about 265 milligrams.[57] To help guard against excessively high blood cholesterol levels, the liver produces less cholesterol when a person is getting cholesterol from food. But this feedback mechanism does not work perfectly. Thus, if a person eats 250 milligrams of cholesterol, the body would not reduce its own production by quite that much, and blood cholesterol would tend to rise.

Only animal products contain cholesterol. All vegetable foods are cholesterol-free. The egg, or to be more precise, the egg yolk, is the single greatest source of dietary cholesterol (see the following table). It provides about one third of our intake. Meat, fish, and poultry contribute another third. Dairy products provide about one sixth. The remainder comes from commercial baked goods, shortening, and other foods.

Sources of Cholesterol in the American Diet[58]

Food	Percent of Dietary cholesterol
Egg yolk	34
Meat, fish, poultry	32
Dairy products	16
Desserts, baked goods	8
Butter, lard, animal shortening	4
Miscellaneous	6
TOTAL	100

Lean beef, pork, lamb, and lobster contain about 100 milligrams of cholesterol per serving, while clams, scallops, oysters, cod, flounder, and other seafoods contain about half that amount. Shrimp, which are practically devoid of fat, are relatively high in cholesterol, containing 171 milligrams per serving (see table on page 72—Cholesterol Content of Common Foods). One large egg contains 275 milligrams of cholesterol, all of which resides in the yolk. While beef is not terribly high in cholesterol, it is often considered a high cholesterol food. This is because beef usually contains plenty of saturated fat. The high fat content promotes high cholesterol levels in the consumer's blood.

Medical researchers have conducted detailed studies on human volunteers to measure the effect of dietary cholesterol on blood cholesterol. University of Minnesota scientists Drs. Ancel Keys, Joseph Anderson, and Francisco Grande found that increasing dietary cholesterol from 50 to 380 milligrams per day, by adding egg yolk to the diet, raises blood cholesterol levels by an average of 16 milligrams per deciliter.[59] In another careful study, Dr. D. Mark Hegsted and his colleagues at the Harvard School of Public Health found that each 100 milligrams of egg yolk cholesterol raises blood cholesterol levels of adult men an average of about 5 milligrams.[60] Above 600 to 800 milligrams a day, however, Hegsted and others found that dietary cholesterol has a smaller and smaller effect on blood levels.[61]

In a more recent study, seventeen Hampshire College students volunteered to eat specially prepared desserts for six weeks. These students were all lactovegetarians and normally consumed only about 100 milligrams of cholesterol daily. For three of the six weeks, one extra-large egg was secretly included in the dessert recipe. Dr. Frank Sacks, of Harvard's Channing Laboratory, tested the students' blood and found that the egg raised total serum cholesterol by 3.9 percent (6.8 milligrams/deciliter) and "bad" LDL cholesterol by 11.8 percent (11.6 milligrams/deciliter).[62] Dr. Sacks concluded that "reduction of cholesterol intake to very low levels is likely to lower serum cholesterol much more than decreasing dietary cholesterol to the moderate levels currently recommended [by the American Heart Association and others]."

The egg industry has been shrinking gradually, partly because people were avoiding cholesterol. To help allay the public's fears, the industry began sponsoring research at the University of Missouri (Dr. Margaret Flynn), University of California at Los Angeles (Dr. Grant Slater), and University of Illinois (Dr. Fred Kummerow). The industry claimed that studies done at all three universities disproved the cholesterol-raising effect of eggs. In fact, the studies were abominably designed and disproved nothing. The National Heart, Lung, and Blood Institute (NHLBI) examined the studies and issued a devastating opinion. Concerning the Missouri study, NHLBI said that:

> Serious design flaws prevent interpretation of the results. The diet instructions were so vague and the control and assessment of diet so poor that it is entirely possible that over all or most of each twelve-week period, any effects of changes in the dietary cholesterol may have been obliterated by the fact that there may have been little or no difference in dietary cholesterol intakes and/or differences in dietary fats.

NHLBI said that the UCLA egg study "suffered numerous serious faults which would be expected to prevent observation of an effect," but "despite the author's conclusions and all the serious flaws in the study, the results do indicate an effect of egg cholesterol on plasma [blood] cholesterol." NHLBI dismissed the University of Illinois study, saying it was "meaningless and should be discarded."

After the dust of the battle settled, the recommendations by government and private health agencies concerning cholesterol stood unchanged: eat less cholesterol. Because cholesterol and saturated fat both raise cholesterol levels, one could choose to make a special effort on reducing fat and be more relaxed about cholesterol, or *vice versa*. But for both fat and cholesterol, the rule of thumb is "the less the better."

To know where you stand on cholesterol, you should get your blood cholesterol level measured—and urge your friends and loved ones to do the same. If you are an adult and your total cholesterol level is 150–180 or below, you could maintain your current cholesterol intake. If it is higher, especially if it is over

225–250, you should make a serious effort to reduce your fat and cholesterol intake.

Cholesterol Content of Common Foods‡[63]

Food	Serving Size	Cholesterol (milligrams)
Egg white	1	0
Milk, skim	1 cup	5
Cottage cheese, uncreamed	1/2 cup	7
Mayonnaise	1 Tbsp.	10
Lard	1 Tbsp.	12
Butter	1 pat	12
Cream, light table	1 fl. oz.	20
Cottage cheese, creamed	1/2 cup	24
Cream, half and half	2 oz.	26
Hot dog	1 (1.6 oz.)	27
Milk, whole	1 cup	34
Butter	1 Tbsp.	35
Ice cream (10% fat)	3/4 cup	40
Cheddar cheese	1.5 oz.	42
Egg noodles	1 cup	50
Cod, flounder, raw	4 oz.	57
Tuna, canned, drained	3 oz.	58
Clams, oysters, scallops	4 oz.	58
Ice cream (16% fat)	3/4 cup	64
Big Mac (McDonald's)	1 (7 oz.)	86
Chicken	4 oz.	98
Pork, lean	4 oz.	101
Beef, lean	4 oz.	103
Sardines, canned	3 oz.	103
Veal, lean	4 oz.	112
Crab, steamed	4 oz.	113
Lamb, lean	4 oz.	114
Shrimp	4 oz.	171
Liver, chicken	1	190
Heart, chicken	3 oz.	196
Egg	1 large	275
Liver, beef	3 oz.	372
Kidney, cooked	3 oz.	680
Brains, raw	3 oz.	1,700+

‡ Vegetable foods never contain cholesterol.

Salt/Sodium

Salt: the white crystals that are present in almost every kitchen, on almost every dining table in the land, look so innocent. But, in this case, looks are deceiving. The high salt content of the American diet promotes high blood pressure and heart disease.

Salt is made up of sodium and chloride, with the sodium portion causing the problems. The human body needs only a few hundred milligrams of sodium each day, but most Americans (and people living in other modern lands) ingest between 4,000 and 10,000 milligrams a day. The National Academy of Sciences has said that Americans should limit their daily sodium intake to 1,100 to 3,300 milligrams. Because the body has developed a wonderful system for conserving sodium, even people who do heavy labor or work in hot climates do not usually need additional sodium.

Natural foods are generally low in sodium, but would more than meet our bodies' needs. Bonnie Liebman, nutritionist at the Center for Science in the Public Interest, calculates that naturally occurring sodium contributes only about 10 percent of the sodium in the average person's diet. An additional 15 percent comes from the salt we use in cooking or add to foods at the table. The great bulk of sodium comes from processed foods, including everything from soup to nuts, cheese to bread, hot sauce to hot dogs.

Salt itself contributes about 90 percent of the sodium added to processed foods, according to the FDA. The rest comes from such sodium-containing additives as monosodium glutamate, sodium benzoate, and sodium phosphate.

The amount of sodium in some processed foods is truly astonishing. A single ten-ounce serving of Campbell's chicken noodle soup contains 1,169 milligrams; a McDonald's Quarter-Pounder with Cheese contains 1,236 milligrams; and one Armour Classic "Lite" beef with broccoli dinner contains 2,120 milligrams. The high sodium prize goes to the Banquet Man-Pleaser cheese enchilada frozen dinner, which contains 4,778 milligrams. This one item by itself exceeds the maximum recommended daily intake of 3,300 milligrams! By contrast, one teaspoon of salt contains 2,000 milligrams of sodium. The following table illustrates how much higher processed foods are in sodium than relatively natural, unprocessed foods.

Sodium in Fresh and Processed Foods

Fresh		Processed	
Beef stew, 1 cup	290	Chef Boy-Ar-Dee beef stew, 1 cup	1,045
Cheddar cheese, natural, 1 oz.	200	Kraft pasteurized process cheese, 1 oz.	446
Chicken breast, roasted, 3.5 oz.	69	Swanson frozen fried chicken breast, 3.8 oz.	620
Corn, cooked, 1/2 cup	1	Del Monte canned corn, 1/2 cup	355
Flounder, cooked with butter, 4.5 oz.	300	Mrs. Paul's flounder with lemon sauce, 4.3 oz.	808
Hamburger, lean, 3.2 oz.	64	Oscar Mayer franks, 2, 3.2 oz.	932
Oatmeal, cooked, 1 oz. (dry)	1	Post Fortified Oat Flakes, 1 oz.	275
Pork, lean, broiled, 2 oz.	40	Eckrich bologna, 2 slices, 2 oz.	526
Rice, cooked, 1/2 cup	2	Minute Rice, Chinese, fried rice, 1/2 cup	635
Green beans, cooked, 1/2 cup	3	Libby's canned green beans, 1/2 cup	343

About the only natural foods that contain significant amounts of sodium are dairy products. Milk contains 120 milligrams per glass, while 1.5-ounce servings of cheese vary from 110 milligrams for Swiss cheese to 770 milligrams for Roquefort cheese. Baked goods contain fairly large amounts of sodium—about 350 milligrams in two slices of bread—and are the greatest source of sodium in many diets.

Many processed foods contain far more sodium than they need for flavoring or other purposes. Companies say they add the appropriate levels of salt to their products "to achieve consumer acceptance," but there is *no* "standard" level of salt in many products. Some major brands of breads, processed meats, frozen foods, canned vegetables, and fast foods contain substantially more salt than other brands. For instance, Ore-Ida Tater Tots contain more than twice as much sodium (550 mg) as Birds Eye Tiny Taters (263 mg) per 3-ounce serving. An 8-ounce serving of Campbell's minestrone soup (960 mg) contains over 400 milligrams more sodium than Progresso minestrone (531 mg). One tablespoon of Seven Seas Viva Italian salad dressing (320 mg) contains more than twice as much sodium as Kraft Golden Blend Italian dressing (150 mg). Consumers probably do not even notice most of these differences. The variation in sodium levels from one brand to another indicates that many manufacturers could reduce greatly the sodium content of their products.

Scientists first suggested a link between high sodium diets and hypertension in the first decade of this century. Since then, the link has been established by numerous studies, yet it is still not completely understood.

High blood pressure, or hypertension, is a condition without any outward symptoms. Rather, it is a silent phenomenon that develops gradually over several decades and increases the risks of stroke, heart attack, and congestive heart failure. Heart attack and stroke are two of the three biggest killers in the United States, accounting for almost three quarters of a million deaths a year. Annual economic costs related to hypertension total over eight billion dollars.

According to the National High Blood Pressure Education Program, about sixty million Americans have definite or borderline high blood pressure. That represents one out of three adult Americans. In addition, many people who do not currently have high blood pressure will develop it later in life. At current rates, by the time they reach sixty-five, more than half of all Americans will have developed high blood pressure.

For some unknown reason, a higher percentage of blacks has high blood pressure than whites. According to the National High Blood Pressure Education Program, in 1980 the death rate due to stroke among people aged thirty-five to seventy-four was two and one-half times as high in blacks as in whites.[64]

Important evidence linking salt to hypertension comes from epidemiological (population) studies. Some population groups or nations have much higher or lower rates of hypertension (and stroke) than others. In the northern part of Japan, 40 to 50 percent of the population has hypertension. These people eat a diet loaded with salty, pickled foods. Other Japanese eat a diet that is still high in sodium, but somewhat lower than their northern relatives. They have a somewhat lower level of hypertension. These findings demonstrate that susceptibility to high blood pressure is not determined solely by genetic background, but is shaped to a great extent by one's environment.

Scientists have also studied the diets and health of people living in isolated areas untouched by Western civilization and processed foods. Mountain-dwelling tribes of the Solomon Islands had essentially no high blood pressure. The same held true for Kalahari Bushmen of southern Africa and Melanesian tribes in New Guinea. Their blood pressure does not even rise gradually with age, as happens to most Americans. However, Solomon Islanders living near seaports obtained salt-laden processed foods from sailors and explorers and did develop high blood pressure.

Critical studies on hypertension have been conducted on human subjects under controlled conditions. In a 1982 British test, nineteen hypertensive patients went on a moderately low sodium diet. When they reduced their sodium intake from 4,000 to 2,000 milligrams per day, their average blood pressure (diastolic—the lower of the two numbers in a blood pressure measurement) declined by 7.6 millimeters. Then the patients were given placebo pills containing no active ingredient. Their blood pressure remained stable. Finally, they were given time-release sodium tablets to bring their daily sodium intake back to about 4,000 milligrams. The higher sodium diet returned their blood pressure to what it had been at the start of the study.[65] Similar studies have also been done in the United States.

The evidence linking high sodium diets to hypertension has led to a strong consensus among public health experts that Americans should consume much less sodium. The Surgeon General of the United States, U.S. Department of Agriculture, U.S. Department of Health and Human Services, Food and Drug Administration, American Heart Association, Food and Nutrition Board of the National Academy of Sciences, and others have all recommended that people cut their sodium intake substantially.

Eating less sodium can help prevent hypertension and alleviate existing hypertension. Though many doctors still prescribe drugs for people with mild high blood pressure, a low sodium diet is the preferred, cheapest, and totally harmless mode of treatment. For people with more severe high blood pressure, low sodium diets can reduce the amount of medication needed. Though low sodium diets can be initially difficult for our taste buds to accept, many people with high blood pressure have managed to treat their condition successfully with diet alone and avoid all the drugs. Many of the drugs (though generally not the common diuretics) trigger frequent side effects, including diarrhea, headaches, drowsiness, and sexual impotence.

To help people reduce their sodium intake, the Center for Science in the Public Interest petitioned the Food and Drug Administration to limit the amount of sodium in processed foods. This request was supported by over five thousand health professionals and students, including leading experts on hypertension. One of these, Dr. Henry Blackburn of the University of Minnesota, said, "The problem is less a scientific than a practical dilemma. The problem is how can the individual avoid excess sodium when so much is added to food before it reaches the table?" Because everyone has a salt shaker, it seems so sensible to include less salt in processed foods and allow consumers to salt their foods to suit their own taste buds.

The FDA's own Select Committee on GRAS (Generally Recognized as Safe) Substances, which evaluated the safety of several hundred food ingredients, concluded in 1979 that salt should *not* be considered "generally recognized as safe." The Committee's report stated:

> It is the prevalent judgment of the scientific community that the consumption of sodium chloride in the aggregate should be lowered in the United States. The Select Committee agrees and favors development of guidelines for restricting the amount of salt in processed foods.

Because of pressures from the food industry and the sheer complexity of the task, the FDA has not sought to restrict sodium levels in processed foods, but has urged industry to reduce levels voluntarily.

Another important step that could be taken would be to list the sodium content on all food labels. In this way, people could compare one brand to another. Congressman (now Senator) Albert Gore, Jr., took up the cudgel on this matter and sponsored legislation to require sodium labeling. Gore said:

> The time for a voluntary approach has passed. Despite strong evidence linking sodium and high blood pressure, only a fraction of the processed food industry has responded. The time has come to ensure that the American people have the information they need to reduce the $8 billion in health care costs that high blood pressure imposes every year.

Though Gore's bill was not voted into law, Gore's involvement lifted the debate to the highest levels in government. The commissioner then of FDA, Arthur Hayes, was, fortuitously, an expert on salt and high blood pressure. Hayes, using the prestige of his office, urged individuals to eat lower sodium foods and urged companies to voluntarily label their products and reduce sodium levels. FDA also ordered that by July 1, 1986, sodium be listed in the nutrition labeling information that is required on many foods and used voluntarily by many companies. What FDA could not do, because of the political stance of the Reagan administration, was require sodium labeling on all foods and reductions in the sodium content of excessively salted foods.

Many manufacturers and retailers have contributed to efforts to reduce sodium levels. Some companies have marketed whole new lines of reduced sodium or no-salt-added products. More and more cooking instructions on packages of processed foods are including salt as an optional ingredient. Numerous supermarket chains developed sodium education programs for their customers. And almost half the processed foods under FDA's supervision now have sodium labeling, though a much smaller percentage of meat and poultry products, which fall under USDA's jurisdiction, have such labeling.

One area that has seen little progress in terms of sodium content is regular processed foods. CSPI nutritionist Bonnie Liebman discovered through her annual surveys that modest reductions in sodium in some products are balanced by a roughly equal number of *increases* in others.

The tremendous interest in sodium is reflected in advertising. Recently I was amazed to see three television commercials in a row touting the low sodium content of products. The first was for the salt substitute "NoSalt." It asked viewers if they were "saltaholics." That was followed by commercials for a low sodium antacid and for shredded wheat, which contains no added salt. These advertisements reach every segment of the population and are perhaps the best portent for a low-sodium future.

People's taste for salt is remarkably adaptable. People who go on low salt diets at first find their unsalted food bland, but their taste buds adjust within a matter of weeks or months. Then they find "normal" processed foods distastefully salty. Everyone's taste buds can make this adjustment. No less an authority than New York *Times* food critic Craig Claiborne, who went on a low salt diet after he found he had high blood pressure, has written a gourmet cookbook to establish once and for all that a low sodium diet can be delicious.

The two best, tastiest, and easiest ways to reduce your sodium intake are to eat natural foods and to hide your salt shaker. Some other suggestions:

- Read labels carefully and choose brands with less sodium.
- Season foods with pepper, curry, garlic, and other spices and herbs instead of salt. Some people fill their salt shakers with curry or other favorite seasonings.
- Buy regular, rather than pasteurized process, cheeses and fresh, rather than processed, meats and poultry.
- Use garlic and onion powder instead of garlic salt and onion salt.
- Leave out the salt when you cook rice, hot cereal, pasta, and frozen vegetables.
- Season vegetables and fish with lemon juice.
- Rinse canned tuna fish under the faucet to wash away some of the added salt.
- Use much less salt than called for in recipes.
- Write a letter to your congressional representative urging him or her to support laws concerning sodium labeling and limits for processed foods.

Sodium Content of Foods

Food/Producer	Serving Size	Sodium (mg)
BEVERAGES		
VEGETABLE JUICES		
Low Sodium V-8 (Campbell)	6 oz.	50
V-8 or Tomato (Campbell)	6 oz.	625
SOFT DRINKS		
Mineral Water (Perrier)	12 oz.	4
Unsalted Club Soda	12 oz.	4
Coca-Cola (Coca-Cola)	12 oz.	14
TAB (Coca-Cola)	12 oz.	30
Club Soda (Schweppes)	12 oz.	47
ALCOHOL		
Gin, Rum, Vodka, Whiskey	1 oz.	0
Table Wine	3 1/2 oz.	5
Beer	12 oz.	25
OTHER		
Water	8 oz.	1 to 30
Coffee, Tea	8 oz.	2
Hot Cocoa Mix (Hershey)	1 oz.	145

Food/Producer	Serving Size	Sodium (mg)
Liquid Slender, Chocolate (Carnation)	10 oz. (1 can)	515

BREADS

Food/Producer	Serving Size	Sodium (mg)
Taco Shells (Old El Paso)	0.7 oz. (2 shells)	100
Sahara Bread, Wheat (Thomas)	1.0 oz. (1 pocket)	187
Brick Oven Whole Wheat Bread (Arnold/Orowheat)	1.6 oz. (2 slices)	190
English Muffin, White or Wheat (Thomas)	2 oz. (1 muffin)	215
Dinner Rolls (Wonder)	2 oz. (2 rolls)	280
White Bread (Wonder)	2 oz. (2 slices)	280
Hot Dog or Hamburger Roll (Wonder)	2 oz. (1 roll)	300
Whole Wheat Bread (Wonder)	2 oz. (2 slices)	320
Plain Bagel (Lender)	2 oz. (1 bagel)	352
Bran'nola Bread (Arnold/Orowheat)	2.4 oz. (2 slices)	355
French Bread (Pepperidge Farm)	2 oz.	360
Real Jewish Rye (Levy's)	2.3 oz. (2 slices)	370
Real Pumpernickel (Levy's)	2.3 oz. (2 slices)	385
Family Rye Bread (Pepperidge Farm)	2.4 oz. (2 slices)	485
Country White (Arnold/Orowheat)	2.4 oz. (2 slices)	490
Pumpernickel (Pepperidge Farm)	2.3 oz. (2 slices)	610

MIXES

Food/Producer	Serving Size	Sodium (mg)
Bran Muffin Mix (Duncan Hines)	1 muffin	165
Cornbread Mix (Aunt Jemima)	1.7 oz. (1/6 pkg.)	516
Hungry Jack Biscuits (Pillsbury)	2 oz. (2 biscuits)	585
Complete Pancake Mix (Aunt Jemima)	1.9 oz., 4" pancakes (3)	643
Bisquick (Betty Crocker)	2 oz. (1/2 cup)	700

CANNED ENTREES

Food/Producer	Serving Size	Sodium (mg)
Refried Beans (Old El Paso)	7.5 oz.	775
Beef Stew (Swanson)	7.6 oz.	890
Chicken Chow Mein (La Choy)	8.0 oz.	924
Pork 'n Beans in Tomato Sauce (Campbell)	8.0 oz.	945
Macaroni 'n Cheese (Franco-American)	7.4 oz.	960

Food/Producer	Serving Size	Sodium (mg)
Spaghetti and Meatballs with Tomato Sauce (Chef Boy-ar-dee)	7.5 oz.	1,010
Beef Ravioli in Meat Sauce (Franco-American)	7.5 oz.	1,030
Texas Chili with Beans (Armour)	7.5 oz.	1,310
Sloppy Joe Beef (Armour)	7.6 oz.	1,700

CANNED VEGETABLES

Food/Producer	Serving Size	Sodium (mg)
Green Beans, unsalted (Libby's Natural)	½ cup, undrained	10
Green Peas, unsalted (Del Monte)	½ cup, undrained	10
Beets, unsalted (Libby's Natural)	½ cup, undrained	60
Green Beans (Green Giant)	½ cup, drained	190
Sweet Peas (Green Giant)	½ cup, drained	201
Whole Tomatoes (Del Monte)	½ cup, undrained	220
Yellow Corn (Le Sueur)	½ cup, drained	230
Beets, sliced (Del Monte)	½ cup, undrained	290
Cream Style Corn (Libby's)	½ cup, undrained	302
Dark Red Kidney Beans (Van Camp)	½ cup, undrained	415
Sauerkraut (Stokely-Van Camp)	½ cup, undrained	825

CEREALS

CEREALS (COLD)

Food/Producer	Serving Size	Sodium (mg)
Wheat Bran	1 Tbsp.	1
Wheat Germ (Kretschmer)	1 oz. (¼ cup)	2
Shredded Wheat (Nabisco)	1 oz. (1 biscuit)	10
100% Natural (Quaker)	1 oz. (¼ cup)	18
Froot Loops (Kellogg)	1 oz. (1 cup)	135
Life (Quaker)	1 oz. (⅔ cup)	160
Sugar Frosted Flakes (Kellogg)	1 oz. (¾ cup)	190
Nutri-Grain, Wheat (Kellogg)	1 oz. (¾ cup)	190
Cap'n Crunch (Quaker)	1 oz. (¾ cup)	193
Grape Nuts (Post)	1 oz. (¼ cup)	195
Wheat Chex (Ralston Purina)	1 oz. (⅔ cup)	200
Raisin Bran (Kellogg)	1 oz. (¾ cup)	205
Special K (Kellogg)	1 oz. (1 cup)	220
Rice Krispies (Kellogg)	1 oz. (1 cup)	285
Corn Flakes (Kellogg)	1 oz. (1¼ cup)	285
Cheerios (General Mills)	1 oz. (1¼ cup)	330
Total (General Mills)	1 oz. (1 cup)	375

CEREALS (HOT, UNCOOKED)

Food/Producer	Serving Size	Sodium (mg)
Quick or Regular Hominy Grits (Quaker)	3 Tbsp.	0

RATING THE NUTRITIONAL VALUE OF FOODS

Food/Producer	Serving Size	Sodium (mg)
Quick or Old Fashioned Oatmeal (Quaker)	1/3 cup	1
Wheatena (Standard Milling)	1 oz.	2
Regular Cream of Wheat (Nabisco)	2 1/2 Tbsp.	10
Quick Cream of Wheat (Nabisco)	2 1/2 Tbsp.	130
Instant Oatmeal (Quaker)	1 packet	252
Instant Grits (Quaker)	1 packet	379

CONDIMENTS

Food/Producer	Serving Size	Sodium (mg)
No Salt (Norcliff Thayer)	1 Tbsp.	0
Vegetable oils	1 Tbsp.	0
Unsalted butter or margarine	1 pat	1
Jam, jelly, pancake syrup	1 Tbsp.	3
Cream, sour cream	1 Tbsp.	5
Hot Taco Sauce (Old El Paso)	1 Tbsp.	30
Butter or margarine	1 pat	38
Mayonnaise (Hellmann's)	1 Tbsp.	80
Relish	1 Tbsp.	107
Mustard (R. T. French)	1 Tbsp.	180
Ketchup (Heinz)	1 Tbsp.	180
Lite Soy Sauce (Kikkoman)	1 tsp.	182
Barbecue Sauce (Open Pit)	1 Tbsp.	250
Soy Sauce (La Choy)	1 tsp.	325
Sherry Cooking Wine (Regina)	1/4 cup	370
Dijon Mustard (Grey Poupon)	1 Tbsp.	445
Miso	1 Tbsp.	927
Lite Salt (Morton)	1 tsp.	1,100
Salt	1 tsp.	2,132

GRAVIES AND SAUCES

Food/Producer	Serving Size	Sodium (mg)
Tomato Paste (Contadina)	4 oz.	46
Tomato Paste (Hunt)	4 oz.	300
Brown Gravy Mix (Pillsbury)	1/4 cup, prepared	305
Homestyle Spaghetti Sauce (Ragu)	4 oz.	470
Tomato Sauce (Del Monte)	4 oz.	665
Spaghetti Sauce (Prego)	4 oz.	670
Tomato Sauce w/Cheese (Hunt)	4 oz.	800
Enchilada Sauce, Mild (Del Monte)	4 oz.	1,090

SALAD DRESSINGS

Food/Producer	Serving Size	Sodium (mg)
Low Sodium Italian (Walden Farms)	1 Tbsp.	1
Low Sodium French Style (Aristocrat)	1 Tbsp.	5
Deluxe French (Wish-Bone)	1 Tbsp.	75

Food/Producer	Serving Size	Sodium (mg)
Thousand Island (Wish-Bone)	1 Tbsp.	130
Golden Blend Italian (Kraft)	1 Tbsp.	150
Creamy Cucumber (Kraft)	1 Tbsp.	200
Chunky Blue Cheese (Kraft)	1 Tbsp.	230
Creamy French (Seven Seas)	1 Tbsp.	265
Viva Italian (Seven Seas)	1 Tbsp.	320

CRACKERS & CHIPS

Food/Producer	Serving Size	Sodium (mg)
Popcorn (no salt or oil)	1 oz.	1
Whole Wheat Matzo (Manischewitz)	1 oz. (1)	10
Fritos (Frito-Lay)	1 oz.	160
Peanuts, salted (Planters)	1 oz.	220
RyKrisps, Natural (Ralston Purina)	1 oz. (4 1/2)	220
Wheat Thins (Nabisco)	1 oz. (16)	240
Potato Chips (Frito-Lay)	1 oz.	260
Ritz Crackers (Nabisco)	1 oz. (9)	270
Cheetos Puffed Balls (Frito-Lay)	1 oz.	280
Cheese Peanut Butter Sandwich (Nabisco)	1 oz. (4)	330
Wheatsworth Crackers (Nabisco)	1 oz. (9)	330
Popcorn (Jiffy-Pop)	1 oz.	453
Premium Saltines (Nabisco)	1 oz. (10)	460
Mister Salty Pretzels (Nabisco)	1 oz. (5 1/2)	685

DAIRY PRODUCTS

Food/Producer	Serving Size	Sodium (mg)
Yogurt, plain or fruit (Dannon)	1 cup	70–125
Milk, whole, lowfat, or skim	1 cup	120–45
Nonfat Dry Milk (Carnation)	1 cup, reconst.	125
Chocolate Milk	1 cup	150
Buttermilk	1 cup	257

CHEESES

Food/Producer	Serving Size	Sodium (mg)
Low Sodium Colby Cheese (Pauly)	1.5 oz.	8
Unsalted Cottage Cheese	1/2 cup	14
Cream Cheese (Philadelphia)	1 oz.	85
Swiss Cheese (Kraft)	1.5 oz.	113
Ricotta Cheese, Whole (Maggio)	3 3/4 oz.	178
Cheddar Cheese (Kraft)	1.5 oz.	270
Part-Skim Mozzarella Cheese (Kraft)	1.5 oz.	330
Parmesan Cheese, Grated (Kraft)	1 oz.	425
Cottage Cheese (Sealtest)	1/2 cup	460
Cheeze Whiz (Kraft)	1.5 oz.	555

RATING THE NUTRITIONAL VALUE OF FOODS

Food/Producer	Serving Size	Sodium (mg)
Blue Cheese (Dorman's)	1.5 oz.	594
American Cheese (Kraft)	1.5 oz.	608
Velveeta (Kraft)	1.5 oz.	645

FAST FOODS

Food/Producer	Serving Size	Sodium (mg)
French Fries (McDonald's)	2.4 oz.	109
Chocolate Shake (Burger Chef)	12 oz.	378
Apple Pie (McDonald's)	3.2 oz.	398
Onion Rings (Burger King)	2.7 oz.	450
Hamburger Sandwich (McDonald's)	3.6 oz.	520
Fried Chicken Rib (Kentucky Fried Chicken)	3.7 oz.	562
Hamburger Sandwich (Wendy's)	7 oz.	774
Cheeseburger Sandwich (Jack in the Box)	3.8 oz.	875
Roast Beef Sandwich (Arby's)	5 oz.	880
Egg McMuffin (McDonald's)	4.9 oz.	885
Super Taco (Jack in the Box)	5.1 oz.	970
Whopper Sandwich (Burger King)	9.2 oz.	975
Big Mac (McDonald's)	7.2 oz.	1,010
Quarter Pounder Cheese (McDonald's)	6.8 oz.	1,236
Chicken Breast Sandwich (Arby's)	7.3 oz.	1,323
Super Supreme Pan Pizza (Pizza Hut)	2 slices	1,640

FISH

Food/Producer	Serving Size	Sodium (mg)
Tuna in Water, White, Low Sodium (Chicken of the Sea)	3 oz.	33
Fish	3 oz., cooked	85–170
Shellfish	3 oz., raw	100–220
Lightly Breaded Fish Sticks (Gorton)	3 oz. (3 sticks)	285
Tuna in Water, White (Chicken of the Sea)	3 oz., drained	400
Pink Salmon (Bumble Bee)	3 oz., undrained	418
Tuna in Oil, White (Chicken of the Sea)	3 oz., drained	536
Crunchy Light Batter Fish Sticks (Mrs. Paul)	3.5 oz. (4 sticks)	795
Light & Natural Flounder (Mrs. Paul's)	6 oz. (1 fillet)	975

Food/Producer	Serving Size	Sodium (mg)
FROZEN FOODS		
DINNERS AND ENTREES		
Original Waffles (Aunt Jemima)	1 1/4 oz. (1 waffle)	261
Stir Fry Cashew Chicken (Green Giant)	10 oz.	965
Zucchini Lasagna (Lean Cuisine)	11 oz.	1,000
Chicken Burgundy (Armour Classic Lite)	11 1/4 oz.	1,060
Chopped Sirloin Beef (Le Menu)	12 1/4 oz.	1,115
Beef Chow Mein (La Choy)	8 oz.	1,226
Chicken Pot Pie (Morton)	8 oz.	1,246
Oriental Scallops (Lean Cuisine)	11 oz.	1,325
Cheese Soufflé (Stouffer)	6 oz.	1,360
Seafood Natural Herbs (Armour Classic Lite)	12 oz.	1,410
Macaroni & Cheese (Swanson)	12 oz.	1,815
Beef w/Broccoli (Armour Classic Lite)	10 1/4 oz.	2,120
King Size Fried Chicken Dinner (Morton)	17 oz.	2,902
Cheese Enchilada Dinner (Banquet)	21 1/4 oz.	4,778
VEGETABLES		
Green Beans (Birds Eye)	3.3 oz.	5
Broccoli (Birds Eye)	3.3 oz.	20
Sweet Peas (Green Giant)	3.3 oz.	80
Chinese Style Vegetables (Birds Eye)	3.3 oz.	315
Sweet Peas in Butter Sauce (Green Giant)	3.3 oz.	404
Broccoli with Cheese Sauce (Birds Eye)	5 oz.	505
Tater Tots (Ore-Ida)	3 oz.	550
Fried Onion Rings (Mrs. Paul's)	2 1/2 oz.	625
Ratatouille (Stouffer)	5 oz.	1,320
PIZZA		
Party Cheese Pizza (Totino's)	6 oz.	635
Pepperoni Pizza (Celeste)	6 oz.	1,298
Sausage French Bread Pizza (Stouffer)	6 oz.	1,320
NATURAL FOODS		
Rice, barley, bulgur and pasta	1/2 cup, cooked	1
Fruit juices	6 oz.	3
Nuts and seeds	1 oz.	3

RATING THE NUTRITIONAL VALUE OF FOODS

Food/Producer	Serving Size	Sodium (mg)
Fruit, fresh, frozen, dried or canned	1 serving	3
Beans, peas, and tofu	1/2 cup, cooked	6
Vegetables, fresh	1/2 cup cooked or 1 serving raw	1–40*
Meat and poultry	3 oz. cooked	30–85†
Eggs	1	69

PACKAGED DISHES

Food/Producer	Serving Size	Sodium (mg)
Hungry Jack Mashed Potato Flakes (Pillsbury)	1/2 cup, prepared	380
Long Grain & Wild Seasoned Rice (Uncle Ben's)	1/2 cup, prepared	420
Scalloped Potatoes (Betty Crocker)	1/2 cup, prepared	570
Complete Cheese Pizza In A Skillet (Chef Boy-ar-dee)	3 1/4 oz., unprepared	610
Stuffing Mix, Chicken Flavor (Stove Top)	1/2 cup, prepared	635
Macaroni & Cheese (Kraft)	3/4 cup, prepared	655
Spaghetti & Meatball Dinner (Chef Boy-ar-dee)	5 1/3 oz., unprepared	900
Hamburger Helper, Chili Tomato (General Mills)	1/5 pkg., prepared	1,310

PROCESSED MEATS

Food/Producer	Serving Size	Sodium (mg)
Bacon (Swift)	0.5 oz. (2 slices)	232
Lower Salt Beef Frank (Best's Kosher)	1.5 oz. (1 link)	270
Lean 'n Tasty Beef Breakfast Strips (Oscar Mayer)	0.6 oz. (2 strips)	404
Pork Sausage (Oscar Mayer)	1.4 oz. (2 links)	446
Beef Frank (Oscar Mayer)	1.6 oz. (1 link)	466
Turkey Roll, White (Land O' Lakes)	2.0 oz.	473
Beef Bologna (Armour)	2.0 oz. (2 slices)	570
Hostess Canned Ham (Swift Premium)	3.0 oz.	929
Cooked Sliced Ham (Eckrich)	2.4 oz. (2 slices)	940

SOUPS

CANNED SOUPS

Food/Producer	Serving Size	Sodium (mg)
Tomato, Low Sodium (Campbell)	10 1/2 oz.	40
Minestrone (Progresso)	8 oz.	531
Tomato (Campbell)	10 oz.	938
Chunky Vegetable (Campbell)	9 1/2 oz.	995

* Celery, spinach, swiss chard, beet greens: 50–65mg.
† Beef and calf's liver, beef kidney: 100–215 mg.

Food/Producer	Serving Size	Sodium (mg)
Lentil (Progresso)	8 oz.	1,031
Chunky Beef (Campbell)	9½ oz.	1,050
Clam Chowder (Campbell)	10 oz.	1,075
Chicken Noodle (Campbell)	10 oz.	1,169

SOUP MIXES

Food/Producer	Serving Size	Sodium (mg)
Low Sodium Chicken Broth (Herb-Ox)	1 packet	10
Cream of Mushroom (Cup-A-Soup)	6 oz.	810
Chicken Flavor Bouillon (Wyler)	1 cube	850
Beef Ramen (La Choy)	8 oz.	872
Beef Flavor Mushroom (Lipton)	8 oz.	995
Chicken Noodle Soup Starter (Swift)	12 oz.	1,451

SWEET BAKED GOODS

READY-TO-EAT

Food/Producer	Serving Size	Sodium (mg)
Plain Donut (Hostess)	1 oz. (1)	135
Cherry Pop-Tart (Kellogg)	1.8 oz. (1)	230
Chocolate Cupcake (Hostess)	1¾ oz. (1)	250
Apple Pie (Hostess)	4½ oz. (1)	540

COOKIES

Food/Producer	Serving Size	Sodium (mg)
Chips Ahoy Cookies (Nabisco)	1.1 oz. (3)	110
Oatmeal Raisin Cookies (Pepperidge Farm)	1.2 oz. (3)	170
Oreo Cookies (Nabisco)	1 oz. (3)	210
Honey Maid Graham Crackers (Nabisco)	1 oz. (4)	210

FROZEN

Food/Producer	Serving Size	Sodium (mg)
Pound Cake (Sara Lee)	1.1 oz. (1/10 cake)	104
Cinnamon Raisin Danish (Sara Lee)	1.3 oz. (1 danish)	130
Cream Cheesecake (Sara Lee)	2.8 oz. (1/6 cake)	161
Coconut Cream Pie (Morton)	4 oz. (1/4 pie)	206
Cherry Pie (Morton)	4 oz. (1/6 pie)	260
Cinnamon Danish w/Icing (Pillsbury)	1.2 oz. (1 danish)	285
Apple Pie (Sara Lee)	4 oz. (1/8 pie)	444

MIXES

Food/Producer	Serving Size	Sodium (mg)
Fudge Brownie Mix (Betty Crocker)	1/16 package	100
Blueberry Muffin Mix (Duncan Hines)	1/12 package	155
Yellow Cake Mix (Pillsbury Plus)	1/12 cake	300
Piecrust Mix (Pillsbury)	1/6 pie	425

Food/Producer	Serving Size	Sodium (mg)
Devil's Food Cake Mix (Betty Crocker)	1/12 cake	425

SWEETS

CANDY BARS

Food/Producer	Serving Size	Sodium (mg)
Milk Chocolate (Hershey)	1 oz. (1 bar)	30
Coconut Granola Bar (Nature Valley)	1 oz. (1 bar)	65
Baby Ruth (Nabisco Brands)	1.8 oz. (1 bar)	100
Snickers (M&M/Mars)	2 oz. (1 bar)	139

PUDDINGS AND GELATIN DESSERTS

Food/Producer	Serving Size	Sodium (mg)
Cherry Gelatin (Jell-O)	1/2 cup	75
Cooked Chocolate Pudding (Royal)	1/2 cup	145
Vanilla Pudding, Canned (Del Monte)	5 oz. (1 can)	285
Instant Chocolate Pudding (Jell-O)	1/2 cup	515

FROZEN DESSERTS

Food/Producer	Serving Size	Sodium (mg)
Sherbet, Raspberry (Light 'n Lively)	1/2 cup	35
Ice Cream, Vanilla (Sealtest)	1/2 cup	78
Ice Milk, Chocolate (Light 'n Lively)	1/2 cup	82

MISCELLANEOUS

Food/Producer	Serving Size	Sodium (mg)
Low Sodium Baking Powder (Featherweight)	1 tsp.	2
Low Sodium Peanut Butter (Peter Pan)	2 Tbsp.	10
Chocolate Flavored Syrup (Hershey)	1 oz. (2 Tbsp.)	20
Chocolate Fudge Frosting, canned (Pillsbury)	For 1/12 cake	80
Egg Beaters (Fleischmann)	2 oz. (1/4 cup)	90
Peanut Butter (Skippy)	2 Tbsp.	150
Bac*Os (General Mills)	1 Tbsp.	165
Seasoned Bread Crumbs (Contadina)	2 Tbsp.	397
Baking Powder (Calumet)	1 tsp.	405
Shake 'n Bake (General Foods)	1/4 envelope	590
Olives, green	10 large	926
Pickle, dill	1 medium	928
Baking soda	1 tsp.	1,360

Vitamins and Minerals

The human body's almost miraculous workings could not proceed without vitamins and minerals. It is from food that we must obtain these life-giving chemicals, which the body itself cannot produce.* Most vitamins and minerals work closely with specific proteins to enable the body to obtain energy from food, build new tissue, and synthesize needed chemicals.

Americans are normally thought of as well-nourished people, but according to government surveys millions are not consuming the recommended levels of vitamins and minerals. According to two top officials of the U.S. Department of Agriculture's Human Nutrition Information Service, Dr. Isabel D. Wolf and Betty B. Peterkin, "50% or more [of 38,000 individuals surveyed] had intakes below the RDA [Recommended Dietary Allowances] for vitamin A, iron, calcium, magnesium, and vitamin B_6; over 30% of the individuals failed to meet the 70% RDA level for these nutrients. Zinc and folacin [a B vitamin] . . . are also known to be short in many diets."[66] Wolf and Peterkin concluded that "U.S. diets do not show up well . . . when either the RDA or [USDA's] Daily Food Guide is used as a standard." This is a rather shocking admission from the government department that has long maintained that Americans are the best-fed people in the world.

Nutrient Deficiencies Among Americans (1977–78)[†]

Nutrient	Percent of Individuals Consuming Less Than 70 Percent of RDA	Percent of Individuals Consuming Less Than 100 Percent of RDA
Protein	3	12
Calcium	42	68
Iron	33	57
Magnesium	38	74
Phosphorus	8	27
Vitamin A	31	50
Thiamin (vitamin B_1)	17	45
Riboflavin	12	34
Niacin	9	33
Vitamin B_6	51	80
Vitamin B_{12}	15	33
Vitamin C	26	40

* The body—or the bacteria in the large intestine—can produce some vitamins, but the quantities are usually too small to allow optimal growth of the individual. Vitamin K is an exception, with the bacteria often able to produce sufficient amounts.

† Nationwide Food Consumption Survey 1977–78, U.S. Dept. Agric., Report No. I-2 (1984).

Our rating system considers the amount of vitamin A, riboflavin (vitamin B₂), niacin (vitamin B₃), ascorbic acid (vitamin C), iron, and calcium in a serving of food. These, of course, are not the only important nutrients, but they are good "indicator" nutrients. That is, if a food naturally (rather than by fortification) contains some of these nutrients, it is likely to contain others as well. In the following pages, we discuss the importance and interesting features of these six vitamins and minerals.

VITAMIN A[67]

If people were quizzed on their knowledge of nutrition, vitamin A would surely be one of the best known nutrients. Many people know that vitamin A is a vital part of the light-detection mechanism in the retina of the eye (hence, another name for vitamin A is *retinol*). Less well known is the vital contribution this vitamin makes to the development of teeth and bones and the health of mucous membranes and skin. Healthy mucous membranes form a vital link in the body's defenses against infection. Vitamin A and beta-carotene, a yellow-orange plant pigment that the body can convert to vitamin A, may help prevent cancer, as discussed later.

Severe and prolonged deficiencies of vitamin A can impair night vision and the eye's ability to readjust rapidly after being struck by bright light (night blindness). Such deficiencies can also cause dry and scaly skin, impaired formation of tooth enamel, reproductive problems, and "dry eye" (xerophthalmia), which is a major and tragic cause of blindness in Third World countries. Regarding "dry eye," the problem has been not so much a shortage of foods that contain the vitamin as dietary patterns that do not include those foods. Vitamin pills, injections, or just eating food rich in vitamin A can quickly cure night blindness and other problems caused by deficiencies.

Liver contains huge amounts of vitamin A, while eggs and dairy products contain modest amounts. Low-fat and skim milk, many breakfast cereals, and various other foods are fortified with this vitamin.

Large amounts of beta-carotene, the plant form of vitamin A, are found in collard greens, broccoli, carrots, sweet potatoes, watermelon, spinach, and many other vegetables and fruits. Small amounts of beta-carotene are sometimes used to artificially color processed foods.

Beta-carotene is a relatively stable nutrient. Only small losses occur when foods are transported, stored, and cooked. Vitamin A, on the other hand, can be destroyed by light. For instance, skim milk, which is always fortified with vitamin A, is often packaged in plastic bottles. Depending upon the brightness of the supermarket lighting and length of exposure, a significant percentage of the vitamin can be lost. Paper cartons offer excellent protection against the light. Interestingly, the vitamin A in whole milk is largely protected from light because it is dissolved in fat globules.

Just how much vitamin A your body needs and how much it can extract from foods, as with other vitamins, depends on the person, the food, and the diet. Fat and protein both increase the absorption of the vitamin from the intestinal tract.

Vitamin A is one of the few vitamins that the body stores. A person can manage without any new vitamin A for many weeks, if his or her reserves have been built up. However, if that person's diet is very low in protein (rarely a problem in the United States), the vitamin cannot be released from the liver into the bloodstream. Because vitamin A is stored in the liver, that organ is one of the best dietary sources. One serving of liver can easily supply a week's worth of vitamin A (though don't eat liver too frequently, because of its high cholesterol content). Though most Americans consume more than enough vitamin A, almost one out of three individuals ingests less than 70 percent of the RDA.

The body's ability to store vitamin A results in occasional vitamin excess problems. One teenager encountered problems after taking 50,000 International Units (IU) each day for two and one-half years. Several infants were harmed by doses of 18,000 to 60,000 IU daily. Symptoms of excesses include painful areas over bones, headaches, insomnia, and the loss of body hair. High-potency vitamin A capsules pose the biggest threat in this regard. Labels on such supplements should warn adults against taking more than 25,000 IU daily. Because large excesses of vitamin A can cause birth defects, pregnant women should not take more than 10,000 IU daily. These doses compare with the Recommended Daily Allowance of 5,000 IU for children and 8,000 IU for pregnant women. In contrast to vitamin A, large amounts of beta-carotene have caused nothing more harmful than temporary yellowing of the skin, a reversible condition that some carrot juice-lovers know well.

The most exciting news related to vitamin A is that diets rich in its precursor, beta-carotene, have been correlated in some studies with a reduced risk of cancer, especially lung cancer. About twenty epidemiological studies conducted in different parts of the world have examined the relationship between beta-carotene and the incidence of lung cancer. While most of the studies were not carefully controlled, they indicate that people who consume relatively small amounts of vitamin A or beta-carotene have an above average risk of cancer. For instance, in a nineteen-year-long study of nearly 2,000 employees of the Western Electric Company, the 488 men who reported eating the least beta-carotene foods had seven times the rate of lung cancer as the 488 men reporting the highest beta-carotene diet.

While cancer experts caution against overinterpreting the studies, they urge people to include rich sources of beta-carotene in their daily diet. One of the more optimistic researchers in this field, Dr. Richard Shekelle, who directed the Western Electric study, believes that:

> The consistency of the epidemiological evidence from diverse populations, the graded nature and temporal sequence of the association, its independence from cigarette smoking, and its coherence with evidence from animals, all suggest that a diet relatively high in beta-carotene may reduce risk of lung cancer even among persons who have smoked cigarettes for many years.

In 1982 the National Academy of Sciences' Committee on Diet, Nutrition and Cancer and in 1984 the American Cancer Society both recommended that people eat more foods, especially vegetables, that provide the body with vitamin A.

Needless to say, even the most hopeful researchers do not suggest that eating a carrot a day will obliterate the risks of smoking cigarettes. They also warn against consuming high doses of the potentially toxic vitamin.

The Vitamin A Scoreboard (below) lists the vitamin A content of a variety of foods. Fortified foods, such as breakfast cereals, are generally not included in this and subsequent Scoreboards; read the label to find out how much vitamin A and other nutrients are added to such products.

Vitamin A Scoreboard

Name	Serving Size	VITAMIN A SCORE	Percent U.S. RDA
Beef liver	3 oz.	10.0	907
Carrot juice	6 oz.	10.0	600
Dandelion greens	1/2 cup	10.0	234
Spinach, raw	2 cups	10.0	178
Carrots	1 medium	10.0	159
Peas/carrots, frozen	1/2 cup	10.0	149
Collard greens, fresh	1/2 cup	10.0	148
Chicken liver	2 oz.	10.0	136
Sweet potato, baked	1 medium	10.0	126
Collard greens, frozen	1/2 cup	10.0	112
Mango	1/2 fruit	10.0	111
Cantaloupe	1/4 medium	9.2	92
Turnip greens	1/2 cup	9.1	91
Kale	1/2 cup	9.1	91
Mixed vegetables, frozen	1/2 cup	9.0	90
Squash, winter, baked	1/2 cup	8.6	86
Red peppers, chopped	1/2 cup	6.7	67

Name	Serving Size	VITAMIN A SCORE	Percent U.S. RDA
Watermelon	10" diameter × 1" thick wedge (half-disc shaped)	5.0	50

RIBOFLAVIN

One of the reasons many dairy foods are so nutritious is that they contain generous amounts of riboflavin (vitamin B_2). In fact, most Americans get almost half of their riboflavin from milk, cheese, and other dairy products.

Some of the first symptoms of riboflavin deficiency are cracks at the sides of the mouth and a soreness and redness of the tongue and lips; the little papillae on the tongue also decline in size. Severe riboflavin deficiency is extremely rare in the United States. Only about one out of eight Americans consumes less than 70 percent of the recommended amount of this vitamin, a smaller fraction than for any other vitamin.[68]

One benefit that the disappearance of the milkman has had is that we are probably getting a little more riboflavin than we used to (assuming we drink the same amount of milk). Riboflavin is rapidly destroyed by light, and when glass bottles of milk sat on our sunlit steps much of the riboflavin was destroyed—as much as 10 percent in thirty minutes and 40 percent in two hours. Paper cartons or dark glass protect the vitamin, though plastic cartons do not (plastic carton manufacturers could add a dye to the plastic to block the light, but so far none has).

Liver is by far the best source of riboflavin, containing about twice the daily recommended amount in a three-ounce serving (before you dive for some liver, though, recall its high cholesterol content). Plain, lowfat yogurt, with about 30 percent of the RDA in an eight-ounce serving, is also an excellent source.

Riboflavin (Vitamin B_2) Scoreboard

Food	Serving Size	RIBOFLAVIN SCORE	Percent U.S. RDA
Beef liver	3 oz.	10.0	209
Chicken liver	2 oz.	10.0	88
Lobster meat, cooked	3 oz.	10.0	31
Yogurt, lowfat, plain	1 cup/8 oz.	9.8	29

Food	Serving Size	RIBOFLAVIN SCORE	Percent U.S. RDA
Whole milk	1 cup	7.8	23
Buttermilk, 1% fat	1 cup	7.6	22
Brewer's yeast	1 Tbsp.	6.8	20
Asparagus	1/2 cup	6.4	19
Vanilla ice milk	1/2 cup	6.0	18
Almonds, shelled	1 oz.	5.2	15
Cream of tomato soup with milk	1 cup	5.0	15
Leg of lamb	3 oz.	5.0	15
Spinach, raw	2 cups	4.4	13
Ham, baked	3 oz.	4.4	13
Swiss cheese	2 oz.	4.2	12
Soybean sprouts	1 cup	4.2	12

NIACIN

Niacin, also called vitamin B_3, helps living cells generate energy. Niacin deficiency—pellagra—leads to skin eruptions; an inflamed mucous membrane, which causes the tongue and mouth to swell and become sore; diarrhea; and irritation of the rectum. Sufferers often experience irritability and depression. In advanced cases of pellagra, delirium, hallucinations, and stupor occur. Pellagra is prevalent among people who have a monotonous diet high in corn. It was widespread in the southern United States until the end of the Depression, when corn meal was fortified with niacin and higher incomes enabled millions of people to eat a more varied diet.

Niacin occurs in many foods, notably liver, tuna and salmon, chicken (light meat contains 50 percent more niacin than dark meat), red meat, and peanuts. In addition, the body can manufacture niacin from tryptophan, one of the amino acids in protein. (Corn-rich diets lead to pellagra because corn protein contains very little tryptophan and because the niacin in corn is not readily available.) That niacin can be obtained in two ways greatly complicated the early investigations into the cause of pellagra.

There has been a resurgence of interest in niacin in recent years, because of speculation that some cases of mental illness are due to deficiencies of the vitamin. Some physicians are treating schizophrenic patients with megadoses of niacin. One or two of the small studies gave promising results, and some individuals may be benefited. However, other studies had negative results. Taken together, the studies suggest that niacin therapy is worth trying but will certainly not be a panacea.[69]

Niacin (Vitamin B$_3$) Scoreboard

Food	Serving Size	NIACIN SCORE	Percent U.S. RDA
Beef liver	3 oz.	10.0	70
Tuna fish, in water	3 oz.	9.9	57
Roaster chicken, roasted with skin	3 oz.	8.1	46
Turkey, roasted	3 oz.	5.7	32
Chicken liver	2 oz.	5.7	32
Salmon, sockeye red, canned	3 oz.	5.3	30
Rump roast, choice	3 oz.	4.4	25
Round steak	3 oz.	4.4	25
Leg of lamb	3 oz.	4.4	25
Kentucky Fried Chicken	1 thigh	4.3	25
Hamburger, 25% fat, regular	3 oz.	4.3	24
Ham, canned	3 oz.	4.2	24
Peanut butter	2 Tbsp.	4.2	24
Pork chop, baked lean with fat	3 oz.	4.2	24
Peanuts, roasted	1 oz.	4.1	24
Veal cutlet, broiled	3 oz.	4.0	23
Shrimp, steamed	3 oz.	2.8	16
Brewer's yeast	1 Tbsp.	3.0	15
Bulgur, cooked	1/2 cup	2.6	13
Baked potato	1 medium	2.3	12

VITAMIN C[70]

The best known vitamin of all is vitamin C, or ascorbic acid—and it is also one of the most unusual. A vitamin, by definition, is a chemical that an animal needs for growth and development, but cannot itself produce adequate quantities. The animal must obtain the chemical from its food. Millions of years ago our early ancestors lost the ability to produce ascorbic acid. From then on, gorillas, monkeys, and humans were fated to require ascorbic acid in their diets —or suffer a disease called scurvy. The inability to produce ascorbic acid can be considered a genetic defect that all primates (and the guinea pig, bulbul bird, and Indian fruit-eating bat) share. Elephants, chipmunks, dogs, and other animals can all produce ascorbic acid within their own tissues and never have to worry about scurvy. For them, ascorbic acid is not a vitamin.

Vitamin C deficiencies can have serious consequences. If a baby suffers a deficiency, the baby's bones do not develop properly and its joints are swollen and tender. In adults, signs of scurvy are most obvious in soft body tissue. Gums become sore, swollen, and may bleed and get infected readily. Tiny blood vessels weaken and may rupture, sometimes leading to anemia. The healing of wounds is severely impaired. Scurvy is very rare in the United States, but isolated cases still occur.

Vitamin C is one of the most fragile nutrients. Both exposure to air (oxygen) and heat can destroy it. To protect vitamin C, you should keep fresh fruits and vegetables refrigerated and avoid chopping them into small pieces. These pieces lose vitamin C and certain other nutrients more rapidly than larger pieces or unchopped produce. Also, if you cook vegetables, do so as briefly as possible. Because vitamin C is water-soluble, it leaches into water during cooking. Steaming is the best way to cook vegetables. Next best is boiling in a small amount of water.

One of the great benefits of refrigeration, during shipping and at stores and homes, is that the cold protects vitamin C. Some cancer experts have theorized that the rate of stomach cancer has declined so dramatically in the United States—down about 75 percent in the last fifty years—because we are getting much more vitamin C in our produce.

Vitamin C rose in status from an ordinary vitamin to a nutritional superstar in 1970 when Dr. Linus Pauling threw the weight of his two Nobel prizes and a systematic survey of the medical literature behind the theory that massive amounts of the vitamin could protect people against the common cold. Several years later, Pauling amended his claim to include inhibition of cancer as another of this vitamin's benefits.

Pauling recommends taking vitamin supplements providing one or two thousand milligrams a day routinely, and at the first sign of a cold taking considerably more. The U.S. Recommended Daily Allowance (U.S. RDA) is sixty milligrams for adults. Probably because of all the media attention given to Pauling's theory, average intake of vitamin C jumped 43 percent between 1965 and 1977–78, according to USDA surveys. This was by far the largest change among 12 nutrients examined.

Much of the medical community pooh-poohed Pauling from the moment he said that vitamin C could prevent colds. In the mid-1970s, several reasonably large studies were conducted to test Pauling's hypothesis more carefully. The studies tended to show that one thousand-milligram-a-day doses of vitamin C reduced the duration and frequency of colds slightly. Such doses represent a seventeenfold excess above the U.S. RDA. Notwithstanding its rather weak overall performance in these studies, vitamin C might conceivably have a more pronounced effect on some individuals, so people who maintain that they have never been bothered by colds since taking vitamin C may be right. And Dr. T. W. Anderson of the University of Toronto, who did several studies indicating either no effect or a modest effect of the vitamin, noted that "even a small reduction in total disability would represent a very large saving to the national economy." Anderson believes that "short-term heroic doses of vitamin C may prove to be justified during acute infection and possibly other forms of stress," but he warned against routinely consuming huge doses.

Proving whether or not vitamin C prevents colds is a minor matter compared to the question of whether it can reduce the risk of cancer or benefit cancer patients. Dr. Ewan Cameron, a Scottish physician, and Pauling gave one hundred cancer patients ten thousand milligrams of vitamin C daily and found that those patients lived an average of ten months longer than patients not taking the vitamin. A subsequent, better-controlled study at the Mayo Clinic did not find any benefit of massive doses. Pauling and the Mayo researchers have debated the quality and meaning of their respective studies. Pauling contends that the Mayo study was very different from his study, because the Mayo patients had received chemotherapy, which might have negated the benefits of the vitamin. Dr. Charles Moertel and his colleagues at Mayo responded by conducting another study, this time on patients who had not had chemotherapy. Again they found that vitamin C did not benefit patients who had colorectal cancer. Again, though, Pauling cited a major difference between his study and theirs. Pauling and Cameron's patients received vitamin C for a number of years, whereas Moertel's patients were given the vitamin for an average of only 2.5 months.

Though more studies will have to be done to determine whether or not vitamin C can benefit cancer patients, it may well serve a preventive function. Several epidemiological studies have found associations between low stomach-cancer rates and diets high in good sources of vitamin C. In addition, animal studies have demonstrated that vitamin C can inhibit the formation of cancer-causing nitrosamines and sometimes cancer itself. On the basis of such studies, both the National Research Council's Committee on Diet, Nutrition and Cancer and the American Cancer Society have recommended that people eat more fruits and other good sources of vitamin C. Eating these foods certainly makes sense, even if they turn out to have no effect on cancer.

While the doctors debate, what should we do? Consuming more than the U.S. RDA of 60 milligrams of vitamin C makes sense, considering the suggestions that large amounts may be beneficial and are unlikely to be harmful. Preferably, the vitamin would come from foods, rather than vitamin pills, because foods contain a wide variety of other nutrients and provide gradual exposure throughout the day, as opposed to occasional blockbuster pills. Some people take several thousand milligrams of vitamin C daily, but I hesitate to endorse that practice, because it might lead to subtle and unrecognized long-term problems. It is possible that a body accustomed to huge daily doses might experience difficulties if the doses are suddenly dropped (such as when the person gets bored taking pills). Persons with chronic diseases, including gout and diabetes, should consult a doctor before experimenting with large doses of vitamin C.

Whatever the outcome of future research on ascorbic acid, Linus Pauling deserves great credit for carefully analyzing long-ignored medical research and almost singlehandedly stimulating dozens of new studies.

The Vitamin C Scoreboard lists some good sources of vitamin C. Note, though, that because vitamin losses often occur, the food you just bought may be higher or lower than what the chart says. Moreover, how long you store and how you cook the food will also affect its vitamin C content. There are also big differences between varieties of foods. For instance, some varieties of apples (such as Northern Spy, Gravenstein, and Willowtwig) have two or three times as much vitamin C as other varieties (McIntosh and Rome Beauty). Also, the vitamin content of a fruit depends in large part upon how much sun it receives. A peach in the middle of a tree, a tomato growing in the shade of a leaf, or turnips growing in a cloudy, rainy year will have comparatively little vitamin C.

Vitamin C Scoreboard

Food	Serving Size	VITAMIN C SCORE	Percent U.S. RDA
Red pepper, chopped	1/2 cup	10.0	255
Green pepper, raw	1/2 cup	10.0	160
Orange juice, frozen	6 oz.	10.0	150
Papaya	1/2 fruit	10.0	142
Broccoli, fresh, cooked	1/2 cup	10.0	140
Collard greens, fresh	1/2 cup	10.0	120
Orange	1 medium	10.0	110
Brussels sprouts, frozen	1/2 cup	10.0	103
Spinach, raw	2 cups	9.3	93
Pink grapefruit	1/2 medium	9.3	93
Kale	1/2 cup	8.5	85
Turnip greens	1/2 cup	8.3	83
Kohlrabi, raw	1/2 cup	8.3	83
Asparagus, fresh	1/2 cup	7.8	78
Cauliflower, fresh	1/2 cup	7.5	75
Cantaloupe	1/4 medium	7.5	75
Strawberries	1/2 cup	7.3	73
Rutabaga, cubed, cooked	1/2 cup	7.1	71
Tomato	1 medium, 3" × 2"	7.0	70
Cabbage, chopped	1 cup	7.0	70
Baked potato	1 medium	5.0	50
Beef liver	3 oz.	3.8	38
Sweet potato	1 medium	2.8	28
Lima beans, fresh cooked	1/2 cup	2.5	25

IRON

North Americans are among the richest and best-fed people in the world, yet many of us suffer from iron deficiency. Iron is vital to good health, because it enables red blood cells to carry oxygen from our lungs to all parts of our body. Infants and pregnant and lactating (nursing) women are especially likely to be deficient (anemic) and require iron tablets or iron-fortified foods. Major surveys conducted in the late 1970s by the Department of Agriculture[71] and Department of Health and Human Services[72] showed that the average eighteen-to-fifty-year-old woman was consuming only about 60 percent of the recommended intake of iron. Only 5 to 10 percent of all women consumed the recommended amount (18 milligrams). Women are often low in iron, primarily because of menstruation, but also because they consume relatively little food compared to men.

You may wonder how people in less affluent countries and earlier eras managed to survive and flourish without the help of Geritol and iron-fortified cereal products. Well, first, many people outside of the United States do not receive enough iron from their food. But another answer is that many people eat and ate better than we do. For example, Sir Jack Cecil Drummond, an English food historian and professor of biochemistry, has calculated that the diet of a fifteenth-century peasant contained 21 milligrams of iron a day.[73] That compares with the 16.5 milligrams that the average American consumed in 1965 in the form of natural and fortified foods. Good sources of iron are listed in the Iron Scoreboard.

The exact amount of iron that is absorbed from a food depends on the form of the iron in the food, the composition of the meal, and the eater's previous intake of iron. For instance, a well-nourished body will absorb only about 5 to 10 percent of the iron in the diet. But when a body is deficient in iron it absorbs 15 to 20 percent of the iron. The nature of the food in which iron occurs is also an important factor in absorption. Iron is absorbed much better from meat than from eggs, beans, and green vegetables. However, if these foods are eaten with meat, ascorbic acid (vitamin C), or other acids, the iron in them will be absorbed slightly better.

Meat has a well-deserved reputation for being a good source of iron, but you do not have to eat meat to get your iron. Vegetarians have every bit as much iron in their blood as do meat-eaters.[74]

Iron Scoreboard

Food	Serving Size	IRON SCORE	Percent U.S. RDA
Beef liver	3 oz.	10.0	42
Clams, raw or steamed	5	10.0	29
Chicken liver	2 oz.	9.0	26
Black beans	1/2 cup	7.5	22
Chick-peas	1/2 cup	6.6	19
Spinach, raw	2 cups	6.4	19
Pumpkin seeds	1 oz.	5.9	17
Round steak	3 oz.	5.8	17
Lima beans, mature	1/2 cup	5.7	17
Ham, baked	3 oz.	5.5	16
Pork chop, baked	3 oz.	5.5	16
Hamburger, 25 percent fat, regular	3 oz.	5.4	16
Rump roast, choice	3 oz.	5.4	16
Sirloin steak, choice	3 oz.	5.3	16
Pork chop, lean with fat	3 oz.	5.1	15
Veal cutlet, broiled	3 oz.	5.1	15
Shrimp	3 oz.	5.1	15
Scallops, steamed	3 oz.	4.8	14
Navy beans, cooked	1/2 cup	4.9	14
Soybeans; tofu	1/2 cup	4.7	14
Bulgur, cooked	1/2 cup	4.3	13
Lima beans, fresh cooked	1/2 cup	4.2	12

CALCIUM

Children, whose bones are growing rapidly, need lots of calcium. Generally that means lots of milk, yogurt, or hard cheese, by far the best sources of calcium. Greens, as well as the bones in sardines and salmon, are also fine sources. To enable the body to absorb calcium, we need adequate vitamin D. Our skin tissue can produce this vitamin by converting cholesterol to vitamin D in the presence of sunlight. Vitamin D is also present in fish liver oil (yuk!) and is added to milk. Calcium comprises about 1.5 to 2 percent of the body's weight.

The combination of too little sunshine, too little vitamin D, and too little calcium causes adult rickets or osteomalacia. Too little calcium by itself can cause osteoporosis, a condition in which bones gradually dissolve and are very fragile. According to a 1984 report from the National Institutes of Health:

> Osteoporosis is a common condition affecting as many as 15 to 20 million persons in the United States . . . Among those who live to be 90 years old, 32 percent of

women and 17 percent of men will suffer a hip fracture, most caused by osteoporosis. The cost of osteoporosis in the United States has been estimated at $3.8 billion annually.[75]

While calcium is best known for its importance in building strong bones and teeth, it is distributed throughout the body and serves many other vital functions. It is necessary for muscle contraction, blood coagulation, and intercellular "cement." Recent research has also identified a possible relationship between calcium and blood pressure. Dr. David McCarron and Cynthia Morris of the Oregon Health Sciences University gave a group of forty-eight people with high blood pressure a daily supplement of 1,000 milligrams of calcium. After eight weeks, the blood pressure of about half the people declined to varying extents.[76]

Significant amounts of calcium are present in only a limited number of foods, and several other factors make it even harder to get. Spinach, Swiss chard, and rhubarb contain moderate amounts of calcium, but they also contain oxalic acid. This acid binds to and reduces the availability of calcium and other minerals. Collards, turnip and mustard greens, and kale, on the other hand, are good sources of calcium and contain little oxalic acid. A high protein diet—typical of North Americans—increases the excretion of calcium from the body.

To some extent, our bodies are smart enough to increase the rate of absorption when calcium supplies are running low. But you do have to help your body by including several servings of food with decent amounts of calcium in your diet every day. Unfortunately, too few of us do that. A shocking 68 percent of the American population consumes less than the Recommended Dietary Allowance of calcium, as set by the National Academy of Sciences. Almost half the population—42 percent—consumes less than 70 percent of the RDA, according to the 1977–78 U.S. Department of Agriculture food consumption survey. Calcium consumption declined by 7 percent between 1965 and 1977–78. Females, once into their teenage years, are especially likely to consume too little calcium.

The National Institutes of Health urges people to consume 1,000 to 1,500 milligrams of calcium a day, from foods when possible, otherwise from calcium tablets. The NIH also emphasizes the importance of estrogen replacement therapy for women who have reached menopause. Women who began estrogen replacement within several years of menopause have a much lower risk of hip and wrist fractures than other women.

Calcium Scoreboard

Food	Serving Size	CALCIUM SCORE	Percent U.S. RDA
Swiss cheese	2 oz.	10.0	54
Yogurt, low-fat, plain	1 cup/8 oz.	7.4	42
Cheddar cheese	2 oz.	7.3	41
Mozzarella cheese, part skim	2 oz.	7.0	37
American cheese	2 oz.	6.2	35
Ricotta cheese, part skim	1/2 cup	6.0	34
Skim milk	1 cup	5.4	30
"Lite" cheese	2 oz.	4.7	26
Salmon, sockeye red, canned, with bones	3 oz.	4.0	22
Collard greens, fresh	1/2 cup	3.2	18
Frozen yogurt, whole milk	4 oz.	3.1	17
Tofu	1 piece, 4 oz.	3.0	15
Turnip greens	1/2 cup	2.4	13
Chick-peas, cooked	1/2 cup	1.4	8
Black beans	1/2 cup	1.3	7

Refined grain products (white bread, spaghetti, white rice), imitation fruit drinks, and breakfast cereals are often "enriched" or "fortified" with some or all of the two minerals and the four vitamins discussed earlier. The refining process, however, removes many other important nutrients that are not replaced. So that these foods are not unduly rewarded for having a few selected nutrients, their ratings are calculated by giving the added nutrients only half-credit. Even with this adjustment, some heavily fortified products are little more than junk foods dressed up as vitamin pills and may have scores higher than their overall nutritional values merit.

CALORIES

If people are concerned about any one aspect of foods, surely it is calories. The surefire path to riches is to write a book on how to lose weight. *The Beverly Hills Diet. The I Love New York Diet. The Scarsdale Diet.* What is your hometown? Now start writing!

Zillions of calorie counters are sold every year, but oversized bellies seem as prevalent as ever, reflecting just how extraordinarily difficult it can be to lose weight. Though there is much disagreement on just how heavy you have to be to be considered "obese," approximately 14 percent of adult men and 20 percent of adult women are 20 percent or more overweight.[77]

Extreme overweight poses not just social and psychological problems, but also significant health problems, particularly when it is of the "potbelly" or "spare tire" variety. It greatly increases the risks of developing diabetes and high blood pressure. In 1984 the American Cancer Society warned that obesity is associated with a 55 percent higher risk of cancer for women and a 33 percent higher risk for men. The cancers linked to obesity include those of the uterus, gall bladder, kidney, stomach, colon, and breast. Obesity is also a suspected risk factor in heart disease.

A panel of scientists convened by the National Institutes of Health recommended in February 1985 that persons 20 percent or more above their desirable weight (an ill-defined measure) should lose weight. For individuals who are twice their desirable weight or 100 pounds overweight, "weight reduction may be lifesaving." The expert panel also recommended that even modestly overweight people should lose weight if they have diabetes, high blood pressure, heart disease, or certain other medical conditions.

Other experts, though, warn that obsessive concern about weight can be as harmful as obesity itself. Witness those suffering from bulimia and anorexia. Dr. William Bennett and Joel Gurin, authors of *Dieter's Dilemma: Eating Less and Weighing More,* charged that the NIH obesity report would "scare the nation, which already is easy prey for worthless weight-loss programs."

Weight control is far too big and complex a subject to cover in a couple of paragraphs, but it is so important that we feel obliged to play Dr. Slimdown and dispense a little advice.

Nutritionists traditionally tell people how easy it is to lose weight. All you have to do is eat fewer calories than you burn up during the day. Unfortunately, this glib advice rarely works. Corpulence seems to be as prevalent as ever, even though government food consumption surveys show that the average American's caloric intake declined by 9 percent between 1965 and 1977–78. For most people, losing or gaining weight is extremely difficult, because the body seems to have a mind of its own. Dr. Bennett and Gurin believe that every body has a specific "setpoint," which is the body's "natural" weight. This setpoint may be affected by the amount of body fat and other factors. Deviating from this weight is difficult, because the body adjusts its metabolic rate—fighting the dieter—to compensate for the changed caloric intake.[78]

One important study concerning obesity showed that workers who have sedentary jobs eat more calories than those whose jobs entail moderate amounts of physical activity.[79] This study highlights the value of exercise in weight control. Not only does exercise use up calories, it also burns up additional calories *after* the period of exercise. The exercise appears to lower the body's setpoint so that it "wants" fewer calories.

Remember the roughage! Roughage, or dietary fiber, occurs in whole grain products, fruits, legumes (beans, peas), and vegetables. These bulky foods cause a full feeling in the stomach and help control one's appetite. Some dieting aids consist basically of synthetic compounds that mimic some of the effects of natural fiber. But why buy artificial concoctions, when you can get all the fiber you need from delicious, natural foods?

Some of the most interesting work on obesity is being done by Richard and Judith Wurtman at the Massachusetts Institute of Technology.[80] The Wurtmans are biochemists who have studied chemicals in the brain that affect behavior, including appetite and eating. One of many chemical messengers in the brain is serotonin, a neurotransmitter that seems to inhibit appetite for carbohydrate. The M.I.T. researchers have found that when rats are fed a high carbohydrate meal, the level of serotonin in their brains rises and the rats eat less carbohydrates at their next meal. Thus, the composition of the diet can affect brain chemistry and behavior. The Wurtmans theorize that the human appetite for carbohydrates may resemble the rats'. If "carbohydrate-craving" people go on a diet and studiously avoid carbohydrates, their serotonin levels may decline and induce a great craving for the forbidden foods. The Wurtmans suggest that people who just love carbohydrates but have a weight problem eat small portions of such foods to keep serotonin levels up and cravings down.

Several factors in our food rating formula reflect the caloric content of food. First, our formula penalizes foods for their content of fat and refined sugar. Fat is the most concentrated source of calories in the diet, 9 calories per gram, compared to 7 calories per gram of alcohol and 4 calories per gram of carbohydrate or protein. Refined sugar is a concentrated form of extra, and "empty," calories. Second, a factor called the "nutrient versus calorie rating" compares the nutrient content to the calorie content. Foods gain points if they are high in nutrients and low in calories and lose points if they are low in nutrients and high in calories.

III

Beyond the Nutrition Scoreboard Formula

The formula we use to rate the nutritive values of foods considers more than a dozen different nutrients. But no one formula can cover every aspect of food. Moreover, even if the formula were expanded, only limited information is available for most brand name foods. Aside from certain nutrients, the formula also leaves out certain factors that are important considerations when we buy food, but that do not lend themselves to being part of a formula. In this chapter, we discuss briefly some of the factors not included in the formula.

Food Additives

The periodic discovery that a chemical widely used in our food may be dangerous has made millions of Americans extremely wary of all food additives. Since 1969, cyclamate, DEPC (a preservative), Violet No. 1 dye (the coloring used to stamp USDA's insignia on inspected meat), and Red dyes Nos. 2 and 4 have been banned, and many others have come under suspicion. Most food additives are safe and some are positively beneficial. However, a few are hazardous, and some of the safe ones may be used to cheat or deceive shoppers —these are the additives that spark concern. If a widely used additive proves to be hazardous, thousands or even millions of people may be harmed.

The rating system does not deduct credit for food additives that are potentially harmful or used to deceive the consumer. Foods containing them should simply not be eaten. Additives to watch out for include artificial colors, BHT, caffeine, saccharin, sodium bisulfite, and sodium nitrite. Salt and sugar, which are usually thought of as ingredients rather than additives, are also major problems. Please refer to Part Two of this book for detailed information regarding most major additives.

Trace Minerals[81]

"Life is a delicate balance of a seemingly infinite number of competing chemical and physiological processes. The trace elements are obviously of great importance to these processes and to that balance." In uncharacteristically poetic words, that is what the U.S. Department of Agriculture said in its 1959 Yearbook about trace elements.

The body needs only tiny, or *trace,* amounts of zinc, copper, manganese, iodine, iron, fluoride, chromium, molybdenum, and selenium, but they are absolutely essential for good health. Most of these elements occur in many foods, so people who eat a balanced diet should not have deficiencies. However, according to Dr. Leon Hopkins, a trace mineral specialist at the Department of Agriculture's Fort Collins, Colorado, laboratory:

> Trace element deficiencies do exist in large numbers of people in this country . . . We cannot assume that animals, including man, are obtaining adequate amounts of the various trace elements for optimum health from plant foods. Soil depletion, increased processing of foods and feeds, and changing eating patterns are forcing us to change our concepts in mineral nutrition.[82]

Traditionally, the sign of a vitamin or mineral deficiency was an obvious physical impairment. Doctors looked for scurvy, rickets, stunted growth, goiter, etc. It was assumed that if a person did not have any of these overt symptoms he or she consumed an adequate amount of vitamins, major minerals, and trace elements. In recent years, however, scientists have begun studying more subtle effects of marginal, but prolonged, deficiencies of trace minerals. These deficiencies may cause diseases that take many years to develop, such as heart disease, or cause such problems as slow healing of wounds, lower resistance to diseases, behavioral changes, and decreased absorption or utilization of nutrients. These deficiencies would have a much greater impact on infants, elders, and infirm people than on the healthy.

Trace minerals are present in natural foods, but certain food processing practices and the priorities of the food industry have led to a precarious situation for many Americans. Refined sugar and flour, which constitute about 40 percent of our diet, do not contribute their share of trace elements. Sugar is devoid of trace minerals. In whole wheat kernels, minerals are concentrated in the germ and bran, and these are the very parts that are removed when grain is processed into white flour. Of the trace elements (manganese, zinc, chromium, copper, iron) lost from whole wheat flour, only iron is restored to "enriched" flour or bread. Furthermore, the food industry and our own laziness have led us to consume more and more convenience and snack foods that are composed of oil, refined flour, and sugar—high in calories, low in trace minerals and other nutrients.

Dr. K. Michael Hambidge, assistant professor of pediatrics at the University of Colorado Medical Center, discovered children in Denver who were deficient in zinc, an essential constituent of many enzymes. These were not starving, ghetto-dwelling children—they were all apparently healthy children from upper- or middle-class families. Most of the children with zinc deficiency were smaller and lighter than other children their age. Dr. Hambidge and his colleagues also found that the children had an abnormally poor sense of taste, a phenomenon that has been tied to zinc deficiency.[83] Shellfish, fish, meat and poultry, eggs, cheese, and liver are some of the better sources of zinc.

Chromium is a little-talked-about mineral that plays several important roles in the body. Chromium is needed for the proper metabolism of food, and chromium supplements have proven beneficial to many diabetics.[84] Supplements of this trace mineral may also help elderly people who have some difficulty metabolizing food, but who do not have frank diabetes, and who often have very low levels of chromium in their tissues.[85] The chromium that occurs naturally in brewer's yeast seems to be the most effective, while some trivalent chromium supplements (such as chromium trichloride) are also effective. According to Dr. Richard Anderson, a Department of Agriculture scientist, commercial chromium containing GTF (glucose tolerance factor) supplements seem to be worthless.

Dr. Walter Mertz, a leading expert on trace minerals at the U.S. Department of Agriculture, believes that chromium may also play a role in the prevention of heart disease. Chromium supplementation reduces levels of the "bad" low-density lipoprotein cholesterol and increases the "good" high-density lipoprotein cholesterol. According to Mertz, "The daily human requirement for chromium . . . is not always supplied by diets habitually consumed in the United States."[86] Good sources of chromium include brewer's yeast, meat, poultry, cheese, and whole grains.

Selenium is another trace mineral consumed by most Americans at less than recommended levels. While large amounts of selenium—like other trace minerals—can be toxic, moderate amounts may protect against cancer. In numerous studies, adding selenium to animals' diets provided partial protection when the animals were exposed to cancer-causing chemicals. In one human study, Dr. Walter Willett and his colleagues at the Harvard School of Public Health correlated low levels of selenium in blood with a subsequent increased risk of developing cancer.[87] Dr. Charles Hennekens, also at Harvard, has begun a multiyear study in which a thousand participants are taking a daily selenium supplement. The rates at which they develop various tumors will be compared to a similar group of people (all dentists) who are taking a placebo.

Selenium intakes vary sharply from region to region in the United States, but few good surveys have been conducted. The average resident of South Dakota, a high-selenium area, is probably consuming about 200 micrograms of selenium per day, whereas most people in Maryland, a low-selenium area, are consuming only about 80 micrograms. Because selenium levels in foods vary so widely, some researchers recommend that people take dietary supplements to boost their selenium intake, while others caution that supplementation has not yet been proven to be beneficial and that excessive amounts can be dangerous. The "estimated safe and adequate daily intake" is 50 to 200 micrograms, with most of us probably down near the lower end. Since many people consume even less than 50 micrograms and since people in parts of China appear to tolerate 750 micrograms without any problem, supplements on the order of 100 micrograms should not pose any problem.[88] Seafoods, meat, poultry, and grains are the food groups that tend to be good sources of selenium.

Organically Grown Food

More and more urban Americans have become interested in the way food is grown. Perhaps the proliferation of tasteless, prepared foods—called "plastic" by some—and the concern about pesticide contamination made this phenomenon inevitable. Many people began growing food organically in their gardens or seeking organically grown food in natural food stores.

Growing food the organic way means using "natural" fertilizers and "natural" means of controlling insect pests. Organic farmers fertilize their fields with manure and compost, rather than the nitrogen-phosphorus-potassium (NPK) fertilizer that is manufactured in a factory. The preference for the natural is not simply a contempt for factories and a romantic vision of Nature. Compost and manure contain trace elements, which can be, but often aren't, added to NPK fertilizer. Compost also provides humus, which is partially decayed vegetable matter that helps hold the soil together. On the other hand, nitrate-rich fertilizer can be used in excess, with consequent pollution of the local water supply.

Some farmers who rely on insecticides gripe that they are on a treadmill. They find that the more insecticide they use, the greater their insect problem is the following year. Insecticides disrupt the balance of nature, kill beneficial insects along with the unwanted ones, and may lead to insects that are resistant to pesticides. Many farmers, not just organic farmers, are reducing their reliance on pesticides, using them in minimal quantities and only when needed (as opposed to prescheduled, massive sprayings).

The best studies of organic farming have been done by Washington University's Center for the Biology of Natural Systems. Barry Commoner and his colleagues, with support from the National Science Foundation, studied middle-sized Midwestern farms, some using traditional and others using organic methods. These researchers found that the organic farms had slightly lower yields than conventional farms, but lower costs. The two factors balanced out, indicating the economic feasibility of organic farming.[89]

The U.S. Department of Agriculture, historically, has been more of a hindrance than a help, treating organic farmers as kooks. However, in the late 1970s, USDA had a task force look carefully at organic farming. The group made numerous favorable and supportive recommendations that focused on research needs, but also urged greater informational assistance for organic farmers and development of more efficient marketing programs.[90] When President Reagan took office in 1981, USDA scrapped this program.

Oregon was the first state to officially recognize and support organic farming. The Oregon State Department of Agriculture adopted regulations in 1974 that defined "organically grown food." The regulations state that organically grown food "has been grown without being subjected to pesticides, synthetic fertilizers or other synthetic chemicals," and "in soil in which the humus content is increased only by the addition of natural matter." Organically processed foods are both grown organically and then *not* treated with preservatives, artificial colorings, artificial flavorings, or any other artificial additive. Organically raised livestock are not given artificial growth stimulants, hormones, or antibiotics, except for the treatment of a specific disease and never within ninety days of slaughter. Such regulations can protect both consumers and honest organic farmers from charlatans, who dishonestly claim to produce organic food. California and Maine have adopted similar regulations.

Because organic farming may result in slightly lower crop yields and is so radically different from what most farmers are now accustomed to, the American agricultural establishment still winces at the word "organic." However, every time fertilizer and pesticide prices shoot up as a result of higher petroleum prices, more farmers go organic. A compromise that many leading researchers are promoting is "integrated pest management" or IPM. This approach seeks to maximize natural means of pest control and minimize pesticides. Farmers do such things as use pest resistant crops, plant before or after insect predators are in the neighborhood, and use the smallest effective amounts of pesticides when they are needed. This is a far cry from the routine sprayings that the chemical companies have recommended.

Currently, we often pay a premium price for organic food, though it is less than one might think. According to a 1980 U.S. Department of Agriculture survey in the Washington, D.C., area of thirty-two foods, organic foods averaged 15 percent more than supermarket foods.[91] The higher costs are due partly to the facts that organic farming may require more labor and yield a slightly smaller harvest than "chemical farming." Another reason is that organic food is handled by small distributors and retailers as a specialty item. Oftentimes, because there are few good distribution systems for organically grown foods, farmers who use organic methods just send their produce or livestock into the marketplace along with nonorganic foods. In such cases, lucky supermarket shoppers unwittingly get an invisible bonus. In the long run, paying a few cents more for organically grown food may be a real bargain. As we are finding out, pesticides kill valuable wildlife in addition to boll weevils; they pollute the environment and lead to chemical-resistant insects; and they pose a risk to farm workers and add a small hazard to our food. The real challenge is to encourage the large farms that produce most of our nation's food to move in the organic direction.

Alcohol

Alcoholic beverages are high in calories due to their alcohol and carbohydrate content, but are almost devoid of nutrients. Also, obviously, they can be inebriating.

Alcohol abuse and alcoholism are problems of monumental proportions in the United States:

- Alcohol is linked to over 20,000 highway deaths and to 100,000 to 200,000 total deaths each year.[92]
- Ten million adults and over three million teenagers have serious drinking problems.
- Alcohol problems cost our nation over $120 billion a year in direct and indirect costs (time lost from work, medical expenses, auto repairs, etc.).[93]
- Alcohol, like sugar, squeezes nutrients out of the diet and has no redeeming nutritional value outside of calories.[94]
- Heavy drinking, combined with cigarette smoking, greatly increases the risk of cancer of the mouth, larynx, and esophagus.
- Excessive imbibing causes brain, heart, and liver damage and high blood pressure.
- Heavy drinking during pregnancy can cause mental and physical birth defects.
- Alcohol is involved in more than 66 percent of the nation's homicides, 50 percent of rapes, and up to 70 percent of sexually aggressive acts against children and adults.[95]

While everyone agrees that heavy drinking is dangerous—to the drinker and to others—the wisdom of even "moderate" drinking is controversial. Some studies suggest that a drink or two a day is actually beneficial, while others suggest it is harmful. Timing, of course, can determine whether a drink is harmful. Even one drink can slow reaction time, so someone stupid enough to have "one for the road" could easily cause a traffic accident.

The most intriguing studies are exploring the effect of drinking on the risk of heart disease.[96] Drinkers tend to have higher HDL-cholesterol levels than nondrinkers. HDL cholesterol is the "good" cholesterol, which correlates with reduced risks of heart disease.

Some studies have found that light drinkers have fewer heart attacks or live longer than either nondrinkers or heavy drinkers, whereas other studies found no difference. Many of the studies are worthless, because former drinkers were mixed together in the group of nondrinkers. The former drinkers category usually includes recovering alcoholics, who have a high risk of early death.

In one of the better studies, conducted by Kaiser Permanente Medical Center in Oakland, California, 3 percent of the "never drinkers" died of heart disease compared to only 1.8 percent of the moderate drinkers. However, when the researchers looked only at *nonsmokers,* they found virtually no difference in the heart disease rates of drinkers and nondrinkers. Dr. Arthur Klatsky, chief investigator of the study, believes that both groups of nonsmokers had similar heart disease rates, because they "are at such a low risk to begin with." The benefits of moderate drinking may be so minor that it only aids those whose cigarette habit has already made them more prone to heart disease.

Others suggest that the alcohol has nothing to do with the increased life expectancy. According to Dr. Charles Hennekens of Harvard, lifelong nondrinkers may be prone to heart attacks not because of their abstinence, but because they have certain personality traits. "The Type A obsessive compulsive who is at increased risk of coronary heart disease may be either rigidly abstaining or drinking heavily. This implies that alcohol has no truly preventive role. Rather, moderate drinking may simply be a marker for a personality type."

The arguments over moderate drinking and heart disease will likely continue for many years. The fact that it is so hard to get good data suggests that any beneficial effect is likely to be small. And, even if a drink a day may reduce the risk of heart disease slightly, few public health experts would dare encourage people to drink, because alcohol has so many potential immediate and long-term disastrous effects.

We have not assigned a nutrient value to alcohol, because its nutritional value is of so little interest compared to its inebriating and addictive effects. However, just as a reminder to both light and heavy drinkers that alcoholic beverages do contain calories, we have included a listing of the average calorie content of various alcoholic beverages.

Calorie Content of Alcoholic Beverages

Beverage	Percent Alcohol by Volume	Serving Size	Calories
Low alcohol beer	2.4	12 ounces	110
Light beer	3.7	12 ounces	97
Regular beer	4.75	12 ounces	150
Table wine	12	4 ounces	100
Dessert wine	19	4 ounces	162
Whiskey, vodka, gin, etc. (80 proof)	40	1.5 ounces (1 jigger)	98

Food for Babies

Expectant mothers and fathers are probably more concerned about nutrition than any other segment of the population. They want to ensure that their baby will enter the world in the best of health. Unfortunately, the concern for good nutrition before birth is sometimes forgotten after birth.

If ordinarily contentious nutritionists can agree upon anything, it is the advisability of breast feeding. Human breast milk is obviously the one food intended specifically for human babies. It is the one food with which humans have evolved over hundreds of thousands of years. It contains antibodies and enzymes that reduce the incidence of infections. It does not cause allergic reactions, as cow's milk formula often does. It is completely digestible. It contains all the right nutrients in the proper balance for the first months of life. And it is inexpensive and convenient. Nursing also fills important psychological needs of both the mother and the baby.

In the last decade, there has been a strong trend back to breast feeding, primarily among college-educated women. They are recognizing that the age-old practice offers psychological and physiological benefits that bottle feeding cannot match.

The one caveat about breast feeding is that human milk is sometimes contaminated with toxic chemicals. Some chemicals, such as PCBs, an industrial pollutant, could conceivably affect a baby's behavior; others might increase slightly the risk of cancer. Some women prepare for breast feeding by switching to a low-fat vegetarian diet months or even years ahead of pregnancy. Such a diet should lead to less contamination, because the highest levels of many toxic substances, particularly chlorinated and brominated hydrocarbons (DDT, aldrin, dieldrin, PCBs, PBBs, dioxin), are usually found in animal fat. Freshwater fish are well-known accumulators of nasty chemicals and should be avoided. Some women also get their breast milk tested for chemical residues.

Then, if their milk is contaminated only slightly or not at all, they continue to breast feed. If their milk is relatively heavily contaminated, they switch to formula after a few days or weeks. The babies benefit from the antibody-rich colostrum that lactating women produce during the first three to five days postpartum and avoid most of the contaminants.

Babies are ready for and need solid foods after about four to six months of nursing. When your baby is ready for solid foods, you can either mash and strain your own or buy commercially prepared foods. By making your own, you can avoid the sugar, starch, and salt that are present in some commercial products. After a few months of this food, your baby's teeth will have started coming in, and you can switch to mashed-up, ordinary table food.

IV

The Nutritional Ratings of Common Foods

The Scoreboards on the following pages list the relative nutritional values of many common foods. In general, the higher the rating the more nutritious the food. Eat more of the foods near the tops of the charts; eat less of the foods that have negative ratings or are near the bottoms of the charts. Small differences in ratings (for example, 34 versus 36) are not really significant.

The ratings give positive credit to protein, unsaturated fat, starch, naturally occurring sugars, dietary fiber, four vitamins, and two minerals. A food loses points for saturated fat, a high total fat content, added sugar and corn syrup, cholesterol, sodium, and high calorie content.

All ratings were calculated for one "average" serving of food. For larger or smaller servings, adjust the ratings appropriately. Thus, while one plum has a score of 12, two plums would receive 24 points. Three cups of coffee, each with a teaspoon of sugar, has a score of −18, triple the rating of one cup. Because a chocolate bar has a score of −42, half a bar would have a score of −21.

You should generally compare a food to others in the same category (dairy, grains, and so on). Because different food categories have such different mixes of nutrients, other comparisons could be misleading.

The ratings of different foods can be added. For instance, a peanut butter and banana sandwich on whole wheat bread would have a score of 78 (two slices of bread = 55, peanut butter = 5, 1/2 banana = 18). While the ratings of food can be added, there is no magic goal to shoot for. A diet adding up to 750 or more points a day is almost certainly balanced and healthful. On the other hand, if your total daily score is in the minus range, or hovering around zero, you really need to work on your diet. Make up charts like the one following to keep track of what you eat. Sample excellent and disastrous diets are shown on the following pages.

HOW DOES YOUR DIET RATE

Food	Serving	Score
Breakfast		
Midmorning		
Lunch		
Afternoon		
Dinner		
After dinner		
	Total	

Make extra copies of charts like this on other sheets of paper.

Brand names are included for illustrative purposes. In general, the most widely distributed, well-known products were selected. That a food was or was not named is in no way intended to imply an endorsement or criticism. If a food you are eating is not listed, use the score of a similar food.

Total daily score	Probable diet quality
750–1,000 points	Terrific
500–750	Good
200–500	Room for improvement
0–200	Needs a lot of work
−200–0	Disastrous

SAMPLE DIETS

Nutrition-conscious Person

	Food	Serving	Calories	Food Rating
Breakfast:	Prunes, uncooked	3 med.	49	26
	Buckwheat pancakes	4, 4" cakes	220	31
	Lowfat plain yogurt w/	1 cup	144	64
	honey	1 tsp.	21	−7
	Grapefruit juice, unsweet.	6 oz.	57	36
Snack:	Green pepper slices	1/2 cup	17	44
Lunch:	Black bean soup	1/2 cup	169	93
	Whole wheat bread	2 slices	122	55
	Cottage cheese, 1% fat	1/2 cup	82	30
	Tomato juice	6 oz.	35	36
Snack:	Peach	1 med.	38	26
Dinner:	Rice, brown	1/2 cup, cooked	116	47
	Tofu (bean curd)	4 oz.	86	31
	Mushrooms	1/4 cup, raw	5	9
	Onions, chopped	1/4 cup, raw	17	12
	Collard greens, fresh	1/2 cup, cooked	31	90
	Broccoli, fresh	1/2 cup, cooked	24	68
	Cabbage, chopped	1/2 cup, raw	11	18
	Bean sprouts, mung	1/2 cup	19	18
	Safflower oil	3 tsp.	120	−9
	Soy sauce	2 tsp.	8	−4
	Cantaloupe	1/4 med.	41	60
	Strawberries	1/2 cup	28	34
	Vanilla ice milk	1/2 cup	112	7
	TOTALS:		1,572	815

A Food Faddist

	Food	Serving	Calories	Food Rating
Breakfast:	Soda pop (1 can)	12 oz.	144	−55
	Peaches, heavy syrup	1/2 cup	100	−10
Snack:	Cheez-its	10 crackers	60	5
Lunch:	White bread, enriched	2 slices	148	45
	Luncheon meat	2 slices (2 oz.)	190	−33
	American cheese	2 oz.	212	−18
	Mayonnaise	1 tsp.	33	−6
	Potato chips	1 oz.	157	15
	Jell-O, flavored	1/2 cup	80	−26
	Soda pop (1 can)	12 oz.	144	−55
Snack:	Hershey's Milk Chocolate	1 bar, 1.5 oz.	185	−42
Dinner:	Hamburger bun, enriched	1	119	36
	Hamburger, reg.	3 oz.	270	−4
	Catsup	1 Tbsp.	16	−1
	Mayonnaise	1 tsp.	33	−6
	Lettuce, iceberg	1 cup	7	11
	Tomato	1/2 med.	20	28
	French salad dressing	2 Tbsp.	32	−12
	Lemonade	6 oz.	81	−20
	Sara Lee Choc. Cake, frozen	1 med. slice	185	−27
	Soda pop (1 can)	12 oz.	144	−55
	TOTALS:		2,360	−230

Beans, Nuts, and Seeds

Though American supermarkets appear to carry virtually every food under the sun, it takes only a glimpse of a grocery store serving recent immigrants from Asia or Africa to discover a multitude of foods that most of us do not recognize or have ever even heard of. Many of the unusual foods are beans, grains, nuts, and seeds. What these foods have in common is that they are the seeds for a new generation of plants. They contain within them, assuming they have not been refined or processed, everything needed to produce an entire plant, be it wheat grass or a hickory tree.

Except in ethnic cooking and as snacks, most beans, nuts, and seeds play a small role in the typical American diet. According to the U.S. Department of Agriculture, the average American eats only about seven pounds of dry beans and eight pounds of tree nuts and peanuts (which is actually a legume, not a true nut) per year. Yet, as inexpensive, concentrated sources of nutrients and energy (calories), these foods cannot be beat. A planted seed is on its own for many days, until it sprouts leaves and starts converting carbon dioxide, water, and light into nutrients. Thus, like a rocket ship, a seed must contain a supply of fuel and the materials needed to convert the fuel into the desired product. The fuel is either oil (soy, peanut, sunflower, sesame, etc.) or starch (chickpea, lima or kidney beans, lentil, rice, wheat, etc.). The materials that make use of this fuel are protein, vitamins, and minerals. Dietary fiber is abundant, as well. The presence of this wide variety of nutrients has made different forms of seeds the mainstay of the diet in many cultures.

Heading the Scoreboard is the black bean (+93). This bean is an everyday food in parts of Africa and Latin America and most popular in North America as a soup. In addition to being delicious, black beans are especially rich in iron and protein. The black bean derives less than 4 percent of its calories from fat, has no cholesterol, and contains only 13 milligrams of sodium per half-cup portion. The other beans near the top of the Scoreboard are similar in that they contain relatively little fat and good amounts of various nutrients.

The foods near the bottom of the Scoreboard are high in fat. Because they are so rich, we usually eat small servings or use them as condiments. Walnuts, for instance, derive 88 percent of their calories from fat. This fat, like that in most nuts and seeds, is relatively high in polyunsaturated oils and low in saturated fat. (The exceptions to this generalization are palm and coconut oils, which are very saturated.)

One of the best ways to introduce children—or yourself—to different beans and grains is to sprout them so you can eat them raw. To start a little sprout garden, all you need is a one-quart jar and a piece of cheesecloth or nylon stocking. Purchase seeds or beans from a food store, not a feed or gardening store, to insure that they are not treated with a pesticide. Soak one tablespoon of alfalfa seeds or wheat berries, or one-third cup of chick-peas, soybeans, or mung beans in a one-quart jar of water for several hours or overnight. Pour off the water. Cover the top of the jar with cheesecloth or stocking and fasten it with a rubber band. Tilt the jar to allow the water to drain off completely. Now, leave the jar on a counter, in a cabinet, or in your dish drainer. Rinse and drain twice a day, morning and evening; if the weather is hot and dry, do this three times a day. Make sure excess water is drained after each rinsing. Harvest the wheat berries after two days, mung beans after three days, alfalfa after four or five days. Place full-grown sprouts in a sunny window for a day to turn them green. Eat and enjoy.

Beans, Nuts, & Seeds Scoreboard

Beans, nuts and seeds are excellent sources of dietary fiber, protein, vitamins, and minerals. While beans are generally low in fat, peanuts and most nuts and seeds are high in both fat and calories.

Food	Serving Size	Nutritional Score
Black beans	1/2 cup, cooked	93
Chick-peas (garbanzo beans)	1/2 cup, cooked	90
Lima beans	1/2 cup, cooked	73
Navy beans	1/2 cup, cooked	61
Lentils	1/2 cup, cooked	57
Kidney beans	1/2 cup, cooked	56
Split peas	1/2 cup, cooked	51
Black-eyed peas	1/2 cup, cooked	49
Soybeans	1/2 cup, cooked	46
Soybean sprouts	1 cup	45
Tofu (bean curd)	1 piece, (4 oz.), 3" × 2¼" × 1"	31
Sunflower seeds, hulled	1 oz.	24
Almonds, shelled	1 oz.	18
Peanuts, roasted	1 oz.	11
Cashews	1 oz.	7
Peanut butter	2 Tbsp.	5
English walnuts	1 oz.	3
Sesame seeds	1 oz.	2

Grain Foods: Bread, Rice, and Pasta

Is bread fattening? Does pasta turn beautiful *signore* into objects of obesity? Does rice zoom to your waistline like a homing pigeon?

No! No! No! Bread, rice, spaghetti and other grain foods have taken a bum rap for years. These foods contain moderate amounts of many nutrients and are fairly low in calories. Believe it or not, they are the very foods we should be eating *more* of.

Americans have been getting fatter and fatter in recent decades. And at the same time we have been eating fewer and fewer grain products. In 1910 the average American ate about 300 pounds of flour and grains in bread, pancakes, cornbread, rice, oatmeal, and other foods. Such foods used to be Americans' major source of protein. The average person is now eating only about 150 pounds of grains a year. Instead of the grain foods, we are eating more sugary and fatty foods, the very culprits that are sculpting our bodies into bulbous shapes.

Twenty years ago, most grocery stores featured mountains of spongy white bread; it is no wonder that bread consumption declined. Puffy white bread may come in handy when you run out of paper towels or need a pillow, but if taste and texture are what you're after, it leaves a lot to be desired.

Supermarkets now carry whole wheat bread, brown rice, wheat germ and other highly nutritious and flavorful grain products. Of course, markets also sell an endless supply of Twinkies, chocolate cake, and other junk foods that contain a bit of white flour along with heaps of sugar and shortening.

Consumer beware: Bakers often use artificial coloring—usually caramel—to make a loaf of bread look darker and more nutritious than it really is. Some dark breads are little more than white breads in disguise. Bakers add caramel coloring to pumpernickel, "wheat bread" (almost all bread is made from wheat), and rye bread to make them look as if they contain more whole grain flour than they really do. Read your labels carefully!

When it comes to nutrition, *whole* grain foods are clearly tops, but *refined* grains are not as bad for you as they are sometimes painted. Refined flour does have less of most vitamins, minerals, and dietary fiber, but it is low in fat and contains about as much protein as whole wheat flour.

When whole wheat flour and brown rice are refined to white flour and white rice, the nutrient-packed germ and fiber-rich bran are removed. They usually end up in feed for livestock. Several of the lost vitamins (riboflavin, niacin, thiamin) and minerals (iron and often calcium) are replaced in the enriching process. But other vitamins (vitamin B_6, vitamin E, folacin, pantothenic acid) and minerals (zinc, chromium, magnesium, copper, manganese, and potassium) are not restored. Now refer to the Grain Foods Scoreboard and note that enriched white bread (+45) scores a full ten points less than whole wheat bread (+55). Likewise, brown rice (+47) has a marginally higher score than enriched white rice (+45) and a substantially higher score than instant white enriched rice (+36).

The Food and Nutrition Board of the National Academy of Sciences issued a report in 1974 that recommended the addition of ten vitamins and minerals to white flour (it is now fortified with four or five nutrients). But the Board acknowledged that even this expanded fortification effort would not make white flour equivalent to whole wheat flour. The report said:

> Because of the increasing recognition of the importance of certain of these trace nutrients in our diets today, it is urged that processors of wheat, in the interest of retaining the maximum amount of all nutrients indigenous to wheat, refine flour no more than is actually required for consumer acceptance and they avoid the use of destructive bleaching and maturing agents wherever possible.[97]

Consumers can encourage bread manufacturers to follow this advice by buying whole wheat bread.

The FDA has recognized that enriching foods with nutrients is a practical way, but not the ideal way of providing good nutrition. Way back in 1943 FDA said that ". . . adequate nutrition could be better assured through the choice of natural foods than through reliance on enrichment . . ." FDA concluded, though, that the nourishing natural foods were not always available and that most consumers did not know enough about nutrition to choose a well-rounded diet from unenriched natural foods.[98]

One of the constituents of whole grains, dietary fiber, made nutritional headlines in the 1970s. Previously dismissed as "just roughage," scientists discovered—or rediscovered—that fiber plays an important role in our health. Unlike vitamins, minerals, and protein, which are worthless until they are absorbed, one form of fiber is valuable because it is *not* absorbed by the body—much of it passes right through.

Insoluble dietary fiber attracts water and promotes larger, more easily passed stools. This reduces the likelihood of getting constipation, diverticulosis, and possibly colon cancer. *Soluble* fiber does not increase stool size, but it does have a modest beneficial effect on cholesterol levels and can help control diabetes. Whole wheat contains about three times as much fiber—mostly of the insoluble type—as does refined flour.

Healthful as whole wheat is, it does contain one potentially undesirable substance: phytic acid. Phytic acid is the storage form of phosphorus in wheat. As the grain germinates, the phytic acid is broken down to release phosphate, which is used by the plant for growth. Phytate in foods—especially high-fiber foods—can be a problem, because it combines with calcium, zinc, iron, and possibly other minerals, reducing their availability to the body. In some Middle East villages, dwarfism due to zinc deficiency is common. The zinc deficiency is thought to be due to diets that consist primarily of *unleavened* whole wheat bread, which is high in phytic acid and fiber. The phytic acid is largely broken down during the leavening/baking process. Most Americans obtain only about 10–20 percent of their calories from grains, and most of this in *leavened* foods, so any adverse effects of phytic acid would be minimal.

Something else to be aware of is that many baked goods are high in sodium, either from salt or baking powder. Bread, rolls, and crackers provide about 25 percent of our total sodium intake. In comparison, salty snack foods like potato chips, popcorn, and pretzels provide only about 2 percent of our sodium. The reason for this huge, and perhaps surprising, difference is that most people eat a much larger volume of bread than potato chips.

Grain foods take a real tumble on the Nutrition Scoreboard when shortening, sugar, and salt are added. Hostess Twinkies (-34), a cupcake (-16), and chocolate cake (-27) are nutritional disasters that should only be eaten occasionally—unless you don't care about your teeth and waistline.

Most people think of a loaf of bread, a bowl of rice, or a dish of spaghetti when they think of grain foods. However, many other types are available and can add variety, flavor, and nutrition to your meals. Some specialty breads score high on the Scoreboard: a good rye ($+46$) or whole wheat pita bread ($+73$) or a sturdy German pumpernickel will give your meals or snacks a hearty change. Bulgur or cracked wheat ($+77$), a Middle Eastern favorite, is the easiest grain in the world to prepare—all you need to do is soak it in hot water. A classic food based on bulgur is tabouli, a delicious dish that is popular on the potluck circuit.

TABOULI

1 1/2 cups cracked wheat (bulgur)
3 tomatoes, finely diced
1 onion, minced
1 large bunch parsley, minced
1/4 tsp. pepper
1/8 tsp. cinnamon

2 Tbsp. chopped mint or
    1/2 tsp. dried mint (optional)
4 Tbsp. oil
2 Tbsp. sharp mustard
2 Tbsp. vinegar
juice of 1 lemon

Soak cracked wheat overnight in 4 cups of water, then press in strainer to remove excess water. Toss thoroughly with all ingredients; taste for seasoning. Chill. Serves six. Tastes great in pita (pouch) bread—whole wheat, of course!

For great nutrition in the morning, a half cup of wheat germ (+120) with sliced fresh fruit and skim or low-fat milk or low-fat yogurt can't be topped. Wheat germ is the most nutritious part of the wheat kernel. It contains most of the goodies: B vitamins, protein, trace minerals, and vitamin E.

As you gulp down more and more grain foods, pay attention to the toppings and sauces you use with them. Gobs of butter will undermine the nutritional value of even the best of breads. Try eating them plain: some flavorful breads, lightly toasted, don't require toppings at all. Yogurt or apple butter makes an interesting spread. If you use butter, margarine, or jelly, spread it on thinly and eat the bread upside down so that the topping hits your taste buds directly. Pasta topped with a tomato sauce and herb seasoning is far better for your arteries than pasta in a rich cream sauce.

The Surgeon General of the United States, the Department of Health and Human Services, and other health authorities have all been urging Americans to eat more grains, beans, potatoes, fruits and green vegetables, as we cut down on sugary foods, fatty meats, whole milk dairy foods, and shortening. Bread used to be our staff of life. In some cultures, rice, bread, or pasta remains the main course for most people. It is in that dietary direction that we should move. Doing so means eating a couple more slices of bread in the morning to replace an egg. For lunch, it means an extra sandwich and no soda pop. For dinner, the spaghetti and meatballs should be heavy on the spaghetti, using the meatballs more as a condiment than the main attraction. Because grains are relatively inexpensive, changes like these will also save you lots of money.

For an almost limitless supply of healthful grain recipes, read: *The Tassajara Bread Book*, by E. E. Brown, Shambhala Publishing, Boulder, Colorado, 1970; *Tassajara Cooking,* by E. E. Brown, Shambhala Publishing, Boulder, Colorado, 1973; *Bread Winners,* by M. London, Rodale Press, Emmaus, Pennsylvania, 1979; *Recipes for a Small Planet,* by E. G. Ewald, Ballantine Books, New York, 1973; *Laurel's Kitchen,* by L. Robertson, C. Flinders, B. Godfrey, Bantam, New York, 1976.

Grain Foods Scoreboard

Contrary to a widespread myth, starchy grain foods are not fattening. Most people would do well to eat more grain foods in place of meat. Grains, especially whole grains, are a nicely balanced, low-fat source of carbohydrates, vitamins, minerals, and protein.

Food	Serving Size	Nutritional Score
Wheat germ	1/2 cup	120
Bulgur (cracked wheat)	1/2 cup, cooked	77
Whole wheat pita (Syrian bread)	1 pouch	73
Whole wheat bread	2 slices	55
Millet	1/2 cup, cooked	52
Brown rice	1/2 cup, cooked	47
Rye bread	2 slices	46
White bread, enriched	2 slices	45
White rice, enriched	1/2 cup, cooked	45
Pearled barley	1/2 cup, cooked	42
Cornbread	2" square	38
Hamburger/hot dog roll, enriched	1	36
Instant white rice, enriched	1/2 cup, cooked	36
Egg noodles, enriched	1/2 cup, cooked	35
Spaghetti or macaroni, enriched	1/2 cup, cooked	32
Pancakes, buckwheat (mix)	four 4" cakes	31
Oatmeal	1/2 cup, cooked	30
Wheat germ	2 Tbsp.	24
Hominy grits	1/2 cup, cooked	23
Cupcake, plain	1	−16
Pound cake	1 medium slice	−18
Chocolate cake	1 medium slice	−27
Hostess Twinkies	1 package	−34

Meat, Poultry, Eggs, and Fish

Meat. The very sound of the word conjures up certain images: strong and masculine, compact and tough. Meat is the all-American food.

In health circles, though, meat is a four-letter word that triggers very different thoughts. It's a food that contributes to major health problems and represents an extravagant style of life in a world of shortages and poverty.

These opposing views of a highly popular food have been fighting it out in biomedical conferences, supermarket aisles, and kitchens from coast to coast.

Beef consumption increased from fifty-five pounds to ninety-five pounds per person per year between 1910 and 1976, with much of the rise coming since 1960. But then several things happened. The price of grain, used to fatten beef cattle, rose dramatically; inflation halved the dollar's value and led to higher beef prices; more people learned that beef was very high in saturated fat, which promotes heart disease. Between 1976 and 1983, Americans cut their beef consumption by 17 percent.

The meat industry is extremely defensive about complaints concerning beef's nutritional value. The industry argues, rightfully, that beef is rich in iron, protein, and B vitamins. In fact, lean meat is highly nutritious, as the score of +51 for a serving of round steak indicates (see Scoreboard on pages 127–28). Most beef, though, contains hefty amounts of saturated fat and cholesterol, which contribute to coronary heart disease and other cardiovascular problems. These diseases account for about one third of all deaths in the United States.

If fat's inclination to promote heart disease and obesity is not enough to scare you away from hot dogs, you should be interested in studies linking high-fat diets to cancers of the breast and colon. The National Cancer Institute, a panel of the National Academy of Sciences, and the American Cancer Society have urged all Americans to reduce their consumption of fat. According to federal surveys, meat (beef and pork) provides about 23 percent of our total fat and 27 percent of our intake of saturated fat, more than any other food group.[99]

As meat is permeated with more fat, nutritional values decline. Thus, rump roast (+26) and sirloin steak (+17) score well below round steak. Hamburger scores even lower (lean at +14; regular fat content at −4). The lower scores are all due to the replacement of nutrient-rich lean meat with fat.

The real nutritional disasters occur when meat is heavily processed. Hot dogs (−20), bologna (−26), and Spam (−35) are loaded with sodium chloride (table salt), sodium nitrite, and fat. Salt increases the risk of high blood pressure (hypertension), nitrite increases slightly the risk of cancer, and fat promotes heart disease and cancer. Processed meats are simply the industry's way of disposing of its garbage—at two dollars a pound.

Although the average hot dog is thought of as a protein food, it has no more protein (about five grams) than the average hot dog bun. A hot dog contains two and a half times as much fat as protein. Looking at hot dogs another way, 80 percent of their calories comes from fat. It is for such reasons that Ralph Nader dubbed the frankfurter "America's deadliest missile."

Typical Composition of the Average Beef Carcass[100]

Grade	Protein	Fat	Nutrition	Price
Prime	14 percent	41 percent	Lower	Higher
Choice	15 percent	35 percent	Medium	Medium
Good	16.5 percent	28 percent	Higher	Lower

After many years of defending "fatfurters," some meat processors are finally trying to improve their products. Several companies now market reduced-fat (20–25 percent by weight instead of 30 percent) hot dogs. Many such products are made from chicken rather than beef. Unfortunately, not only is the fat content still rather high, but many of these lower-fat products are higher in sodium than regular frankfurters. The chicken hot dog's −7 score beats the score of regular hot dogs, but it's not terrific, especially compared to chicken (+68).

The beef industry's slight decline in the past decade is remarkable considering the proliferation of fast-food restaurants. Thousands of McDonald's, Wendy's, Burger Kings, and others sell billions of hamburgers a year. While the hamburgers served at fast-food restaurants are probably hygienic, they tend to be loaded with fat, both from the meat and the sauce that is usually slapped on the "specialty" sandwiches. CSPI nutritionist Bonnie Liebman surveyed the fast-food scene in 1983 and discovered that a Wendy's triple cheeseburger was so high in fat that it deserved to be dubbed the "coronary bypass special." Each serving had more than two solid ounces of fat! Wendy's regular hamburger sandwich had a bit more fat than protein, while the Roy Rogers sandwich actually had 20 percent more fat than protein. It is no exaggeration to say that fast-food restaurants are major contributors to this nation's toll of heart disease and cancer. Fortunately, restaurants have been broadening their product line so that it is oftentimes possible to get a nice salad, baked potato, or corn on the cob.

Pork, like beef, is rich in nutrients and comes in either lean or fatty varieties. Pork is one of the best sources of riboflavin and thiamin. Ham (+28) tends to be relatively low in fat, but it is cured and preserved with sodium chloride and sodium nitrite. Thus, ham contains far more sodium than is desirable. Read the label, though, because brands with somewhat reduced sodium are now available. A great deal of pork also goes into hot dogs (−20), pork sausage (−19) and luncheon meat (−33), all high in both sodium and fat. These ingredients are a problem for the 60 million Americans suffering from high blood pressure. On your next shopping trip, *don't bring home the bacon* (−5)!

While beef consumption has declined and pork consumption has stayed about the same, chicken consumption has increased by about 20 percent since 1976. Chicken is, or at least starts out, lean and nutritious (+68 if skinless; +42 if roasted and eaten with the skin). Frying, of course, adds to the fat content and the calorie count, unless you remove the skin and breading before dining. Nutritionist Bonnie Liebman has calculated that a standard serving of Chicken McNuggets oozes with an amount of fat equivalent to five pats of butter. More than half the calories in this product come from fat. One chicken breast from Kentucky Fried Chicken contains the equivalent of three pats of butter.

Whether chicken will remain as nutritious in the future as it has been is the big question. Modern chicken farms—almost like factories—raise sedentary chickens on a diet of grain and chemicals. As a result, today's "agribusiness" chicken is significantly fattier than an "old-fashioned" barnyard chicken.

From chickens come eggs, and from eggs (−7) come controversy. Basically a healthful food containing a variety of nutrients, the egg would be fine were it not for its cholesterol content. The protein-rich white scores +11, while the fat- and cholesterol-rich yolk rates −18. Two thirds of an egg's calories come from the fat, and an average large egg contains about 275 mg of cholesterol. If you know that your cholesterol level is reasonably low—150–180 or below for an adult—you could continue eating eggs at about your normal rate. But if you are trying to reduce your cholesterol level, eggs, or at least egg yolks, are the place to start cutting back.

If you must have your omelette on Sunday morning, you can cut your cholesterol intake in half by discarding the yolks from half the eggs. You can also replace some or all of the egg ingredient with egg substitutes, such as Eggbeaters (+27). What to do with your extra yolks? The Stanford Heart Disease Prevention Program suggests that you "put the hard-boiled yolks in your bird feeder. Or give an occasional extra yolk to your dog. Or beat up uncooked yolks with some water and brush on the leaves of your houseplants." Or you can toss them down the drain.

Beef liver and chicken liver are remarkably nutritious foods. Beef liver's virtues are legendary: a two-ounce serving supplies the entire day's requirement for vitamin A and riboflavin. Beef liver also supplies 28 percent of the U.S. RDA for protein, 46 percent of the U.S. RDA for niacin, 28 percent of the U.S. RDA for iron, and 24 percent of the U.S. RDA for vitamin C. It is also low in fat and sodium. As the sportscasters say, that is *some* food. Some people boost the nutritional value of their hamburgers and meat loaf by grinding a quarter pound of liver in with one pound of ground beef.

Liver would get the "Super Food" award had it not one real flaw. A three-ounce serving of beef liver has 50 percent more cholesterol than one egg. Thus, if you are at all concerned about cholesterol, you should not eat liver too frequently.

Liver has sometimes been criticized for collecting pesticides and toxic chemicals. However, according to the U.S. Department of Agriculture, liver actually contains *less* of those chemicals than muscle meat. The reason for this is that liver contains little fat, while red meat is often high in fat, and many toxic chemicals accumulate in fat. Liver is higher than red meat in only a couple of contaminants.

For variety in healthful eating, many people include fish as a regular part of their diet. Fish is nutritious, a high-protein food that never contains much saturated fat—unless it is cooked or seasoned with butter, or fried in a fast-food restaurant. You can avoid unnecessary sodium or fat by paying attention to a few tips:

- Canned tuna fish is available either water packed (+75) or oil packed (+40). Oil-packed tuna contains about twice the calorie and ten times the fat content of the water-packed variety.

- Shrimp (+52), oysters, scallops (+52), clams (+43), lobster (+72), and crab (+46) are fine low-fat foods, if boiled or baked, but dipping them in bread crumbs and deep frying them adds lots of fat and calories. Shrimp, incidentally, is moderately high in cholesterol, though a 3-ounce serving still contains only about half as much as does an egg, 128 versus 275 milligrams.

- Some fish, including salmon (+67), mackerel, and herring, are naturally oily. Between 40 and 60 percent of their caloric content comes from oil. Cod (+50), flounder (+54), haddock, halibut, ocean perch, pollack, and sole all contain less than 20 percent of their overall calories as fat.

- Avoid McDonald's "Filet o' Fish" and similar fast-food fried fish sandwiches. "Filet o' Fish" contains two and one-half times as much fat as a regular McDonald's hamburger.

Many fish are naturally very low in fat. Of the oilier varieties, only 11 to 27 percent of the fat is saturated, as compared to about 48 percent in beef and 44 percent in pork. In addition, fish fat appears to provide a special benefit. Recent studies have found that fish oil contains unusual types of fatty acids that are especially capable of preventing heart attack and stroke. The fatty acids are polyunsaturated "omega-3" fatty acids (eicosopentaenoic acid [EPA] and docosahexaenoic acid [DHA]). They seem to prevent blood clots as well as reduce cholesterol buildup in the arteries. Eskimos eat a tremendous amount of fish and they have an extremely low risk of heart disease. A recent study done in Holland, though sponsored in part by the U.S. Government, found that the more fish middle-aged men ate, the lower their risk of heart attack death. According to the authors, "Mortality from coronary heart disease was more than 50 percent lower among those who consumed at least 30 grams (about one ounce) of fish per day than among those who did not eat fish."[101]

Some health food companies are now producing capsules with omega-3 fatty acids to enable people to consume significant amounts without adding salmon to every meal. The limitations of the capsules is that they are fairly expensive, dilute, and caloric (100–200 calories to get 3–6 grams of the fatty acids).[102]

Before you rush out and fill your freezer with oily fish, you should know that many environmental contaminants, such as DDT, dioxin, and PCBs collect in the oil. These chemicals, chlorinated hydrocarbons, are suspected of causing cancer and birth defects. Most likely to be contaminated are the fattier freshwater fish, such as carp, lake trout, catfish, and yellow perch, as well as fatty migratory species, like bluefish. Least likely to be contaminated are saltwater fish, such as salmon, shellfish, and freshwater fish grown on farms or caught in unpolluted mountain streams.

If you want to eat fish and not worry about the fat or the contaminants, choose cod, haddock, flounder, sole, turbot, ocean perch, halibut, tuna, pollack, clams, scallops, or other lean species.

Millions of Americans are drifting away from meat and discovering that more vegetarian diets are nutritious, delicious, and relatively inexpensive. While there is no nutritional reason to give up meat entirely, you might want to get a copy of a good vegetarian cookbook, such as *Laurel's Kitchen* or *Moosewood Cookbook*, and give vegetarianism a whirl for a meal, a day, a week, or longer. Many people who switch to a plant-food-based diet—for ethical, health, or other reasons—say they feel much better than they ever did before.

Meat, Poultry, Egg, and Fish Scoreboard

The foods near the top are excellent sources of iron, protein, and other nutrients. Lower-scoring foods tend to be high in calories, cholesterol (eggs), fat (red meat), or sodium (processed meats).

Red meat scores are for cooked, semitrimmed cuts. (If more than half the removable fat is trimmed away, scores would improve; if less than half is removed, the scores would fall).

Next time instead of frying these foods, try baking, broiling, or poaching them.

Food	Serving Size	Nutritional Score
Beef liver, fried*	3 oz.	119
Chicken livers, simmered*	2 livers (1.8 oz.)	90
Tuna, water packed (no salt added)	3 oz.	75
Lobster, cooked meat	3 oz.	72
Chicken, roasted, skinless	3 oz.	68
Salmon, pink, fillet	3 oz.	67
Turkey, roasted	3 oz.	62
Flounder, baked	3 oz.	54

Food	Serving Size	Nutritional Score
Scallops, steamed	3 oz.	52
Shrimp, steamed	3 oz.	52
Salmon, sockeye red, canned (with salt)	3 oz.	52
Round steak	3 oz.	51
Cod, broiled	3 oz.	50
Crabs, steamed meat	3 oz. (1 cup)	46
Veal cutlet, broiled	3 oz.	44
Clams, raw or steamed	5 clams (2.5 oz.)	43
Chicken, roasted with skin	3 oz.	42
Tuna, oil packed, drained	3 oz.	40
Leg of lamb	3 oz.	34
Shrimp, fried, breaded	3 oz.	31
Ham, baked	3 oz.	28
Chicken, fried, breaded	2 oz., 1 thigh	27
Eggbeaters	1/4 cup	27
Rump roast	3 oz.	26
Pork chop, baked	3 oz.	25
Canadian bacon	2 slices (2 oz.)	21
Sirloin steak	3 oz.	17
Hamburger, 20 percent fat, lean	3 oz.	14
Ham, smoked	2 slices (2 oz.)	12
Egg white	1 large egg white	11
Pork chop, baked, lean with fat	3 oz.	8
Cotto salami	2 slices	5
Hamburger, 25 percent fat, regular	3 oz.	−4
Bacon	2 slices (1/2 oz.)	−5
Egg*, hard-boiled	1 large	−7
Hard salami	2 oz.	−18
Pork sausage	3 links (2 oz.)	−19
Hot dog	1 (1.5 oz.)	−20
Beef bologna	2 slices (2 oz.)	−26
Luncheon meat	2 slices (2 oz.)	−33
Spam	3 oz.	−35

* Liver and eggs are rich in vitamins, minerals, and protein, but liver is high in cholesterol and egg yolks are rich in cholesterol and fat.

Dairy Foods

Since the first people took milk from cows and goats way back when, dairy products have been a mainstay in the diets of many cultures. The variety of dairy foods is increasing rapidly, as scientists reshape traditional products. But as with other categories of food, some dairy foods are more nutritious than others.

Whole milk, with an average of about 3.7 percent butterfat, is the quintessential dairy food. It rates +28 on the Scoreboard. As the dairy industry is fond of reminding us, milk is one of the best sources of calcium, riboflavin, and protein. An eight-ounce glass contains about 19 percent of our daily requirement for protein, 29 percent of the calcium we need, and 24 percent of the riboflavin. Milk also contains some vitamin A and thiamin. Milk's one serious flaw is that it contains a significant amount of saturated fat. Milk and other dairy products provide 15 to 20 percent of our total fat and about 29 percent of our saturated fat.[103] You can play it safe by buying low-fat milk (1 percent butterfat), skim milk (0 percent), or buttermilk made from skim milk. Nonfat dry milk and skim milk have all of milk's nutrients at a lower cost, with fewer calories, and without any fat.

Another problem relates to lactose, the main carbohydrate in milk. All children and many Caucasian adults have an enzyme in the small intestine that breaks lactose into its two component sugars, glucose and galactose, which are then absorbed into the bloodstream and used for energy. Most blacks and Orientals lose that enzyme during childhood and are not able to digest the lactose. Instead, bacteria in the large intestine metabolize the lactose. This causes flatulence (intestinal gas), diarrhea, and stomachaches. It may, at first, seem unusual to white Americans that a large percentage of humans cannot drink milk comfortably, but in fact, few adult mammals drink milk (the domestic cat is one obvious exception). Before lactose intolerance was recognized, powdered milk was a staple in America's foreign aid program. Latin American, African, and Asian recipients who could not drink milk used the free powder for whitewashing houses, as a laxative, or simply threw it away. As discussed in Part Two of this book under "lactose," there are ways consumers can reduce the lactose content of milk.

The foods outranking whole milk on the scoreboard all contain less fat and fewer calories. A cup of skim milk (+55), for instance, contains only 85 calories (compared to the 150 in whole milk) and virtually no fat. Mixed with banana in a blender, it is a perfect refresher for diet-conscious people.

Consumption of whole milk has declined dramatically in the past thirty years, from about thirty-five to twenty-one gallons per person per year. However, low-fat milk consumption has more than doubled, to about eleven gallons per person. The switch to low-fat milk probably reflects greater concern for health, as well as the lower price. The overall reduction in consumption is due in part to the ubiquitous soft drink machine. Also, our population is gradually aging, and oldsters drink less milk than youngsters.

A new form of milk, called UHT milk, may be entering our stores and our lives in the 1980s. "UHT" stands for ultra high temperature, a pasteurization process that eliminates the need for refrigeration. It can be stored in a sealed container, but once exposed to air it needs normal refrigeration. Shelf-stable whipping cream has been available for several years. The taste of such products is said to leave something to be desired.

Unflavored low-fat yogurt (+64) is at the top of the Scoreboard. Yogurt is made by adding a bacterial culture to milk, usually low-fat milk. As the bacteria multiply, they convert some of the lactose (milk sugar) to lactic acid. The acid curdles the milk and adds flavor. Yogurt has all the nutrition of the milk, but can be stored for a much longer time. Lactose-intolerant people, who cannot drink milk, usually can eat yogurt without a problem. If you've never had yogurt, try a cup—you're in for a pleasant, refreshing surprise.

Yogurt rates higher on the chart than skim milk primarily because most producers add nonfat dry milk solids, which boost its nutrient content. But note what happens when plain low-fat yogurt is flavored with fruit preserves: the score nosedives from +64 to +27. The drastically lower score reflects the ounce or more of refined sugar that has replaced some of the cultured milk. Your best and yummiest yogurt bet is to slice your own fresh fruit into a dish of plain, low-fat yogurt.

Americans have been saying "cheese" more than ever. Cheese consumption rose gradually from five pounds per person in 1920 to ten pounds in 1950. Then, in the past thirty years, cheese consumption doubled again. Most of the increase is probably attributable to the proliferation of franchised restaurants that offer pizza and cheeseburgers. Also contributing to the increase is the popularity of ovo-lacto vegetarianism, a diet that includes eggs and dairy products.

Cottage cheese is one of the best foods around. Note that low-fat (1 percent butterfat) cottage cheese (+30) easily outpoints regular cottage cheese (+17). A half-cup serving contains about one third of our daily protein requirement and 17 percent of our riboflavin requirement. However, a half-cup serving of cottage cheese has only one fourth as much calcium as a glass of milk. Mix cottage cheese with blueberries, sliced banana, diced peaches, or pineapple, if you want a touch of sweetness.

Hard cheeses are not as nutritious as cottage cheese, because of their high content of fat, saturated fat, and sodium. But they still are rich sources of protein, riboflavin, calcium, and vitamin A. A two-ounce serving of Swiss cheese (+13), for instance, contains 30 percent of the daily dose of protein, half the calcium requirement, and 13 percent each of the vitamin A and riboflavin allotments—not bad for two ounces of food. The worst cheese, according to our rating system, is American cheese (−18). The Stanford Heart Disease Prevention Program discourages people from eating American and other hard cheeses, noting that one ounce of such cheeses contains a whole tablespoon of fat. Also near the bottom of the chart is cream cheese (−11). It is loaded with fat and would have scored even worse, but for the fact that portion sizes are small. A cottage cheese and lox sandwich would be more nutritious than cream cheese and lox, but I am not sure how good it would taste. If you crave cream cheese, try spreading just a very thin layer on your bagel.

Ice cream (−22) is the least nutritious of the milk-derived products. A three-ounce serving contains relatively little calcium (7 percent of the U.S. RDA), vitamins, and protein. On the other hand it contains hefty amounts of saturated fat and sugar. Depending on its richness, ice cream contains between 10 and 18 percent butterfat. Ice cream is fine for special occasions, but should not be an everyday food.

For those who love hard cheeses and frozen desserts, reduced-fat versions of old favorites are becoming more common. For instance, while whole-milk mozzarella cheese scores −1, part-skim mozzarella ranks a much more respectable +19. Likewise, vanilla ice cream scores −22, while ice milk, which contains about one-third as much fat and one-third fewer calories, scores +7. Frozen low-fat yogurt is nutritionally similar to ice milk.

Natural dairy products contain more sodium than most other natural foods. For instance, low-fat milk contains 130 milligrams of sodium. An apple contains only 1 milligram. However, processed cheeses are the real sodium culprits. Cheez Whiz has 885 milligrams per 1.5 ounce serving, and American cheese has over 800 milligrams for the same size serving. People on low-sodium diets need to be especially careful about processed dairy foods.

The dairy industry would like people to gobble up all dairy foods from ice cream to cream cheese (and manages to get this message to schoolchildren from coast to coast). Our job as smart eaters is to separate the best from the worst, the calcium from the cream. The Nutrition Scoreboard approach should help you do it.

Dairy Foods Scoreboard

The best dairy foods are the low-fat milks, yogurts, and cottage cheeses. While all dairy foods are good sources of protein, calcium, and riboflavin, the lower-scoring foods are high in saturated fat or sodium.

Food	Serving Size	Nutritional Score
Yogurt, low-fat, plain	8 oz., 1 cup	64
Skim milk	8 oz.	55
Buttermilk, 1 percent fat	8 oz.	46
Low-fat milk, 2 percent fat	8 oz.	43
Yogurt, low-fat, vanilla or coffee	8 oz.	37
Soy milk	8 oz.	33
Cottage cheese, 1 percent fat	½ cup	30
Whole milk, 3.7 percent fat	8 oz.	28

Food	Serving Size	Nutritional Score
Chocolate milk, 2 percent fat	8 oz.	27
Yogurt, low-fat, fruit preserves	8 oz., 1 cup	27
Ricotta cheese, part skim	1/2 cup	26
Low-fat American cheese	2 oz.	26
Mozzarella cheese, part skim	2 oz.	19
Cottage cheese, 4 percent fat	2 oz.	17
Yogurt, whole milk, plain	8 oz., 1 cup	15
Swiss cheese	2 oz.	13
Vanilla ice milk	1/2 cup	7
Frozen yogurt, vanilla	1/2 cup	6
Ricotta cheese, whole milk	1/2 cup	−1
Mozzarella cheese, whole milk	2 oz.	−1
Orange sherbet	1/2 cup	−2
Frozen yogurt, fruit	1/2 cup	−2
Whipped cream	1 Tbsp.	−3
Sour cream	1 Tbsp.	−4
Cream, light	1 Tbsp.	−6
Cheddar cheese	2 oz.	−10
Cream cheese	1/2 oz., 1 cubic inch	−11
Butter	1 pat	−13
American cheese	2 oz.	−18
Vanilla ice cream	1/2 cup	−22

Nondairy Beverages

The difference between a healthful meal and a deficient one often lies in the drink that washes it down. One excellent choice is orange juice (+47), which is rich in vitamin C and has small amounts of vitamin A and B vitamins, or another pure fruit juice. Drinks like these can make a major contribution to the nutritional value of a meal. Canned tomato juice (+36) with generous amounts of vitamins A and C and V-8 juice (+26) miss the honor roll, because of their high sodium content.

Of course, not everyone drinks a nutritious beverage all the time. Soft drinks and coffee, which are dispensed by zillions of vending machines and promoted by enormous advertising expenditures, are often drunk in place of nutritious alternatives. In 1982 the average American drank twenty-four gallons of coffee and forty gallons of soda pop, as well as twenty-four gallons of beer, according to the U.S. Department of Agriculture. That compares to about twenty-seven gallons of milk.

Coffee and tea contain no nutrients, but do contain caffeine, which, being a stimulant of the central nervous system, can keep you awake and make you jittery if you are sensitive or drink too much. The caffeine has also been linked to birth defects and fibrocystic breast disease (benign breast lumps). Women who are troubled by breast lumps or are pregnant should abstain from caffeine-containing beverages and drugs or consume only minimal amounts. The score for coffee and tea is knocked from 0 to -6 by the addition of a teaspoon of sugar and to -18 if you also add a tablespoon of light cream.

Decaffeinated coffee is becoming increasingly popular, because more and more people are concerned about the adverse effects of caffeine. Decaffeinated coffee contains only about one twentieth as much caffeine as regular coffee. The virtual absence of caffeine is a real benefit, but there is controversy over the chemical, methylene chloride, that some companies use to remove the caffeine. Methylene chloride is a chlorinated hydrocarbon, a family of chemicals many of whose members have caused cancer. A 1985 study gives every reason to believe that this chemical, too, promotes cancer. Only minuscule amounts of methylene chloride survive the processing and the addition of hot water in your cup, but it certainly makes sense to avoid the suspicious substance. High Point, Taster's Choice, and Nescafé are several brands made without methylene chloride.

Numerous studies have suggested that coffee may be bad for the heart, while others did not detect a problem. The most recent study, published in 1985 by scientists at Stanford and the University of Washington, was also one of the most sophisticated. This study found that coffee intakes exceeding two or three cups a day were strongly correlated with increased levels of two blood chemicals associated with heart disease.[104]

Coffee is under suspicion for another reason: a couple of studies have linked coffee to increased risks of cancers of the pancreas and bladder, though other studies did not detect such a link. In a recent study on coffee and cancer of the urinary bladder, Yale scientists concluded that their "results suggest that about one quarter of bladder tumors in Connecticut might be attributable to drinking more than one cup of coffee per day."[105] About eleven thousand Americans die annually of bladder cancer.

While Yale was focusing on the urinary bladder, Harvard epidemiologists were studying the pancreas. In a study published in 1981, Dr. Brian MacMahon and his colleagues estimated that "the proportion of pancreatic cancer that is potentially attributable to coffee consumption to be slightly more than 50 percent."[106] Pancreatic cancer, which is almost always fatal, accounts for about twenty-three thousand deaths per year.

That coffee may promote cancer did not come as a complete surprise to cancer specialists. It is well-known that chemical reactions occur at high temperatures—such as those at which coffee beans are roasted—and often lead to the formation of carcinogenic agents.

Now who wants that second cup of coffee?

Whether or not coffee contributes to heart attacks has been a hotly debated question for two decades. There are plenty of warning signs that coffee isn't very good for the heart. For instance, caffeine can cause heart arrhythmias, and coffee intake correlates with increased levels of the "bad" type of cholesterol. A 1983 Norwegian study of over fourteen thousand men and women found a strong relationship between coffee consumption and cholesterol levels. But other studies have not found that coffee consumption is higher in heart attack victims than other people. (The fact that Norwegians boil their coffee may account, in part, for the results of that study.)

After reviewing a variety of conflicting evidence, Drs. Robert I. Levy and Manning Feinleib, both then at the National Heart, Lung, and Blood Institute, concluded that:

> there is no definitive proof that the ingestion of coffee increases the risk of cardiovascular disease . . . Although the data as an independent risk factor for coronary artery disease are mixed, they do suggest that coffee plays a role in association with other existing factors, such as hypertension.

I think it makes sense for people who have heart disease to avoid coffee (and caffeine) altogether, while others should drink no more than a cup or so of coffee a day.[107]

Coffee consumption has been declining steadily in the past thirty years, especially among young people, but Americans are in no danger of dehydration. The soft drink industry has been more than happy to provide us with beverages. Soft drink consumption, per capita, increased fourfold between 1950 and 1982 and doubled between 1968 and 1982. A survey taken in August 1970 by *Boys' Life* magazine revealed that the average Boy Scout reader consumed more than three 8-ounce servings of soda pop a day, while 8 percent of the boys drank two quarts or more a day! This much soda supplies between one third and one fourth of a boy's daily caloric requirement—and squeezes a good fraction of nutritious foods out of the diet. Though exact figures are not available, Americans probably spend in the neighborhood of $30 billion a year on carbonated soft drinks. That is almost 10 percent of our total food bill.

There isn't much good to say about soda pop—it rates −55 on the Scoreboard—though the National Soft Drink Association brags about all the "liquid" that soft drinks provide. Water aside, soda pop contains sugar (which adds to your waistline and dental bills), acid (which can also eat away at teeth), artificial colorings (some of which are suspected of causing health problems), caffeine, and a few other goodies, none of which are nutritious.

Per capita consumption tripled between 1962 and 1983, from 142 twelve-ounce servings to 438 servings.[108] Even toddlers are gulping the stuff. According to a 1981 study, 40 percent of one and two year olds average nine ounces of carbonated and noncarbonated soft drinks a day.[109] Soft drinks provide about 8 percent of all calories in the average American's diet. The calories come from the ten teaspoons of sugar in a typical twelve-ounce cola drink. The "empty calories" in soft drinks both squeeze out more nutritious foods from the diet and promote tooth decay.

Caffeine has been a traditional ingredient of cola beverages, Dr. Pepper, and many other brands. Caffeine, be it in coffee or Coke, is a stimulant and hardly belongs in a food which is consumed in such volume by so many children. Dr. Candace Pert, a National Institute of Mental Health expert on psychoactive drugs and how they affect the brain and behavior, believes that caffeine affects children. "I have seen the reaction of my own children to two or three glasses of cola containing caffeine—their behavior changes drastically. Maybe a little psychoactive kick for the kids is not a bad thing at all. But then again, maybe it changes their brain so that future development is affected."[110] The Food and Drug Administration has shown no interest in acceding to requests by several consumer groups to ban caffeine from soda pop.

When caffeine became the center of controversies, soft drink companies saw an opportunity to carve out another niche in the marketplace and grab more shelf space in supermarkets. Following 7-Up's introduction of Like caffeine-free cola, all the major soft drink companies quickly followed suit. The absence of caffeine makes the products a little less objectionable, but the net effect of the new varieties is probably that more people are drinking more soda pop.

Noncarbonated soft drinks have never been as popular as soda pop, but many chemists, especially at General Foods, have spent their lives developing such products. Kool-Aid, the first popular imitation fruit drink, has been fortified with vitamin C to fend off the "junk food" insults, but it is still filled with artificial colorings and flavorings and enough sugar to place it at -21 on the Scoreboard. Two of General Foods' more sophisticated imitation fruit drinks are Awake (-3) and Tang (-9). While these beverages have some vitamin C, they generally lack other vitamins and minerals that were not specifically added; they also contain artificial colorings.

To drink nutritiously, the best thing to do is to keep a variety of your favorite, healthful beverages in your refrigerator or on your shelves. Start with water (from the tap or bottled), salt-free club soda, caffeine-free teas, and fruit and vegetable juices. Mixtures of club soda and fruit juice are great refreshers.

Nondairy Beverages Scoreboard

Most beverages made from fruits and vegetables are high in vitamins A and C and natural sugars; they also contain modest amounts of other vitamins and minerals. While some low-scoring beverages may be fortified with one or two vitamins, they are generally high in added sugar or contain artificial sweetener or coloring.

Food	Serving Size	Nutritional Score
Carrot juice	6 oz.	48
Orange juice, unsweetened	6 oz.	47
Tomato juice	6 oz.	36
Grapefruit juice, unsweetened	6 oz.	36
Pineapple juice, unsweetened	6 oz.	31
V-8 juice	6 oz.	26
Apple juice	6 oz.	23
Grape juice, frozen	6 oz.	15
Pineapple-grapefruit juice	6 oz.	11
Water	8 oz.	0
Coffee or tea[1]	6 oz.	0
Salt-free club soda	8 oz.	0
Tab, other diet sodas[2]	12 oz., 1 can	−1
Awake	6 oz.	−3
Cranberry Juice Cocktail	6 oz.	−6
Welch's grape juice drink	6 oz.	−6
Tang	6 oz.	−9
Hawaiian Punch	6 oz.	−13
Hi-C	6 oz.	−15
Welchade Grape Drink	6 oz.	−19
Lemonade	6 oz.	−20
Kool-Aid, presweetened	6 oz.	−21
Gatorade	12 oz., 1 can	−34
Coca-Cola, other sodas[1]	12 oz., 1 can	−55

[1] Certain varieties contain caffeine, which may cause insomnia, breast lumps, and reproductive problems.

[2] Diet sodas contain saccharin, an artificial sweetener that increases the risk of cancer, or aspartame, a sweetener that needs to be better tested.

Vegetables

When it comes to vegetables, most Americans are culturally deprived. And I was no exception. Raised on mashed potatoes, peas (+45), carrots (+48), and corn (+41), I usually ignored the dozens of other choices—some having strange names and bizarre shapes—that can be found lurking in grocery store produce displays.

Fresh vegetables have so many nutritional virtues it is difficult to know where to begin. If you are tired of hearing about health problems caused by familiar foods, you can take comfort in the fact that virtually all vegetables are nutritious, the only difference being that some are moderately nutritious, while others are extremely nutritious. None score below zero on the Nutrition Scoreboard, and some superstars have scores of 90 or more. Except for the avocado—and it is technically a fruit—fresh vegetables contain virtually no fat and absolutely no cholesterol. They are also extremely low in sodium and not burdened with added sugar. The only negative note is that vegetables are often contaminated with tiny amounts of pesticides.

All vegetables boast some dietary fiber, are usually loaded with vitamins and minerals, and contain some protein. They are low in calories, usually fairly low in price, and delicious. Many of the vegetables at the top of the chart are excellent sources of vitamins A and C, which may help prevent cancer, according to the National Academy of Sciences.

With all these virtues, why are most veggies such strangers to most people? There are probably many reasons, but some must have to do with the changing nature of our food system. Years ago, most everyone had a garden and grew everything from asparagus to zucchini. We were also a nation of cooks, not of TV-dinner junkies or fast-food fanatics.

Television commercials and magazine ads rarely encourage us to eat fresh vegetables. Instead, they push processed foods, which are highly profitable to manufacturers. The farming business, as competitive as it is, doesn't generate the profits that would allow growers to buy many thirty-second prime-time television spots for kale.

Also, unlike packaged foods, fresh vegetables don't come with cooking instructions emblazoned on their skins. Even though vegetables are amazingly easy to prepare—and can often be eaten raw—it does take a bit of mental effort to learn how to use them. I have found the old standby, *Joy of Cooking*, indispensable. Once you have mastered the basic methods of preparing vegetables, you should turn to vegetarian cookbooks for more exotic, exciting ways to prepare them.

Despite the glories and variety of fresh vegetables, consumption (excluding potatoes) has averaged about 90–100 pounds per person for fifty years, with only a modest upswing to 110 pounds in the last decade. Consumption of processed vegetables grew steadily from about 30 pounds in 1920 to 131 pounds in 1979, but has since declined to 115 pounds. Fresh potato consumption nosedived from 200 pounds per person in 1910 to only about 55 pounds per person in recent years. On the other hand, we are eating more and more processed (chips, dehydrated, or frozen) potatoes.

Weight watchers can dive into a plate of vegetables like a child dives into a cookie jar. A standard half-cup serving of most nonstarchy vegetables contains only 20 to 30 calories. Even a small baked potato has less than 100 calories. You could eat four cups of brussels sprouts or broccoli and still consume fewer calories than you would get from one ounce of cheddar cheese (125 calories).

Children who turn up their noses at the mere mention of vegetables are missing out on real treats. Many of these fussy eaters will eat crisp, raw vegetables. Another way of interesting your children in vegetables is to help them grow a small garden. Children are thrilled as they follow the miraculous development of a tiny seed into a mature plant. And few children will not eat the tomato, peas, or swiss chard that they themselves grew. If you cannot have a garden, have your children help prepare and cook fresh store-bought vegetables.

Leafy green vegetables are among the most nutritious and easiest to prepare. These include spinach (+93), kale (+71), collards (+90), and mustard greens. They contain much or all of your daily requirements of vitamins A and C. Kale, for instance, contains 90 percent of the vitamin A requirement and 85 percent of the vitamin C requirement in a 22-calorie half-cup serving. Wow! Greens also contain significant amounts of iron, calcium, riboflavin, niacin, and fiber.

Forget about canned varieties of greens; they are usually soggy, salty abominations. Also forget the stereotype that only blacks and Southerners eat greens; people of every color and of many nations relish their flavor.

Spinach, chard, and lettuce can be eaten raw, but other greens need to be cooked. Mustard greens, aptly named, taste best if cooked long enough (about thirty-five minutes) to eliminate their sharp taste. You can cook them in a couple of inches of water, but they taste best and retain most of their vitamins if they are steamed. Cooking supply, hardware, and some grocery stores usually have inexpensive devices that convert any pot into a steamer.

Collard and turnip greens, kale, and spinach contain 10 to 16 percent of the U.S. RDA of calcium. However, spinach leaves contain oxalic acid, a chemical that can combine with much of the calcium and prevent it from being absorbed.

Romaine lettuce, which has a deep green color, easily outshines iceberg lettuce. Romaine has three times as much calcium, iron, and vitamin C and six times as much vitamin A as iceberg. The score of romaine is 17, iceberg 11.

To most of us, potatoes are less foreign than greens. But many people think sweet potatoes can only be eaten on holidays and that white potatoes are fattening. Banish those misconceptions. A medium sweet or white potato contains only about 125 calories; a very large one may have 200 calories.

Both white potatoes (+71) and sweet potatoes (+82) contain 33 percent of the U.S. RDA of vitamin C (it was this vitamin in white potatoes that prevented the Irish from developing scurvy). Sweet potatoes also contain large amounts of vitamin A. Both are good sources of dietary fiber—if you eat the skin.

Squash is a relative stranger to most tables. It comes in as many varieties as Kool-Aid but is far tastier and more nutritious. The two basic types are summer squash (+22), such as zucchini and yellow, and winter squash (+70), such as acorn, butternut, and the best of them all, buttercup. Summer squash can be eaten raw, steamed, baked, or sautéed. It is light and watery. Winter squash needs to be baked or boiled and is relatively solid and starchy—somewhat like a sweet potato. Cooking winter squash is child's play: slice in half and put face down on a greased pan, or put in a pan with enough water to cover the bottom, in a 375-degree oven for sixty minutes.

A half cup of baked winter squash has 86 percent of the U.S. RDA of vitamin A, 13 percent of vitamin C, 8 percent of riboflavin, and 4 percent of iron—all this with just 65 calories.

One of the best ways to experiment with vegetables is to make an old vegetarian standby, rice and sautéed vegetables. You can use any number of chopped vegetables, including such familiar ones as broccoli (+68), green pepper (+44), onion (+12), and mushrooms (+9) and some more unusual ones like red cabbage, rutabaga (+54), and zucchini. Just place the lightly cooked vegetables on top of a bed of brown rice and enjoy. (See recipe).

"RICE & VEGETABLE NIRVANA"

. . . A fantastic main course . . . this recipe makes 4 servings.

A) The Rice. Prepare 4 cups of brown rice (1 1/3 cups rice, 2 2/3 cups water). After water boils, cook about 45 minutes in a covered saucepan. Add 1/3 cup of raisins a few minutes before removing from heat. Add curry or other spice if you desire.

B) The Veggies. Take out a large frying pan (several inches deep) and a cutting board. Cut up the following and cook gently (cover the pan) for 10 or 15 minutes in a bit of oil and the vegetables' juices:

    6 medium sized carrots (cut into disks or strips)
    2 green peppers
    1 pound of fresh broccoli
    3 tomatoes (cut in sixths or eighths)

Don't be limited by this recipe; add celery, bean sprouts, cauliflower, apple, or what have you. Season with your favorite spices or a bit of soy sauce.

C) Serving. Serve the veggies on a bed of rice. For your beverage try orange, tomato, or grapefruit juice, water, or low-fat milk. Also, be sure to have heated up a fresh loaf of whole-wheat bread.

For dessert have cantaloupe or watermelon. Brace yourself for an incredibly delicious, nutrition-packed meal.

One delightful way to familiarize yourself with a vegetable is to cook it in different ways. Make a dinner with some raw, some steamed, and the rest stir-fried. You can also whip up a fancier dish using a cookbook recipe.

Perhaps the most underrated, best-rounded (excuse the pun!) vegetable of all is the pea. It, like other vegetables, is low in fat and sodium. A serving contains between 10 and 25 percent of the U.S. RDA of vitamins A and C, thiamin, riboflavin, and niacin. And, unlike most vegetables, it is a good source of protein. Finally, fresh peas can be eaten raw as a deliciously sweet snack. While the egg industry has been advertising eggs quite heavily, nutritionist Patricia Hausman believes that the pea industry has missed the boat. Consider this nutritional comparison of one egg to a serving of green peas:

The Incredible, Edible Pea[111]

Nutrient	1 large egg (hard-boiled)	3/4 cup green peas, cooked
Calories	79	100
Fat, grams	6	less than 1
Cholesterol, milligrams	275	0
Protein, g	6	6
Vitamin A, Intl. Unit (IU)	260	717
Thiamin, mg	0.04	0.31
Riboflavin, mg	0.14	0.17
Niacin, mg	0.03	2.4
Vitamin B_6, mg	0.06	0.26
Vitamin C, mg	0	17
Iron, mg	1.0	1.9
Phosphorus, mg	90	141
Calcium, mg	28	33
Potassium, mg	65	326
Magnesium, mg	6	47

One of the shortcomings of most fast-food chains is that most meals are woefully deficient in vitamin A. McDonald's has admitted that a meal of a milk shake, order of fries, and two hamburgers supplies only 6 percent of one's daily vitamin A requirement. More and more franchised restaurants are installing salad bars, an innovation that deserves applause. You can pile as much carrots, chick-peas, broccoli, beets, tomatoes, and other vegetables on your tray as you want. Don't be shy about going back for seconds or thirds.

To ensure that you will not spend the rest of your life content with canned vegetables and oblivious to the joys of artichokes (+23), promise yourself that you will explore the produce counter and try one new vegetable a week.

Vegetables Scoreboard

Most vegetables are great sources of vitamins—especially A and C—and minerals and usually taste best either raw or just lightly cooked. Try a new vegetable today!

Vegetable	Serving Size	Nutritional Score
Spinach, fresh	2 cups, raw	93
Collard greens, fresh	1/2 cup, cooked	90
Sweet potato	1 med., baked	82
Dandelion greens	1/2 cup	72
Potato	1 med., baked	71
Kale, fresh	1/2 cup, cooked	71
Winter squash (acorn, butternut)	1/2 cup, baked	70
Broccoli, fresh	1/2 cup, cooked	68
Asparagus, fresh	1/2 cup, cooked	67
Spinach, frozen	1/2 cup, cooked	65
Mixed vegetables, frozen	1/2 cup, cooked	63
Lima beans, fresh	1/2 cup, cooked	61
Potato	1 med., baked	60
Broccoli, frozen	1/2 cup, cooked	59
Brussels sprouts, fresh	1/2 cup, cooked	58
Tomato	1 medium	56
Rutabaga	1/2 cup, cooked	54
Lima beans, frozen	1/2 cup, cooked	53
Carrot	1 medium	48
Green peas, frozen	1/2 cup, cooked	45
Green pepper	1/2 cup	44
Sweet corn, fresh (on the cob)	1 ear, cooked	41
Cauliflower, fresh	1/2 cup, raw	36
Cabbage, chopped	1 cup, raw	36
Okra	1/2 cup, cooked	34
Yellow corn, canned[1]	1/2 cup, drained	34
Sweet peas, canned[1]	1/2 cup, drained	33
Asparagus, canned[1]	1/2 cup, drained	23
Artichoke, fresh	1/2 bud	23
Green beans, fresh	1/2 cup, cooked	22
Summer squash (zucchini)	1/2 cup, cooked	22
Turnips	1/2 cup, cooked	21
Potatoes, french fried	10	19
Bean sprouts, mung	1/2 cup	18
Eggplant	1/2 cup, cooked	18
Parsley, fresh chopped	2 Tbsp.	18
Lettuce, romaine	1 cup	17
Green beans, canned[1]	1/2 cup, drained	17
Celery	four 5" pieces	17
Beets, canned[1]	1/2 cup, drained	15
Sauerkraut, canned[1]	1/2 cup, drained	14

Vegetable	Serving Size	Nutritional Score
Onion, chopped	1/4 cup, raw	12
Water chestnuts, Chinese	4	12
Lettuce, iceberg	1 cup	11
Mushrooms, fresh	1/4 cup, raw	9
Avocado[2]	1/2 medium	6
Radishes	2 medium	3
Dill pickle	1 medium	−3

[1] Canned vegetables are usually high in salt.
[2] Avocado is the only high-fat vegetable.

Fruits

Fruit—juicy, vitamin-packed, and delicious—is nature's answer to Twinkies and candy bars. Delicious as fruit is, it is amazing to me that Americans eat much less fruit today than our grandparents and great-grandparents ate in the early years of this century. According to the U.S. Department of Agriculture, which keeps detailed records on practically everything that has ever been grown and eaten in this country, Americans ate an average of 140 pounds of fresh fruit (other than melons) per person in 1915. Fruit consumption dropped to 73 pounds in 1972, but since then we have gone on a fruit binge that has raised consumption to 92 pounds in 1983. For some types of fruits, the decline has been remarkable. For instance, we eat only about one third as many apples as our ancestors did in the early 1900s.

Despite the trend downward in fresh fruit consumption, people now eat larger amounts of fruit in processed form. Processed citrus fruit—mainly in the form of frozen orange juice—was almost unknown fifty years ago; now we consume about 90 pounds per person per year.

Fruit juices are healthful foods, but several interesting studies have highlighted special benefits of whole fruit.[112] Scientists fed volunteers equal amounts of oranges or apples, either in the form of whole fruit or fruit juice. During the next few hours, they measured the volunteers' blood sugar levels and asked about their state of hunger. In both cases blood sugar levels rose soon after the sugar-rich "meal." Two hours later, though, the fruit juice drinkers experienced relatively low blood sugar levels and greater feelings of hunger than the eaters of fruit. The scientists attributed these differences to the lack of fiber in the juice and the liquid's more rapid transit time through the body. G. B. Haber of the Royal Infirmary in England, concluded that "these effects favor overnutrition and, if often repeated, might lead to diabetes mellitus." Anyone concerned about gaining weight ought to favor fruit over fruit juice. There's certainly nothing time-consuming about washing an apple

(+23) or quartering an orange (+49). A convenient breakfast favorite requires only the slicing of one or more kinds of fresh fruit into some plain, low-fat yogurt.

Perhaps the most characteristic quality of fruit is sweetness, which reflects the presence of natural sugars. These sugars include fructose, sucrose (table sugar), glucose (dextrose, corn sugar), and many other less common sugars.

The vitamin C content of fruit and fruit juice varies enormously. Among the best sources of vitamin C (per serving) are oranges (+49), strawberries (+34), cantaloupe (+60), and grapefruit (+42). The average apple (+23) contains only a modest amount of vitamin C, about 5 percent of our daily need.

While fruit is famous as a source of vitamin C, it contains other vitamins and minerals as well. A serving of watermelon (+68), for instance, supplies half our daily requirement of both vitamins A and C, along with 10 to 20 percent of our iron requirement.

The only form of fruit I recommend avoiding is the canned, packed-in-heavy-syrup variety, which is high in calories but largely devoid of taste and texture. At the bottom of the Scoreboard, rating −10, is a serving of peaches canned in heavy syrup. In the last few years, some companies have decreased, or eliminated entirely, the amount of syrup sugar used in the canning process. However, they can do little to restore the texture and flavor of the fresh product.

Although fruit may have lost ground to ice cream, cupcakes, and other heavily processed foods as the dessert of choice in the American diet, perhaps we can help turn the tide by setting an example for the rest of the public. A bowl full of several varieties of colorful, ripe fruit is as tasty and pleasing to the eye as anyone could want in a dessert. As for snacks, apples, bananas (+36), and tangerines (+26) are convenient and delicious. Try a piece of fruit for breakfast and a fresh fruit salad for lunch to round out your own and your family's menu plans.

Fruits Scoreboard

Fruit	Serving Size	Nutritional Score
Watermelon	10″ diameter × 1″ thick (half-disc shaped) slice	68
Papaya	1/2 medium	60
Cantaloupe	1/4 medium	60
Mango	1/2 medium	52
Orange	1 medium	49
Grapefruit	1/2 medium	42
Banana	1 medium	36
Honeydew melon	7″ × 2″ slice	35

Fruit	Serving Size	Nutritional Score
Strawberries	1/2 cup	34
Pear	1 medium	29
Raspberries	1/2 cup	27
Peach	1 medium	26
Prunes, uncooked	3 medium	26
Tangerine	1 medium	26
Apple	1 medium	23
Blueberries	1/2 cup	21
Pineapple	1/2 cup	18
Cherries	1/2 cup	17
Pomegranate	1/2 fruit	14
Plum, red	1 medium	12
Grapes	1/2 cup	10
Peaches, heavy syrup	1/2 cup	−10

Breakfast Cereals

In 1983 Americans purchased over 2 billion pounds of cold cereals at a cost of $3.6 billion, according to market analyst John C. Maxwell, Jr. A few products—Puffed Rice and Cream of Wheat—are little more than starch and air. At the other extreme, some products—Product 19, Concentrate, Kaboom, and Total—have been fortified so heavily that they are as much vitamin pills as breakfast cereals. The nutrients are clearly added as a marketing gimmick, but are still beneficial to those cereal-eaters who have a marginal intake of one or another vitamin or iron.

In a couple of cases, the amount of nutrient added to the cereals may pose a slight risk. Kellogg's Product 19 and Most are fortified with 100 percent of the U.S. Recommended Daily Allowance of vitamin D, the vitamin that helps prevent the bone disease called rickets. A recent National Institutes of Health panel stated flatly that no one should consume more than twice the RDA of this vitamin a day without a doctor's recommendation. Two servings of either Kellogg product would put the consumer well over the safe limit. Inasmuch as milk is fortified with vitamin D and rickets is virtually unknown, vitamin D should not be added to cereals.

Many popular cereals—Sugar Frosted Flakes, Lucky Charms, Super Sugar Crisp—are heavily fortified with nutrients, but in addition contain so much sugar that they would be better called breakfast candy. In fact, a 1974 statement by the Food and Nutrition Board of the National Research Council said that sugar-coated cereals "do not contain sufficient cereal to warrant their classification as a breakfast cereal. They more properly belong in the category of snack foods . . ." Finally, a few cereals are not overly sugared, not sprayed with vitamins, and not overly processed: oatmeal, wheat germ, Shredded Wheat, Grape-Nuts, Wheatena, and Nutri-Grain.

The heaps of inexpensive nutrients that are added to many cereals can fool our nutritional rating formula. Therefore, we have ranked products according to their sugar content, one index of their quality. If the cereal contains more than about 20 percent sugar, avoid it, regardless of how many nutrients it contains. According to the U.S. Department of Agriculture, sugar-coated cereals accounted for about 9 percent of children's (one to ten years old) daily sugar intake.[113] These cereals, especially when eaten as snacks without milk, contribute to tooth decay. Avoid also the cereals that are sprayed with artificial coloring. Coloring adds to the cost and subtracts from the safety; it does not add to the nutritional value. Most of the child-oriented, dyed cereals contain 30–50 percent sugar.

After you exclude the highly sweetened and colored cereals, you are on your own. You can buy a fortified product or you can stick to the "natural" cereals. Wheat germ is one of the best of the naturals, because it consists entirely of the most nutritious part of the wheat berry. All-Bran and 100% Bran are the best sources of dietary fiber.

If you buy a fortified product, you could be paying dearly for vitamins you do not need. For instance, one of the biggest gyps in the marketplace is General Mills' heavily advertised Total. Total is exactly the same product as Wheaties—also made by the Big G—except that it has been fortified with about two cents' worth more vitamins per twelve-ounce box. At the store you pay about sixty cents more for those vitamins. General Mills has reaped millions of dollars of profits from this one little trick. Total is one reason why some cynics say that the Big G stands for the Big Gyp.

In response to the public's concern about artificial foods, the cereal industry has introduced new "natural" cereals, like Nutri-Grain, Quaker 100% Natural, Alpen, Heartland, Nature Valley Granola, and Kellogg's Country Morning. Far from being innovations, these products are actually just well-packaged, higher priced versions of cereals that have been sold for years in health food stores. They are good in that they represent a tacit admission by the food industry that "natural" foods still do have a place in the supermarket, along with all the processed novelties. They are made largely from whole grains, nuts, and seeds. Unfortunately, however, the cereal companies have added large amounts of sugar to many of the so-called natural cereals. Quaker's 100% Natural is approximately one-fifth sugar and should really be called Quaker 80% Natural. The rule still holds: avoid high-sugar cereals, even ones made with whole grains. Some of the natural cereals are also rather high in fat, often highly saturated coconut oil.

Cereal companies are constantly engaged in a great War for Shelf-space. They have been producing every variety of cereal their chemists and advertising agents could think of. Total is nothing but heavily fortified Wheaties. Trix is nothing but colored and sweetened Kix. The impetus for the War for Shelf-space was that companies realized that the cereal market is a flexible and impulsive one. The greater the number of company X's cereals on a supermarket shelf, the greater the likelihood that the shopper will select a company X product.

Another reason for all the new sugary cereals is television. Cereal companies saw television for what it is: a "salesperson" that can reach into every home and persuade the children to ask Mommy or Daddy to buy a certain product. Companies then devised products that were specially geared to the child market and mentality. Smurfs, Pebbles, and others are tied in directly to popular television shows. Most of these products are loaded with sugar and coloring.

In August 1974, health professionals joined the attack on sugar-coated cereals. More than six hundred nutritionists, dentists, dietitians, doctors, and nutrition students, along with twenty-two citizens' groups and professional associations, petitioned FDA to set a "standard of quality" for breakfast cereals. Cereals containing less than 10 percent sugar could be marketed as they are. But products containing more than 10 percent sugar would have to bear a label statement reading: "Contains __% Sugar; Frequent Use Contributes to Tooth Decay and Other Health Problems."

The petition quoted FDA assistant commissioner Dr. Lloyd Tepper, who at a 1973 Senate hearing criticized sugar-coated cereals. Dr. Tepper said:

> I don't think you have to be a great scientist to appreciate the fact that a highly sweetened, sucrose-containing material, which is naturally tacky when it gets wet, is going to be a troublemaker. And I would not prescribe this particular food component for my own children, not on the basis of scientific studies, but because I do not believe that prolonged exposure of tooth surfaces to a sucrose-containing material of this sort is beneficial.[114]

The breakfast cereal industry claimed that its products were safe and the FDA denied the petition, but the demand for better labeling certainly struck a responsive chord with consumers. Partly to prevent FDA from adopting tough regulations, cereal companies voluntarily began listing sugar contents on product labels. However, few people know how to decipher the information, which is listed as grams of sucrose and other sugars per serving of cereal. If you don't have your calculator with you in the supermarket, you may want to copy the following table.

Calculate the Sugar Content of Your Cereal

If one ounce of your cereal contains this many grams of sucrose and other sugars . . .	your cereal contains this percentage sugar:	and this many teaspoons of sugar per 1-ounce serving:
0 grams	0 percent	0
2 grams	7.1 percent	1/2
4 grams	14.1 percent	1
6 grams	21.2 percent	1 1/2
8 grams	28.2 percent	2
10 grams	35.3 percent	2 1/2
12 grams	42.3 percent	3
14 grams	49.4 percent	3 1/2
16 grams	56.4 percent	4
18 grams	63.5 percent	4 1/2

The cereal industry responded to critics by sponsoring studies on the relationship between cereals and tooth decay. The Kellogg Company ran double-page newspaper ads in 1977 that trumpeted the results of the studies: "Fact: Ready-to-eat cereals do not increase tooth decay in children." Kellogg cited three studies, one of which had been published only in abstract form. The other studies were sponsored by Kellogg and General Mills and were cleverly designed so that no effect of cereals on cavities could have been detected.

In a letter to the *Journal of the American Dental Association,* in which the Kellogg-sponsored study was published, National Institute of Dental Research scientist Herschel Horowitz, D.D.S., found the study "weak" and the conclusions "not justified." Another dentist called it "unacceptable on any reasonable scientific or epidemiological grounds."

The General Mills-funded study was also seriously flawed, because, among other reasons, it did not distinguish presweetened from other cereals. While these studies were scientifically worthless, industry's p.r. people use them to good advantage.

How to Choose a Cereal

The best way to judge the quality of a breakfast cereal is to read carefully the list of ingredients on the label. If sugar is listed first, avoid the product, regardless of how many nutrients have been added. Select cereals that contain whole grains and little or no sugar. Here are two labels:

Wheatena
INGREDIENTS
100% toasted wheat. Contains no added salt, sugar or preservatives.

Waffelos
INGREDIENTS
Sugar, Wheat Flour, Corn Flour, Coconut Oil, Oat Flour, Rice Flour, Salt, Sodium Ascorbate (Vitamin C), Artificial Flavor, Niacinamide, Reduced Iron, Caramel Color, FD&C Yellow #5, Artificial Color, Vitamin A Palmitate, Pyridoxine Hydrochloride (Vitamin B_6), Riboflavin (Vitamin B_2), BHT (a Preservative), Thiamin Mononitrate (Vitamin B_1), Vitamin D_2, and Vitamin B_{12}.

What's wrong with Ralston-Purina's Waffelos?

1) Sugar is listed first, which means that it is the major ingredient. It makes up 46 percent of the product.

2) It contains refined, instead of whole grain flours.

3) It contains artificial colors, artificial flavors, and BHT, a preservative of questionable safety.

What's right with Wheatena? It is made with whole wheat and does not contain added sugar, salt, or artificial anything. It is also relatively inexpensive, 90 cents per pound compared to $2.26 per pound for Waffelos.

Cost of Breakfast Cereals

Kellogg's Corn Flakes 24 ounce box	$1.51	$1.01 per pound
Kellogg's Sugar Frosted Flakes 25 ounce box	$2.49	$1.59 per pound

You pay almost 60 percent more for sugar-coated cornflakes than for plain, old-fashioned cornflakes. You pay extra for a product that is not as good for your body.

While sugar-coated cereals are not ideal foods, we should remember that they are certainly not the only foods that contribute to our high intake of sugar. The average person consumes far more sugar from soda pop than from cereals.

Breakfast can be a psychedelic experience. Don't believe for a minute that eating anything but a packaged cereal, an egg, or a doughnut would violate the U.S. Constitution. Breakfast can be a time to use up some of the leftovers in the refrigerator. Or make a toasted cheese or peanut butter sandwich on whole wheat bread. My own favorite is a bowl of chopped fresh fruit drowned in tangy, homemade yogurt along with several pieces of whole wheat toast.

Breakfast Cereals[115]

Cereal (1 oz. serving)	Grams Sucrose & Other Sugars	Percent Sugar by Weight	Teaspoons of Sugar per Serving
Wheat Germ	0	0	0
Oatmeal	0	0	0
Farina	0	0	0
Wheatena	0	0	0
Instant and Regular Ralston	0	0	0
Shredded Wheat	0	0	0
Quaker Puffed Rice, Puffed Wheat	0	0	0
Cheerios	1	4	1/4
Wheat, Corn and Rice Chex	2	7	1/2
Nutri-Grain, Corn, and Wheat	2	7	1/2
Kix	2	7	1/2
Special K	2	7	1/2
Corn Flakes	2	7	1/2
Grape Nuts	3	11	3/4
Wheaties, Total	3	11	3/4
Crispy Rice	3	11	3/4
Product 19	3	11	3/4
Corn Total	3	11	3/4
Country Corn Flakes	3	11	3/4
40% Bran	5	18	1 1/4
All-Bran	5	18	1 1/4
Bran Chex	5	18	1 1/4
Life	6	21	1 1/2
Most	6	21	1 1/2
Brown Sugar & Honey Body Buddies	6	21	1 1/2
Kaboom	6	21	1 1/2
Natural Fruit Flavor Body Buddies	6	21	1 1/2
100% Bran	6	21	1 1/2
Nature Valley Granola (toasted oat mixture)	6	21	1 1/2
Quaker 100% Natural Cereal (brown sugar and honey)	6	22	1 1/2
Heartland (Coconut)	6	22	1 1/2
Familia	7	23	1 3/4
Vita-crunch (regular)	7	24	1 3/4
Frosted Mini-Wheats	7	25	1 3/4
C. W. Post (plain)	7	25	1 3/4
Natural Valley granola (cinnamon and raisin)	7	25	1 3/4
Quaker 100% Natural (apple and cinnamon)	7	25	1 3/4

Cereal (1 oz. serving)	Grams Sucrose & Other Sugars	Percent Sugar by Weight	Teaspoons of Sugar per Serving
Fruit & Fibre (w/dates, raisins and walnuts)	7	25	1 3/4
Nutri-Grain with raisins	7	25	1 3/4
Heartland (raisin)	7	26	1 3/4
Vita-crunch (raisin)	8	27	2
Post Raisin Bran	8	28	2
Bran Buds	8	28	2
Cracklin' Bran	8	28	2
Vita-crunch (almond)	8	28	2
C. W. Post (raisin)	8	28	2
Quaker 100% Natural (raisins and dates)	8	28	2
Nature Valley granola (fruit and nut)	8	28	2
Country Morning	9	31	2 1/4
Buc Wheats	9	32	2 1/4
Raisin Bran (Ralston-Purina)	9	32	2 1/4
Honey and Nut Cornflakes	9	32	2 1/4
Graham Crackos	10	35	2 1/2
Golden Grahams	10	35	2 1/2
Banana Frosted Flakes	10	35	2 1/2
Raisins, Rice and Rye	10	35	2 1/2
Crispy Wheats 'N Raisins	10	35	2 1/2
Honey Nut Cheerios	10	35	2 1/2
Powdered Donutz	10	35	2 1/2
Marshmallow Krispies	10	35	2 1/2
Frosted Rice	11	39	2 3/4
Sugar Frosted Flakes	11	39	2 3/4
Lucky Charms	11	39	2 3/4
Cocoa Puffs	11	39	2 3/4
Honeycomb	11	39	2 3/4
Alpha-Bits	11	39	2 3/4
Sugar Corn Pops	12	42	3
Fruit Brute	12	42	3
Cookie Crisp (oatmeal and chocolate chip flavors)	12	42	3
Raisin Bran (Kellogg's)	12	42	3
Trix	12	42	3
Crazy Cow	12	42	3
Cap'n Crunch	12	42	3
Cocoa Pebbles, Fruity Pebbles	13	46	3 1/4
Boo Berry	13	46	3 1/4
Count Chocula	13	46	3 1/4
Cookie Crisp (vanilla)	13	46	3 1/4
Franken Berry	13	46	3 1/4
Froot Loops	13	46	3 1/4

Cereal (1 oz. serving)	Grams Sucrose & Other Sugars	Percent Sugar by Weight	Teaspoons of Sugar per Serving
Waffelos	13	46	3 1/4
Super Sugar Crisp	14	49	3 1/2
Apple Jacks	14	49	3 1/2
Sugar Smacks	16	56	4

Note: raisins, dates, and other fruit contribute to the sugar content of certain cereals.

Top Ten Selling Cold Cereals[116]

1983 Share

	Pounds	Dollars
Corn Flakes (Kellogg)	6.8 percent	4.7 percent
Cheerios (General Mills)	5.5 percent	5.8 percent
Sugar Frosted Flakes (Kellogg)	5.2 percent	4.8 percent
Raisin Bran (Kellogg)	4.6 percent	4.1 percent
Chex (Ralston Purina)	4.3 percent	4.4 percent
Shredded Wheat (Nabisco)	4.0 percent	3.1 percent
Rice Krispies (Kellogg)	3.6 percent	3.9 percent
Raisin Bran (General Foods)	3.0 percent	2.5 percent
Cap'n Crunch	2.9 percent	3.5 percent
Grape-Nuts (General Foods)	2.5 percent	1.9 percent

Desserts

After a delicious, hearty meal our taste buds often yearn for a bit of sweetness to add the crowning touch to a pleasurable experience. The dessert is usually the weakest part of the meal, as far as nutrition goes, and this is nothing new. Foods rich in sugar and fat—cakes, pies, ice cream, and cookies—have been traditional desserts for generations.

As the Scoreboard shows, with some care we can greatly improve the nutritional value of our desserts and still please our taste buds. In many homes, an after-dinner fruit bowl is a tradition. A peach (+26), apple (+23), or a bowl of strawberries (+34) is a way of getting sweetness along with some fiber, vitamins, and minerals. Two of the tastiest treats—cantaloupe with a small scoop of ice cream (+49) and a cold wedge of watermelon (+68)—are also among the most nutritious.

Canned fruit is a reasonable backup when fresh fruit is unobtainable. However, look for it packed in juice or water, rather than in a thick sugar syrup. The rating of peaches canned in water is +18, but the rating in heavy syrup is −10. Heavy syrup reduces the rating of pineapple from +17 to 0. Unsweetened applesauce scores +17, but the sweetened variety scores −10.

Many of the commercial products that are sold as desserts are nutritional disasters. Morton coconut pie, those flip-top cans of imitation pudding, and gelatin desserts contain little besides sugar, water, oil, artificial coloring and flavoring, and a flock of chemical additives to hold them together. Jell-O and other gelatin desserts, despite their longstanding place in the market, are among the worst foods. They are mainly sugar and contain artificial flavoring. They do contain a little gelatin, but it is such a low quality protein that it is almost worthless. All in all, a gelatin dessert has no redeeming nutritional value and certainly deserves its score of −26 for a 1/2 cup serving. A homemade gelatin dessert, made with fresh fruit, fruit juice, and plain gelatin, is a distinct improvement.

It is not just store-bought desserts that have low ratings. Homemade brownies, chocolate cake, and apple pie also have disaster-zone scores, because they contain so much sugar, fat, and sodium. It is partly from products like these that so much sugar and other refined sweeteners (about 125 pounds per year per person) sneak into our diet. The fat in most packaged desserts is butterfat, lard, or other saturated fat . . . the type that promotes heart disease. However, if we substitute whole wheat flour for white flour and use less fat, salt, and sugar, homemade desserts can be much more nutritious than Betty Crocker's.

Desserts Scoreboard

Most desserts are high in fat, sugar, and calories. Next time, try fresh fruit for a change!

Dessert	Serving Size	Nutritional Score
Watermelon	10" diameter × 1" thick (half-disc shaped slice)	68
Cantaloupe	1/4 medium	60
Strawberries	1/2 cup	34
Peach	1 medium	26
Apple	1 medium	23
Peaches, canned in water	1/2 cup	18
Applesauce, unsweetened	1/2 cup	17
Pineapple, canned in juice	1/2 cup	17
Blueberry muffin	1 muffin	8
Vanilla ice milk	1/2 cup	7
Frozen yogurt, low-fat, vanilla	1/2 cup	3
Pineapple, canned in heavy syrup	1/2 cup	0
Frozen yogurt, low-fat, fruit	1/2 cup	−1
Angel food cake	1 med. slice	−1
Orange sherbet	1/2 cup	−2
Chocolate pudding	1/2 cup	−7

Dessert	Serving Size	Nutritional Score
Pears, heavy syrup	½ cup	−8
Sponge cake	1 med. slice	−10
Peaches, heavy syrup	½ cup	−10
Applesauce, sweetened	½ cup	−10
Brownies w/nuts	1¾" square	−12
Frozen yogurt, whole milk	4 oz.	−14
Apple pie a la mode	med. slice with small scoop of ice cream	−15
Cupcake, plain	1	−16
Pound cake, old-fashioned	1 med. slice	−18
Vanilla ice cream	½ cup	−22
Jell-O, flavored	½ cup	−26
Sara Lee chocolate cake, frozen	1 med. slice	−27
Chocolate éclair	1	−30
Coconut	1 piece (1" × 2" × 1½")	−36

Snacks

Eleven o'clock in the morning, you get the hungries and crave a snack. The kids come home from school, take off their coats and ask for a snack. Sitting up late watching the tube, the stomach rumbles and you reach for a snack. Snacks constitute an ever growing part of our eating pattern and the food producers recognize this. Not only have they responded by producing a mind-boggling array of products—ranging from bite-size candies to Screaming Yellow Zonkers and Fiddle Faddles—but they have packaged them in single-serving portions for vending machines everywhere and advertised the dickens out of them. Unfortunately, most commercial snacks are nutritional abominations: high in sugar, high in saturated fat, high in salt; low in vitamins, minerals, fiber, and protein.

Snacks do not have to be junk. As the Scoreboard shows, a handful of nuts has a score ranging from 9 for peanuts, 18 for almonds, to 28 for soynuts. When you buy nuts and seeds, try to get them without all the salt.

Bring an extra apple (23), peach (26), or banana (36) to work or school to help you make it through the afternoon. They contain some fiber and vitamin C; in addition, peaches contain vitamin A. Raisins rate well (28), partly because of their iron content, but they contain lots of sugar that can stick between your teeth and promote tooth decay.

For a late night snack, try a bowl of wheat germ, chopped banana, and skim milk—it is exceptionally satisfying and offers well-balanced nutrition. Popcorn

(+19) is fine, at least until it is coated with butter and sprinkled with salt; after all, popcorn is whole kernel corn. The worst thing you can do to popcorn is soak it in sugary syrup, which is basically what Cracker Jack is.

Jelly beans (−38) and hard candies are composed primarily of sugar and corn syrup, artificial coloring and artificial flavoring. Enough said.

Candy bars contain a considerable amount of sugar and oil and have the low scores that we would expect. Unfortunately, we cannot calculate scores for many candies, because the producers do not disclose enough nutrition information. Unlike hard candies, most candy bars contain milk, nuts, or other ingredients that do provide a little nutrition. The "goodies," however, are outweighed greatly by the "baddies." Candy bars are made primarily of fat and sugar. Thus, the score of a Hershey bar (−42) reflects the high sugar and fat content, rather than the nutritious milk. If I were hanged by my thumbs until I said something good about candy, I might mention that Snickers (1.8 oz.) has modest amounts of protein, calcium, and niacin (about 5 percent of the recommended daily allowance), which come from the milk, peanuts, egg white, and vegetable protein. But as soon as my thumbs recovered, I would announce loudly that Snickers is filled to the brim with sugar, fat, and calories (240 per bar).

One strange line of food products is "health food candy." An apparent contradiction in terms, such products are certainly more candy than healthy. Despite the words "natural," "carob," "bio," and "nutrition" in their names, CSPI nutrition director Bonnie Liebman recently found that they, too, are loaded with fat and sugar (though labels never indicate what percentage of the carbohydrate is sugar).

Carob is a powder produced by grinding the pulp of the podlike carob tree. To some palates it is a dead ringer for chocolate. Carob lacks the caffeine that cocoa contains, but a chocolate bar contains so little caffeine (6 milligrams compared to the 110 milligrams in a cup of coffee) that the difference is negligible. Carob also is very low in fat. Manufacturers, though, usually negate that advantage by adding gobs of saturated palm oil to the candies. Joan's Natural Honey Bran Carob Bar (by Estee) contains about 40 percent fat (by weight), more than any other candy bar Liebman could find. One of Joan's 3-ounce bars provides 509 calories!

One of the worst of the "health food candy" crop is Jack La Lanne's Honey-Coconut Bar, which brags about "100% Natural Goodness." Its first five ingredients include four forms of sugar: fructose corn syrup, turbinado sugar, corn syrup solids, honey. This candy, like several others, is fortified with five vitamins and two minerals to distract attention from the sugar.

Finally, in the high protein category are products like Tiger Milk Nutrition Bar. Its label claims "goodness from nature." It contains numerous synthetic nutrients, and its two prime ingredients are corn syrup and brown sugar.

Snacking on sugar-containing foods is the quickest way to develop tooth decay. The classic study demonstrating this was conducted thirty years ago on patients in a mental hospital in Vipeholm, Sweden.[117] This carefully controlled study proved that eating sugary foods frequently between meals causes much more tooth decay than eating the same foods only at meals. If you care about your teeth, eat snacks that do not contain sugar and indulge your sweet tooth only at mealtimes. Why pay for your dentist's trip to Bermuda?

There is nothing inherently wrong with eating between meals. Many nutritionists even recommend lots of little meals in place of three big ones. But it is easy to fall into the habit of eating junky snacks that push nutritious foods out of our diet, contribute to tooth decay, and add on the pounds. The number one, most important way to insure healthful snacking is to keep a variety of nutritious snacks around the house, school, cafeteria, clubhouse, or office. Ditto for parties—don't feel compelled to buy the junky "party" foods that smile down from supermarket shelves. Popcorn, nuts, roasted soybeans, raw carrots and green peppers, slightly steamed broccoli and cauliflower, and fruit are convenient, delicious, and fun to eat.

Snacks Scoreboard

Try to keep nutritious snacks—hot or cold, crisp or mushy—around your home and workplace so you won't be tempted to eat junk foods. Most packaged chips and similar snacks add salt, unwanted calories, and questionable preservatives to your diet. Crisp raw vegetables, fresh fruit, and moderate amounts of nuts and seeds all make great snacks!

Snack	Serving Size	Nutritional Score
Carrot	1 medium	48
Green pepper	1/2 cup	44
Banana	1 medium	36
Dried apricots*	2 medium	31
Raisins*	1 box (1.5 oz.)	28
Soynuts, salted	1 oz.	28
Sunflower seeds, hulled	1 oz.	24
Apple	1 medium	23
Dates, pitted*	3	22
Pretzels, three-ringed, salted	3 pretzels	19
Popcorn, plain	2 cups	19
Almonds, shelled	1 oz.	18
Celery	four 5" pieces	17
Ry-Krisps	2 triple crackers	15
Potato chips	1 oz.	15
Corn chips	1 oz.	13
Graham crackers	2 crackers, 2 1/2" square	12

Snack	Serving Size	Nutritional Score
Saltine crackers	4 crackers	10
Jumbo peanuts (in the shell)	10	9
Popcorn, buttered and salted	2 cups	6
Cheez-its	10 crackers	5
Pringles potato chips	1 oz.	4
Peanuts, salted	15/8 oz.	1
Dill pickle	1 medium	−3
Sugar wafers	2	−3
Popsicle	1	−27
Marshmallows	4	−28
Hostess Twinkies	1 package	−34
Hunt's Vanilla Snackpack pudding	1 can, 5 oz.	−34
Jelly beans	10	−38
Hershey's milk chocolate	1 bar (1.5 oz.)	−42

* Go easy on the dried fruits! Their natural sugars are sticky and can promote tooth decay.

Condiments

Don't forget the toppings and garnishes! This Scoreboard will help you determine the scores of such items as a hot dog with mustard or french fries with catsup.

An easy way of adding to the taste and nutritional value of your food is to sprinkle a tablespoon or two of wheat germ (+12) on it. Wheat germ is an especially good source of thiamin and trace minerals. It "works" on ice cream and breakfast cereals and in meat loaf and hamburgers. Brewer's yeast (+41) can also be used to squeeze extra thiamin and other B vitamins into a meal . . . but it has a pungent presence, so use it sparingly.

Catsup, which consists primarily of tomatoes, contains small amounts of vitamins A and C. Catsup's score of −1 for one tablespoon would be significantly higher if some of the vitamin C were not destroyed in the processing and if it did not contain so much sugar. The presence of perhaps 10 to 20 percent added sugar in catsup is one of many ways that sugar has sneaked into our diet. Some health food stores offer low-sugar or low-salt catsup, which, because of strange government regulations, must be labeled "imitation catsup."

Honey (−7) rates even slightly worse than sugar (−6), because for all practical purposes it is a highly concentrated solution of sugar. Honey contains trivial amounts of vitamins and minerals; the rest is water. Honey makes food sticky and can contribute to tooth decay. Aside from its taste, the best thing about honey (to all those killjoy nutritionists) is its high price—this keeps people from eating too much of it. The average annual consumption of honey is only one pound per person, as compared to about 125 pounds of refined sugars.

The one special group of people who should avoid honey is infants under one year. The California health department has linked honey to infant botulism, a disease that is scary, though rarely fatal. The symptoms start with irritability, lethargy, and "floppy baby syndrome" and may end with respiratory paralysis.[118] The California health department has reported that, "The number of babies hospitalized with infant botulism in California has increased dramatically in early 1984 compared to comparable periods in previous years . . . a special note of concern is the large proportion of these patients who have been fed honey." Treating a single sick baby can cost well over $100,000. The American Academy of Pediatrics, the Food and Drug Administration, and even the Sue Honey Association have warned against feeding honey to infants, but FDA refuses to require label warnings.

Blackstrap molasses (+2) does not rate too badly, despite its high sugar content, because it contains significant amounts of minerals. One teaspoon of blackstrap molasses provides one sixth of the recommended intake of calcium, magnesium, and iron, as well as 60 percent of the body's potassium requirement. If blackstrap molasses is too hard to swallow, a lighter kind of molasses has one third as much of the several nutrients.

On the salty side, soy sauce is largely salt (thus its score of −2), but it has a more interesting flavor than salt so smaller amounts can be used. Some companies are producing reduced-sodium soy sauces that can be a reasonable compromise between flavor and sodium.

Mayonnaise has a low score, −6, although it contains polyunsaturated vegetable oil. Recall that our formula penalizes foods if they are high in fats and oils. Of the calories in mayonnaise 98 percent come from oil, and the points lost for this more than balance the modest credit received for polyunsaturated oil. Americans average 37 to 40 percent of their calories from fats, as compared to the recommended 20 to 30 percent.

The secret of diet margarine (−3) is that water replaces some of the vegetable oil. It may be cheaper to use a thin spread of regular soft margarine (−5). Reduced calorie salad dressings also use various tricks—more seasonings, more additives—to allow water to replace much of the oil.

One of the challenges of preparing healthful meals is to devise tasty, nutritious condiments. Plain yogurt (+4) can replace many uses of sour cream (−4). When you are eating whole wheat pancakes, squish some fresh berries and yogurt on them, instead of pouring on the syrup or butter. Use lemon juice instead of salt and butter on vegetables. Let your nutritionally educated instincts and imagination be your guides when seasoning other foods.

Condiments Scoreboard

Carefully choose condiments—they can easily add unwanted salt, fat, or sugar to your diet.

Condiment	Serving Size	Nutritional Score
Brewer's yeast	1 Tbsp.	41
Tomato sauce	1/4 cup	13
Wheat germ	1 Tbsp.	12
Yogurt, plain	1 Tbsp.	4
Molasses, blackstrap	1 tsp.	2
Lemon juice	1 tsp.	2
Low-calorie Italian salad dressing	1 Tbsp.	0
Mustard	1 tsp.	−1
Catsup	1 Tbsp.	−1
Soy sauce	1 tsp.	−2
Cream, half and half	1 Tbsp.	−2
Imitation mayonnaise	1 tsp.	−3
Diet margarine	1 tsp.	−3
Whipped cream	1 Tbsp.	−3
Salt	1/4 tsp.	−4
Sour cream	1 Tbsp.	−4
Coffee creamer	1 Tbsp.	−5
Soft margarine	1 pat	−5
Cool Whip	1 Tbsp.	−5
Jelly	1 tsp.	−6
Mayonnaise	1 tsp.	−6
Olives, green, canned	4 med.	−6
Pancake syrup	1 Tbsp.	−6
Margarine, stick	1 pat	−6
French salad dressing	1 Tbsp.	−6
Cream, light	1 Tbsp.	−6
Sugar	1 tsp.	−6
Honey	1 tsp.	−7
Cranberry sauce	1 Tbsp.	−7
Blue cheese salad dressing	1 Tbsp.	−12
Butter	1 pat	−13
Safflower oil	1 Tbsp.	−13
Corn oil	1 Tbsp.	−17
Italian dressing	1 Tbsp.	−18
Soybean oil	1 Tbsp.	−19
Peanut oil	1 Tbsp.	−23
Snowdrift shortening	1 Tbsp.	−26

Notes

1. "Cancer Facts and Figures," Am. Cancer Soc., 1984.
2. Ibid.
3. National Heart, Lung, and Blood Institute.
4. Ibid.
5. Ibid.
6. "The Treatment and Control of Diabetes: A National Plan to Reduce Mortality and Morbidity," National Diabetes Advisory Board (NIH Pub. No. 81-2284, 1980).
7. Ibid.
8. "The Prevalence of Dental Caries in United States Children 1979–1980," National Institute of Dental Research (NIH Pub. No. 82-2245, 1981).
9. "Drug Topics," p. 32, July 2, 1984.
10. "Advancedata," National Center for Health Statistics (August 30, 1979).
11. *Science 185*, 932 (1974).
12. *Cancer 17*, 486 (1964).
13. See references cited in *J. Am. Med. Asso. 251*, 1160 (1984).
14. Washington *Post*, March 8, 1979, p. E1.
15. "Voodoo Science, Twisted Consumerism," CSPI (1982).
16. Pers. Comm., T. J. Thom, Epidemiology and Biometrics Research Program, National Heart, Lung, and Blood Institute (July 11, 1984).
17. *New Engl. J. Med. 312*, 1053 (1985).
18. *J. Am. Med. Asso. 247*, 877 (1982).
19. Calculated from *Vital & Health Statistics*, Series 11, No. 231, p. 14 (March 1983).
20. *Nutr. Rev. 39*, 11 (1981); *J. Nutr. 111*, 244 (1981).
21. "The Nutritional Significance of Dietary Fiber," Fed. Am. Soc. Exp. Biol., May 1977.
22. *Brit. Med. J. 1*, 274 (1973).
23. *Brit. J. Surg. 58*, 695 (1971).
24. *Brit. Med. J. 2*, 450 (1971).
25. *J. Am. Diet. Asso. 60*, 499 (1972).
26. *Am. J. Clin. Nutr. 37*, 763 (1983).
27. *Geriatrics 36*, 64 (1981).

28. *Am. J. Clin. Nutr. 34*, 824 (1981).
29. *Nutrition Action*, p. 5, June 1984.
30. *Diabetes Care 3*, 38 (1980).
31. *Sugars in Nutrition*, ed. Sipple, H. L. and K. W. McNutt, Academic Press, New York (1974).
32. *Human Nutrition: Clinical Nutrition 37C*, 31 (1982).
33. *Hearings*, Senate Select Committee on Nutrition and Human Needs (March 5, 1973).
34. "The Prevalence of Dental Caries in United States Children," NIH Publication No. 82-2245, Dec. 1981.
35. "Dental Treatment Needs of United States Children," NIH Publication 83-2246, Dec. 1982.
36. *Consumer Reports*, March 1984.
37. *Gut 25*, 269 (1984).
38. *Lancet i*, 870 (1970).
39. *Nutrition Action*, p. 11, Dec. 1980.
40. *Pediatrics 74*, 876 (1984).
41. Symposium on Diet and Behavior, Am. Med. Asso. and Intern. Life Sci. Inst., Arlington, Va. (Feb. 1985).
42. J. L. Rapoport in *J. Psychiatric Research 17*, 2 (1982–83); entire issue devoted to nutrition and behavior.
43. *New Engl. J. Med. 309*, 1147 (1983).
44. Meiers, R., in *Orthomolecular Psychiatry*, ed. D. Hawkins and L. Pauling (W. H. Freeman & Co., 1973).
45. *Biol. Psychiatry 17*, 125 (1981).
46. *Mayo Clinic Proc. 58*, 491 (1983).
47. "National Food Consumption Survey, 1977–78, U.S. Dept. Agr., p. 62 (Sept. 1980).
48. *J. Lipid Res. 26*, 194 (1985).
49. "National Food Review," No. 26, U.S. Dept. Agr. (1984); Agriculture Handbooks No. 8-5, 8-9, 456, U.S. Dept. Agr.
50. *Am. J. Clin. Nutr. 17*, 281 (1965).
51. *Ann. Intern. Med. 74*, 1 (1971).
52. *J. Am. Med. Asso. 251*, 351, 365 (1984).
53. *J. Am. Med. Asso. 247*, 2674 (1982).
54. *New Engl. J. Med. 310*, 805 (1984).
55. *The Story of Heart Disease*, East, T., Dawson & Sons, London (1958).
56. *Hearing*, Subcommittee on Nutrition, Senate Committee on Agriculture, Nutrition, and Forestry, October 2, 1979.
57. "Dietary Intake Source Data: United States, 1976–1980," DHHS Pub. No. (PHS) 83-1681.
58. "Advancedata," No. 54, National Center for Health Statistics, (Feb. 27, 1981).
59. *Metabolism 14*, 759 (1965).
60. *Am. J. Clin. Nutr. 17*, 281 (1965).
61. R. I. Levy, testimony for National Heart, Lung, and Blood Institute, Nutrition Subcommittee, Senate Agriculture Committee (May 22, 1979).
62. *Lancet i*, 647 (1984).

63. *J. Am. Diet. Asso. 61*, 134 (1972); U.S. Dept. Agr. Handbook No. 8 updates.
64. Pers. Comm., Carol Haines, NHBPEP, National Heart, Lung, and Blood Institute (August 13, 1984).
65. *Lancet i*, 351 (1982).
66. *Food Tech.*, p. 82 (July 1984).
67. *Int. J. Cancer 15*, 561–65 (1975); *Lancet i*, 1185–89 (1981); *J. Dairy Sci. 64*, 2031 (1981); *Nutrition Action 9*, (1) 12–13 (1982); *J. Am. Med. Asso. 247*, 1317 (1982); *Acta Paediatr. Scand. 54*, 49 (1965); Nat. Acad. Sci., *Diet, Nutrition, and Cancer*, Ch. 9 (1982); *Nutr. Rev. 40*, (9) (1982); *Lancet i*, 319 (1985).
68. *Food Tech.*, p. 82 (July 1984).
69. "Diet as Therapy," M. A. Lipton in *Nutrition & Behavior*, ed. S. A. Miller. Franklin Institute Press, Philadelphia (1981).
70. *Proc. Nat. Acad. Sci. 68*, 2678 (1971); *Vitamin C and the Common Cold*, Pauling, L., W. H. Freeman (San Francisco) (1971); *J. Am. Med. Asso. 231*, 1073 (1975); *Nutrition Today*, pp. 6, 14 (Jan.-Feb. 1977), p. 6 (March-April, 1977); *New Engl. J. Med. 301*, 687, 1399 (1979), *302*, 694 (1980); *312*, 137, 178 (1985).
71. "National Food Consumption Survey 1977–78," Preliminary Report No. 2, p. 2 (Sept. 1980).
72. "Vital and Health Statistics," Series 11, No. 231, p. 24 (March 1983).
73. *The Englishman's Food*, J. C. Drummond. Jonathan Cape, London, p. 467 (1958).
74. *Am. J. Clin. Nutr. 2*, 73 (1954).
75. *J. Am. Med. Asso. 252*, 799 (1984).
76. *Science 225*, 705 (1984).
77. "Advancedata," National Center for Health Statistics (August 30, 1979).
78. *The Dieter's Dilemma*, Bennett, W. and J. Gurin, Basic Books (1982).
79. *Am. J. Clin. Nutr. 9*, 530 (1961).
80. *The Carbohydrate Craver's Diet*, Wurtman, J. J., Houghton Mifflin, New York (1983).
81. "Trace Elements in Human Nutrition," WHO Tech. Report Series No. 532.
82. Paper given at the 1971 annual meeting of the American Association for the Advancement of Science.
83. *Pediatrics Res. 6*, 868 (1972).
84. *Metabolism 15*, 510 (1966).
85. *Metab. 17*, 114 (1968); *J. Chron. Dis. 15*, 941 (1962).
86. *Science 213*, 1332 (1981).
87. *Lancet ii*, 130 (1983).
88. *Nutrition Action*, p. 5 (Dec. 1983).
89. Center for the Biology of Natural Systems, Rep. No. CBNS-AE-7; Washington Univ., St. Louis, Mo. (1976).
90. "Report and Recommendations on Organic Farming," U.S. Dept. Agr. (July 1980).
91. "National Food Review," p. 31, (Summer 1981).
92. "Third Report to Congress," Nat. Inst. on Alcohol Abuse and Alcoholism (1978).
93. "The Effectiveness and Costs of Alcoholism Treatment," U.S. Office of Technology Assessment (1983).

94. "Second Special Report on Alcohol and Health," Nat. Inst. on Alcohol Abuse and Alcoholism (1974).
95. *The 1982 Report on Drug Abuse and Alcoholism*, J. Califano, Office of the Governor, Albany, New York (1982).
96. *Nutrition Action*, p. 10 (March 1984); *J. Am. Med. Asso.* 253, 285A (1985).
97. *Proposed Fortification Policy for Cereal-Grain Products*, Nat. Acad. Sci., Washington, D.C. (1974).
98. Ibid.
99. "Advancedata," No. 54, Nat. Center for Health Stat. (Feb. 1981).
100. Figures from USDA Handbook No. 8.
101. *New Engl. J. Med.* 312, 1205, 1253 (1985).
102. *Nutrition Action*, p. 8 (Sept. 1984).
103. "Advancedata," No. 54 (Feb. 27, 1981).
104. *J. Am. Med. Asso.* 253, 1407 (1985).
105. *Amer. J. Epidem.* 117, 113 (1983).
106. *New Engl. J. Med.* 304, 630 (1981).
107. R. I. Levy, Feinleib, M. in *Heart Disease: A Textbook of Cardiovascular Medicine* (Saunders Co., 1980); *New Engl. J. Med.* 308, 1454 (1983); *J. Am. Med. Asso.* 253, 1407 (1985); *J. Am. Med. Asso.* 226, 540 (1973).
108. National Soft Drink Association, "Sales Survey 1983."
109. *Food Tech.* (Feb. 1981).
110. *Nutrition Action*, p. 8, August 1981.
111. *Composition of Foods*, Agriculture Handbook 8–1, 8–11, U.S. Dept. of Agr.
112. *Lancet*, ii, 679 (1977); *Am. J. Clin. Nutr.*, 31, 738 (1978); *Am. J. Clin. Nutr.*, 34, 211 (1981).
113. Wotecki, C. E., "Recent Trends and Levels of Dietary Sugars and Other Caloric Sweeteners," in *Metabolic Effects of Utilizable Dietary Carbohydrates*, Reiser, S., ed., p. 21, Marshall Dekker (1982).
114. *Hearing*, Senate Select Committee on Nutrition and Human Needs, p. 559–60 (April 1973).
115. Manufacturers' stated values; U.S. Dept. of Agriculture 1980 study of granola-type cereals.
116. Data compiled by John C. Maxwell, Jr., who is a managing director of A. G. Becker & Paribas, and reprinted with permission *(Advertising Age,* May 28, 1984).
117. *Acta Odont. Scand.* 11, 232 (1954).
118. "FDA Drug Bulletin" (July 1981).

APPENDIX I

The *Nutrition Scoreboard* Formula

Each factor in the formula used to rate the nutritional values of foods is discussed below. The coefficients in each factor were selected after considering the approximate health significance for an average American of each constituent. The values for U.S. Recommended Daily Allowances (U.S. RDA) are those used by the Food and Drug Administration for the purposes of nutrition labeling.* They differ slightly from the Recommended *Dietary* Allowances set by the National Academy of Sciences. Our calculations are done on a per-serving basis, rather than per-ounce, per-hundred grams, or per-calorie basis, because we are interested in how much nourishment there is in the portion of food that we actually eat. Information about the nutritional values and composition of the foods was obtained from companies, food packages, government publications, and by our own calculations.

PROTEIN SCORE =

    Animal protein: 33.1 × gm protein/45
    Vegetable protein: 33.1 × gm protein/65
    Mixed protein: 33.1 × gm protein/53

---

* U.S. Recommended Daily Allowances
for persons over 4 years of age.
(established by the U.S. Food and Drug Administration)

Nutrient	RDA	
Protein	45	grams†
Vitamin A	5,000	International Units (IU)
Riboflavin (Vitamin B_2)	1.7	milligrams
Niacin (Vitamin B_3)	20	milligrams
Vitamin C	60	milligrams
Calcium	1,000	milligrams
Iron	18	milligrams

† If the protein quality in a food is not as high as that of casein
(milk protein), the U.S. RDA is 65 grams.

The number of points a food gets for protein is based on the percentage of the adult U.S. RDA of usable protein that the food supplies. The U.S. RDA for protein is 45 grams. This is slightly more than one and one-half ounces (one ounce contains 28.35 grams) of pure protein. Because of its generally lower quality, the recommended daily intake of vegetable protein is 65 grams (about 2.3 ounces of pure protein). The most animal protein found in a standard serving of food is 27 grams in 3 ounces of lobster meat. This amount receives 20 points. Food containing less protein receive proportionately fewer points.

CARBOHYDRATE SCORE =

(1) complex carbohydrates: (gm complex carbohydrates/31) $\times$ 25
+
(2) dietary fiber: 1.6 $\times$ gm dietary fiber
+
(3) natural sugars (dairy, fruit): (gm natural sugar/27) $\times$ 10
+
(4) added sugars: $-0.66 \times$ gm added sugars

The formula rewards starchy foods by awarding 25 points to the food that contains the most complex carbohydrate per serving: one-half cup of chick-peas, containing 31 grams of starch and fiber. Other foods get proportionately less.

The second portion of the carbohydrate-rating formula scores for fiber. Chick-peas, the highest rated food, receives 4 points for its content of fiber.* Foods containing less fiber receive proportionately fewer points.

Next, the formula rates natural sugars. While natural sugars may be chemically indistinguishable from refined sugars, natural sugars did not pose any significant problem when they provided the sole source of sugar. Moreover, the calories provided by natural sugars are virtually always accompanied by vitamins, minerals, or protein. All fruit and dairy products have sugar scores based on the 27 grams of sugar found in a serving of watermelon, which is awarded the maximum of 10 points.

Refined sugars provide most of the sugar that we consume. The formula penalizes refined sugars 0.66 points per gram.

FAT SCORE =

(1) $-1/3 \times$ gm total fat
+
(2) $-1.67 \times$ gm saturated fat
+
(3) $-0.36 \times$ gm monounsaturated fat
+
(4) (gm polyunsaturated fat)$^{1/2}$

---

* Traditionally, the "crude fiber" content of foods has been measured by a harsh chemical method that does not simulate the conditions of our gastrointestinal tract. The more accurate "dietary fiber" content is somewhat different. Because most published values are for "crude fiber," we have had to use them in our calculations.

The fat factor considers both the quantity and quality of the fat in a food. Foods are first penalized one third of a point for every gram of fat, regardless of the type. In addition, 1.67 points are subtracted for every gram of saturated fat, up to a maximum of 20 points. (A 2-ounce serving of cheddar cheese loses the maximum for its 12 grams of saturated fat.) For each gram of monounsaturated fat, 0.36 points are subtracted (the maximum loss is 5 points in the case of Spam, which has 14 grams of this type of fat in a 3-ounce serving). Finally, polyunsaturated fats are given positive credit. Because the impact of large amounts of polyunsaturated fats in the human diet is unknown, credit is limited by using the square root function.

CHOLESTEROL SCORE = $-0.027 \times$ mg cholesterol

The *Nutrition Scoreboard* formula penalizes foods of animal origin for their cholesterol content. The cholesterol content in a 3-ounce serving of beef liver is penalized 10 points. An egg loses 7 points for its cholesterol, and one chicken liver loses 5 points. Most fish and dairy products contain only small amounts of cholesterol and lose only two or three points.

SODIUM SCORE = $-$mg sodium/143

The formula penalizes foods for their sodium content. One of the highest sodium foods is a 10-ounce serving of canned turkey vegetable soup, which contains about 1,050 milligrams of sodium. This amount of sodium is penalized the maximum of 7.5 points. Foods containing less sodium lose proportionately fewer points.

VITAMINS AND MINERALS

VITAMIN A SCORE = International Units of vitamin A/500.

The formula gives a maximum of 10 points to foods containing 100 percent of the U.S. RDA for vitamin A.

RIBOFLAVIN SCORE = $20 \times$ mg riboflavin

The *Nutrition Scoreboard* formula gives its maximum of 10 points for riboflavin to yogurt and proportionately less to other foods. (Liver is so high in riboflavin that if the ratings were based on liver, no other food would get more than 1 point credit.)

NIACIN SCORE = $0.88 \times$ niacin

The niacin factor rates food on a scale of 0 to 10, with the 11.3 milligrams found in a 3-ounce serving of canned tuna fish getting the maximum of 10 points. (Only liver has more niacin per serving than tuna; as with riboflavin, we have not based the scoring on liver, because it would skew the scores of all other foods sharply downward.)

Vitamin C Score = 0.167 × mg vitamin C

Our formula awards foods with 10 points if they contain 100 percent or more of the U.S. RDA (60 milligrams) of vitamin C. Other foods get proportionately less credit.

Iron Score = 1.89 × mg iron

Perhaps the best source of iron is a serving of clams, to which we award 10 points for its 5.29 milligrams. That is almost one third of the U.S. Recommended Daily Allowance of 18 milligrams.

Calcium Score = 0.018 × mg calcium

The U.S. Recommended Daily Allowance for calcium is 1,000 milligrams. Swiss cheese contains the most calcium per serving, 544 mg in 2 ounces. Our formula gives Swiss cheese 10 points for its calcium content and proportionately less to other foods.

Nutrient vs. Calorie Score =
(15 (protein score + vitamin scores + mineral scores) − calories)/50

This factor adds the scores for protein, four vitamins, and two minerals and subtracts the actual caloric content of the food. For instance, this factor awards a glass of skim milk 8.6 points, a glass of whole milk 6 points, canned peaches in heavy syrup −1.6 points, and a tablespoon of corn oil −4.8 points.

This factor differs from traditional "nutrient density" calculations, which add up the protein, vitamin, and mineral content of a food and *divide* by the number of calories. Nutrient density does not reflect portion size. Moreover, a low-calorie, nutrient-poor food may have the same nutrient density as a high-calorie, nutrient-rich food. By using the *difference* between nutrients and calories, the relative amounts of nutrients and calories are more clearly defined.

Total Nutritional Score =

The scores for each of the factors are totaled, then multiplied by a scaling factor of 2 to obtain the final nutritional score.

APPENDIX II

1983 Advertising Budgets of Major Food Companies

Company	1983 Advertising Budget*
Beatrice Companies	$603 million
General Foods	$386 million
Nabisco Brands	$368 million
PepsiCo Inc.	$356 million
McDonald's Corp.	$311 million
Ralston Purina Co.	$286 million
Coca-Cola Co.	$282 million
General Mills	$269 million
H. J. Heinz Co.	$202 million
Consolidated Foods Corp.	$196 million
Pillsbury Co.	$191 million
Kellogg Co.	$176 million
Quaker Oats Co.	$148 million
Campbell Soup Co.	$126 million
Mars Inc.	$120 million
Nestlé	$115 million
CPC International	$97 million
Hershey Foods Corp.	$68 million
Wendy's International	$64 million
Carnation Co.	$54 million

* Ref.: *Advertising Age* (September 14, 1984). These figures include the costs of buying time or space for television, radio, newspaper, magazine, and billboard advertising. They do not include cable television, direct mail, trade shows, promotion staffs, coupon deals, and many other "unmeasured" forms of advertising.

APPENDIX III

Job Changes Between Government and Industry

One of the ongoing problems in our government is conflicts of interest. All too often our top government officials used to work at the industries they are now supposed to regulate. While working in industry does enable one to know a great deal about the inner workings of that industry, in practice it usually means that the government official has a mind-set that favors industry. Likewise, when they are planning to leave government, many officials look to industries that they have had experience regulating for future, lucrative job possibilities.

The lawyers are the main travelers through the revolving door. They work for government for a few years, getting a good education at taxpayers' expense, then easily slide over to a nice job in a big law firm. It is always refreshing, but unfortunately rare, to see the occasional government official going back to a university or research institute or taking a job with a nonprofit organization.

While a potential conflict of interest does not guarantee that any shenanigans have been going on, it is important that citizens know who their government officials are (and where they go when they leave government) in order to keep some check on conflicts.

The list on the following pages includes many top FDA and USDA officials who either came from or went to a regulated industry since the early 1970s. Many attorneys who now work at Washington law firms, but whose clients are unknown, are not listed. Also not included are most of the junior government officials who made the leap to or from industry.

FOOD AND DRUG ADMINISTRATION

Government Official	from/went	Corporate Job
Charles Edwards, Commissioner	came from	Booz, Allen, & Hamilton (consulting firm)
	went to	Becton, Dickinson & Co. (medical supply company)

APPENDIX

Government Official	from/went	Corporate Job
Sherwin Gardner, Dep. Commissioner	went to	Grocery Manufacturers Association
William Goodrich, General Counsel	went to	President, Institute of Shortening and Edible Oils
James Grant, Deputy Commissioner	went to	Special Assistant to the Chairman, CPC International (Skippy peanut butter, Hellmann's mayonnaise, etc.)
Jerome Halperin, Deputy Director, Bureau of Drugs	went to	Vice-President, Ciba-Geigy Corp.
Peter Hutt, General Counsel	came from and went to	Covington & Burling law firm; representing ITT-Continental Baking, Milk Industry Foundation, Institute of Shortening and Edible Oils, Grocery Manufacturers of America, etc.
John Jennings, Dir. of International Affairs	went to	American Pharmaceutical Association
Ogden Johnson, Director, Division of Nutrition	went to	Hershey Co.
Stephen McNamara, Assoc. General Counsel	went to	Cosmetics, Toiletries and Fragrances Association
Mark Novitch, Deputy Commissioner	went to	Vice-President, Upjohn Co.
Stuart Pape, Spec. Assistant to the Commissioner	went to	Patton, Boggs & Blow law firm, representing National Soft Drink Association
Howard Roberts, Dep. Dir., Bureau of Foods	went to	Vice-President, National Soft Drink Association
Robert Schaffner, Director, Office of Product Technology	came from	Libby, McNeill & Libby

Government Official	from/went	Corporate Job
Richard Silverman, Assoc. Chief Counsel for Enforcement	went to	R. J. Reynolds (Chun-King, Hawaiian Punch)
Malcolm Stephens, Assistant Commissioner for Regulations	went to	President, Institute of Shortening and Edible Oils
C. D. Van Houweling Dir., Bureau of Veterinary Med.	went to	National Pork Producers Council
John Walden, Asso. Commissioner for Public Affairs	went to	Proprietary Association (drug industry)
Virgil Wodicka, Director, Bureau of Foods	came from went to	Ralston Purina; Libby, McNeill & Libby; Hunt-Wesson private consultant to industry

U.S. Department of Agriculture

Government Official	from/went	Corporate Job
Earl Butz, Secretary	came from	Director, Ralston-Purina
Clifford Hardin, Secretary	went to	Vice-President and Director, Ralston-Purina
Edward Hekman, Administrator, Food and Nutrition Service	came from	President, Keebler Biscuit Co.; Director, Grocery Manufacturers of America
Robert G. Hibbert, Director of Standards and Labeling, Food Safety and Inspection Service	went to	General Counsel, American Meat Institute
Steven Laine, Director of Public Affairs	came from	International Foodservice Manufacturers Association; Cling Peach Advisory Board
Robert Long, Assistant Secretary	came from	Bank of America (which has huge land holdings)

Government Official	from/went	Corporate Job
Caro Luhrs, M.D., Medical Advisor to the Secretary	went to	Director, Pillsbury Co.
Richard Lyng, Assistant Secretary; Deputy Secretary	went to	President, American Meat Institute
	came from	American Meat Institute
C. W. McMillan Ass't. Secretary	came from	President, National Cattlemen's Association
	went to	Lobbyist for the meat and other industries
Clyde Merriman, Assistant Sales Manager of Commodity Exports	went to	Louis Dreyfus (grain dealer)
Harry Mussman, Admin., Animal and Plant Inspection Service	went to	National Food Processors' Association
Clarence Palmby, Assistant Secretary	went to	Continental Grain Co.
Clifford Pulvermacher, Export Marketing Service	went to	Bunge Corp. (grain dealer)
George Shanklin, Assistant Sales Manager of Commodity Exports	went to	Bunge Corp.
Ewen Wilson, Deputy Ass't. Secretary for Economics	came from	American Meat Institute

Selected Bibliography

Deliciously Low, Harriet Roth (New American Library, 1983). How to tickle your tastebuds while eating nutritiously; a gourmet cookbook.

Diet for a Small Planet, Frances Moore Lappé (Ballantine, 1982). A beautifully integrated discussion of nutrition, agribusiness, and world hunger.

Diet, Nutrition, and Cancer, National Academy of Sciences Committee on Diet, Nutrition and Cancer (National Academy Press, Washington, D.C., 1982).

Eat Your Heart Out, Jim Hightower (Crown Publishers, 1975). The story of agribusiness by someone who had investigated it for five years and was elected Texas Commissioner of Agriculture in 1982.

Jane Brody's Nutrition Book, Jane Brody (New York Times Books, 1981). A wonderful compendium of information on nutrition and health written by the New York *Times*'s personal health columnist.

Present Knowledge in Nutrition, 5th Edition, Nutrition Foundation (New York and Washington, 1984).

Salt: The Brand Name Guide to Sodium Content, Michael Jacobson, Bonnie Liebman, and Greg Moyer (Warner Books, 1985). Everything you wanted to know about sodium and health . . . plus the sodium content of over five thousand foods.

The Pritikin Promise: 28 Days to a Longer, Healthier Life, Nathan Pritikin (Simon and Schuster, 1983). If you want the details on the basic possible diet, this book is for you.

The Supermarket Handbook, Nikki and David Goldbeck (New American Library, 1976). A wealth of information on all kinds of foods and cooking.

2
EATER'S DIGEST

V

An Overview of Food Additives

Introduction

The lists of ingredients on food labels read like the index of a chemistry textbook. A popular powdered "citrus" drink contains:

> sugar, citric acid, gum arabic, natural and artificial orange flavors, cellulose gum, calcium phosphate, sodium citrate, ascorbic acid, hydrogenated vegetable oil, vitamin A, artificial colors and butylated hydroxytoluene.

A nondairy coffee creamer is concocted from:

> corn syrup solids, partially hydrogenated vegetable oils (coconut oil, cottonseed oil, soybean oil, palm oil, or safflower oil), whey, sodium caseinate, dipotassium phosphate, sodium silicoaluminate, artificial colors, mono- and diglycerides, lecithin, BHA, propyl gallate, citric acid, artificial flavor.

A popular canned frosting contains a scientifically balanced blend of:

> sugar, hydrogenated vegetable oil (soybean, cottonseed, coconut, or palm) with BHA and BHT, water, dextrose, corn syrup, pecans, artificial flavor, salt, acetylated monoglycerides, mono- and diglycerides, potassium sorbate, pectin, polysorbate 60, xanthan gum, corn starch, artificial color and Yellow No. 5, lecithin, citric acid.

If you ever asked yourself, "What is all that stuff?!" this section of *The Complete Eater's Digest* is for you.

The artificially colored, emulsified, stabilized, and preserved foods that line supermarket shelves are a far cry from the fresh meat and vegetables that can still be found around the fringes of the store. Today's foods contain hundreds of millions of dollars' worth of several thousand food additives. The average American consumes approximately 5 pounds of these chemicals per year. (If you include salt and sugar as additives, the poundage soars to 140 per year.)

"Just what are all these chemicals?," "Why are they used?," "Are they safe?" are questions that everyone wonders about when they read food labels. The labels themselves are usually not very informative. "BHT added" says nothing about the chemical's safety nor that it may not be necessary in the food. Is gum arabic a sticky substance used to prevent the contents of a package from rattling about? What good is it to persons who don't have Ph.D.'s in toxicology to know that a food contains propyl gallate without also being told that this additive is suspected of causing cancer and may actually serve no useful purpose in that food?

For answers to our questions about food additives, we have had three basically unappetizing choices. We could read the popular books and articles, usually entitled something like "Poisons in Your Pantry," that paint a uniformly dismal, and often misleading, picture of our adulterated food supply and condemn almost every chemical created by God or man. Or we could write to the manufacturer of a food or chemical and wait for the inevitable response that runs something like this: "Consumers of our product are well protected; all of the ingredients in our products have been evaluated and deemed safe both by our own scientists and by the United States Food and Drug Administration." Or we could write directly to our Federal Protectors in Washington, the Food and Drug Administration (FDA) and U. S. Department of Agriculture (USDA), and receive a pamphlet that is superficial, outdated, and packed with reassurances about safety. USDA's Food Safety and Inspection Service (FSIS) soothingly states:

> Although limited amounts of food additives are necessary to guarantee adequate food supplies for a growing population, their use is strictly controlled by laws that assure consumers that foods are safe to eat and accurately labeled . . . Before any substance can be added to food, its safety must be assessed in a stringent approval process . . . Additives are never given permanent approval. FDA and FSIS continually review the safety of approved additives to determine if approvals should be modified or withdrawn.

Eater's Digest offers what I hope you will find to be objective, satisfying answers to your questions about food additives. Your author has been closely monitoring the safety of food additives for over a decade. In writing this book, the author investigated the history, function, regulation, and safety of scores of common additives. He reviewed the scientific literature, interviewed scientists, scrutinized government reports, and corresponded with numerous manufacturers.

The primary focus of the discussion of each food additive can be summarized in one word: safety. If a chemical additive was tested and found to be safe, as many have been, I have had no hesitancy to state that reassuring fact in this book. On the other hand, if reliable scientific studies indicated that a chemical may be harmful, or if a chemical has not been adequately studied, I want you and other consumers to know about it. The hazardous and poorly tested additives are obviously the ones that we should avoid.

To help clean up our food supply, over the past decade the Center for Science in the Public Interest (CSPI) and I have filed official complaints with the government about possible hazards associated with several food colorings, sodium nitrite, sodium bisulfite, brominated vegetable oil, caffeine, BHT, and propyl gallate. Other additives may also be hazardous or serve no useful function in many foods. This sounds like a lot of dangerous chemicals, but, fortunately, the vast majority of additives is safe.

Why Are Additives Used?

Cooks were adding chemicals to their dishes long before General Foods and Coca-Cola set up their prolific chemistry labs. Brine and smoke preservatives, seaweed and starch thickeners, herb and spice flavorings, plant extract colorings, and flavor enhancers made from dried fish have been used for ages. Just about every naturally occurring substance within reach has been added to food at one time or another in humankind's perpetual effort to delight the taste buds.

Today, new food additives, created by the powerful combination of imaginative chemistry and aggressive food technology, have replaced Nature as the good fairy that fills our insatiable food wishes. Do people desire strawberry-flavored creamy topping that can be frozen or refrigerated and that will not melt or wilt when placed on a pie months later? If so, it is thickening agents, artificial flavoring, preservatives, natural and artificial colorings, and synthetic emulsifiers to the rescue! Do campers fancy orange beverages but not the chore of lugging around fresh, spoilable oranges, weighty bottles of juice, or melted frozen concentrate? Then bring forth the powdered, colored, flavored, preserved, fortified, instantly dissolving fruit of a chemistry laboratory! The food and chemical industries have proven that almost any "food" that one can describe can be created in a laboratory.

Food additives have made possible more convenient foods, entirely new kinds of foods, and, in some cases, more economical foods. Consider bread: do you recall the days when we discarded half-loaves that had become stale or moldy? That was before emulsifiers were used to prevent staling and before preservatives were used to retard the growth of mold. Adding such substances to dough greatly extends the shelf life of bread and saves consumers the time and expense of buying bread every day or discarding spoiled bread. (The *taste* of bread, of course, is something else.)

Antioxidants, as well as other kinds of preservatives, can lower manufacturing costs by permitting a company to produce, store, and ship extra-large batches of food at a time and to stock up on ingredients when their cost is low.

The intelligent use of additives can overcome shortcomings or annoying properties of traditional foods in many more ways than extending shelf life. Does ice cream melt too fast or develop an undesirable texture when it melts and then is refrozen? If so, add a vegetable gum stabilizer to hold it together and prevent ice crystals from forming. Does salt cake up? Add a silicate to keep the grains from sticking together. Is the meat tough and tasteless? Try a dash of tenderizer and a sprinkling of monosodium glutamate. Do dried apricots turn brown? Just gas them with sulfur dioxide. The chemical cabinet contains remedies for almost every food problem.

Some additives promote nutrition. Although they are not always thought of as food additives, minerals and vitamins are used to fortify common foods with nutrients that at one time were deficient in many individuals' diets. Fifty years ago, the addition of iron and niacin to flour and iodine to salt helped prevent anemia, pellagra, and goiter. Valuable vitamins and minerals lost in the production of white flour and white rice are partially replaced in "enriched" products. Factory-made foods, such as sugary breakfast beverages and cereals can be made more nutritious by adding an assortment of vitamins, minerals, and proteins.

Aside from modifying familiar foods, the vast array of food chemicals has enabled manufacturers to create entirely new kinds of food. For busy people—or lazy people—ready-mix cakes, powdered juice bases, frozen dinners, dehydrated potatoes, and similar products, which are created, cooked, dried, powdered, or frozen at a distant factory, are timesaving miracles. Most of these easy-to-prepare dishes would not be possible or palatable without the generous use of flavorings, thickening agents, colorings, emulsifiers, and other additives.

So far, we have been discussing food additives in functional terms, in much the way a company would respond to a consumer's inquiry as to why chemicals X, Y, and Z are present in a certain food. The answers are simple and straightforward. Chemical X improves the food's shelf life; chemical Y adds to the nutritional value of the food; chemical Z creates a smoother texture. Without denying the value of understanding the purposes additives serve on this technical level, we must proceed from the laboratory to company headquarters and answer the question "Why are food additives used?" on a more basic, economic level.

Some food additives make foods tastier, others make foods cheaper, others make foods more or less nutritious; all food additives help companies make money, and that, in a nutshell, is why additives are usually used.

A steady stream of articles and ads in food industry magazines, such as *Food Engineering, Food Product Development, Processed, Prepared Foods,* and *Food Technology,* reveals the corporate mind-set and industry secrets. "Tomato flavors and solids replacers can be used with or without tomato powder to create a variety of tomato-based products." Learn how, with calcium and algin, to "make fruit in a variety of believable forms. Colors and flavors may be added to the mixes, of course, to achieve specific results."

One of the oldest ways that merchants have of enhancing profits is to substitute an inexpensive ingredient for an expensive one. This frequently, but not always, decreases the food's nutritive value. Makers of ice cream substitute air and thickening agents for cream. Synthetic vanillin replaces expensive vanilla as a flavoring. Turkey packers use phosphate additives to hold in added water, for which the consumer pays turkey prices. Cheap protein or starch binders replace a fraction of expensive meat in frankfurters, chili con carne, and frozen or dehydrated factory-prepared dinners.

The whole spectrum of food additives, including such "good guys" as vitamins and minerals, can be used to improve a firm's profit picture. Let's examine several major categories of food additives, focusing, as a sales department might, on their effect on corporate earnings.

Nutrients: criticizing the fortification of foods with vitamins and minerals is almost like slamming motherhood. But fortification must be recognized for the sales gimmick that it usually is; it is the food industry's equivalent to Hollywood's sex symbols. Some foods, such as white flour and white rice, have been stripped of much of their natural nutritional value; then, to the accompaniment of much advertising and self-congratulation, manufacturers add back a few of the nutrients. Some companies are adding nutrients to breakfast cereals and cupcakes and advertising that the foods are nutritious. Nutrient-rich, yes; but not necessarily the kind of foods we should be eating. Most of these foods, such as General Foods' Super Sugar Crisp cereal, just to pick one old standby, are little more than vitamin-coated candy. The vitamins that companies add do not cancel out the detrimental effects of sugar, salt, and certain other ingredients. Moreover, manufacturers frequently charge exorbitant prices for fortified products. Total, for instance, is simply a more heavily vitamin-coated form of Wheaties. For its generosity in adding an extra penny or two's worth of vitamins to twelve ounces of cereal, General Mills adds about sixty cents to the retail price.

Flavor enhancers: the food industry spends millions on chemicals that accentuate the natural taste of foods. These chemicals, monosodium glutamate, maltol, ethyl maltol, disodium guanylate, and disodium inosinate, do bring out the flavor. At the same time they enable a company to reduce the amount of expensive, natural ingredient in its product.

Thickening agents and stabilizers: some companies have the integrity and patience to follow a traditional recipe and produce a food that has a satisfying texture and consistency. Others use inferior ingredients or poor manufacturing techniques and rely on food additives to avoid a watery, lumpy, or crystalline product. This is most obvious in ice cream and yogurt: some manufacturers need a shopping list of additives, others not a single one.

Antioxidants: these chemicals are added to oil-containing foods to prevent the oil from going rancid and spoiling the food. "Enter the ageless age" advertised one manufacturer of the synthetic and controversial antioxidant butylated hydroxyanisole (BHA). Rancid-proof foods enable a manufacturer to produce and ship larger quantities at a time, cutting down on costs. Merchants never lose their investment on a slow-moving item if the item never loses its apparent freshness (whether it loses its vitamins is another question).

Meat analogs: for a time it appeared that the 1970s would be remembered as the decade in which imitation meat replaced real meat. Food engineers have devised ways of processing soy protein that give it something close to the taste, appearance, texture, and nutritive value of meat. They are currently at the beef stew and meat loaf stage, but are working toward the era of imitation steaks.

The profit potential of imitation meat is described in blunt terms in trade magazine advertisements:

> Meat is beautiful. Delicious. High in protein. Scarce. And Expensive. TPP brand (textured protein product) looks like meat. Can be flavored like meat. It's high in protein like meat. But it's plentiful, and just a fraction of the cost of meat.

When meat prices soared in the midseventies, imitation meat products flooded the supermarkets and institutional food-services industry. However, when meat prices dipped, they lost favor in most places. They still can be found in a few foods, though, including some brands of canned chicken soup, where they give the impression that the soup is brimming with chicken.

The Japanese are way ahead of Americans when it comes to artificial protein foods. A traditional Japanese food, kamaboko, is based on surimi, a paste made from inexpensive fish. The paste can be mixed with various flavorings, stabilizers, and colorings to create foods that look and taste remarkably like crab and other seafood. Not surprisingly, a number of restaurants, according to New York *Times* writer Nancy Jenkins, have been caught peddling surimi-based crab legs as the real thing.

The most effective way that a manufacturer has of converting food additives to money is to use them to develop a new product. Additives enable a white-coated food technologist to translate a marketing concept into an actual product. The vast variety of industry-developed, government-approved additives makes possible foods that are immune to germs, that retain their consistency for months or years, whose artificial coloring does not fade in storage, that contain oil that will never go rancid, or that have unusual textures or shapes.

Innovative products mean money because they don't have any competition for a significant period of time. In this period they can become established as *the* brand to buy. The relative lack of competition enables a manufacturer to set as high a price as the public lets it get away with. Check the price per ounce of such new items as party snacks, dehydrated or frozen meals, vitamin-enriched breakfast cereals, and canned toppings or puddings. Then check the labels for the lists of ingredients that made these products possible. The prices are usually extraordinarily high compared to traditional foods (even steak!) despite the low cost of the major ingredients (vegetable oil, water, sugar, flour, emulsifiers, thickeners).

Eventually, of course, competitors will arrive, but by that time the research department should have developed a new food that makes the last one obsolete, and the cycle can begin anew. Edible obsolescence. Consider the vegetable industry. First there were fresh vegetables; then they were put in cans. Next, freezing the vegetables was innovative and profitable, but the market got crowded and profits declined. Companies began pushing new angles: plastic boiling bags, "international" flavors, and so on. Because consumers are not out in the streets demanding these new products, sales departments must shift into gear with heavy advertising expenditures to create the demand. And so it goes in the food biz.

The Scope of Our Focus

Almost three thousand different substances are intentionally added to our foods. These substances range from sugar, billions of pounds of which are used annually, to citric acid and mono- and diglycerides, millions of pounds of which are used annually, to flavorings, some of which are produced in amounts of only tens or hundreds of pounds per year. They range from the salt that seasons our soups to the wax that coats our cucumbers. Because this book would never have been completed if each and every one of the additives were evaluated, our emphasis is on the major additives. Included are almost all the additives mentioned on food labels: emulsifiers, thickening agents, colorings, preservatives, flour treatment agents, and acids. Excluded are most natural and synthetic flavorings (there are well over a thousand), spices, and the thousands of accidental, but important, contaminants: pesticides, hormones, antibiotics, and processing aids. Let's touch on these substances briefly before moving on.

Several hundred different species of plants or extracts of plants are used as spices and, under the law, are food additives. Most of these substances, such as cloves, vanilla extract, and thyme, have been in use for ages and are probably innocuous. Few herbs and spices, however, have been studied in the laboratory.

Until scientists conduct tests, we cannot state with any assurance that these substances are safe. The suggestion that the spice cabinet may contain hazardous compounds is more than just an idle worry. Sassafras, which was used to flavor root beer, was found to contain a cancer-causing chemical and in 1960 was banned from foods, except when the offending ingredient, safrole, is removed. In 1968 another flavoring, oil of calamus, was found to cause cancer and was banned from food. (See the discussion of "artificial flavoring" in Chapter VI.) Black pepper and cinnamon are two widely used natural substances now being studied for possible slight health risks.

In these days of large, mechanized farms, a sizable fraction of our farm-grown food is contaminated with potentially dangerous chemicals. Grains are cultivated in heavily fertilized fields, which may also have been sprayed with weed killers; after harvest the grain may be treated with insecticides or fungicides. Cattle and poultry may eat fodder that contains antibiotics to prevent disease and spur their growth. Packaging materials, be they burlap sacks, treated papers, or detergent-washed cans, may further contaminate the food.

Manufactured foods encounter many different objects and chemicals before they reach the dinner table and are little purer than farm produce. Fortunately, though, manufacturing contaminants are rarely as biologically active as pesticides and hormones. Small amounts of the materials and machinery used to produce, transport, or store prepared foods or food ingredients may wind up in the final product. All of these detergents, solvents, lubricating oils, defoamers, adhesives, plasticizers, resins, rubber catalysts, textile fibers, plastics, and preservatives, of which there are thousands, are considered by the Food and Drug Administration to be food additives.

Pesticides, hormones, antibiotics, and processing materials may persist in active form even after food is cooked and digested. They are never listed on labels as additives because they are never intended to be in the food and do not serve a functional purpose in the food. For more extensive discussions of these substances, please refer to books listed in the Bibliography (page 371–73).

Safety: The Number One Priority

In the never-ending search for the Great New Product, food technologists reach deep into their bag of food additive tricks or invent new ones if necessary. If some of these chemicals have not been exhaustively tested and exonerated of every foreseeable hazard, well, that is just a tradeoff the public will have to make if it wants the timesaving conveniences and tasty new products that the food and chemical industries can create. As described more fully in the coming pages, many additives have been systematically tested. Some chemicals have not been well studied for their ability to cause cancer. Even fewer have been tested on pregnant animals to see if they cause birth defects. And rarely is an additive tested for possible interactions with other chemicals one might ingest.

While we are on the subject of safety, we ought to examine briefly two extreme positions. First, there are the "Poisons in Your Pantry" type books. All too often, the authors fall into the trap of needing to find something wrong with *every* chemical used in food. Sometimes the reasoning is so tortured that a chemical is indicted just because its manufacturer also produces explosives or pesticides; obviously, the safety of one product has no bearing on the safety of the other. Other times, these writers condemn a chemical because its safety has not been proved with total, absolute certainty. We must recognize that no chemical can be proved absolutely safe—scientists can gather good evidence that a chemical is not harmful, but cannot prove that a chemical will be perfectly safe for all persons under all circumstances. The best we can get, and the least we must settle for, is solid evidence that a hazard does not exist. Other traps that erstwhile critics fall into are citing ancient scientific reports that have since been disproved, citing unreliable scientists, or taking accurate quotes out of context.

On the other side of the fence, the $400-billion-a-year food industry fills our magazines, newspapers, and air waves with a constant stream of propaganda about "the world's safest food supply" and criticizing those who dare question our foods' safety. One standard argument, in a nutshell, runs:

> People, natural foods, and water are made of chemicals.
> All of these things are safe.
> Food additives are chemicals.
> Therefore food additives are safe.

The Manufacturing Chemists Association's pamphlet entitled "Good Morning! Your 'Breakfast Chemicals' " lists some of the chemicals that occur naturally in coffee, eggs, milk, and other foods, then editorializes cheerily:

> So, you see, not only your favorite foods—but your best friends, too—are chemicals!

Monsanto, which produces many food additives, and General Foods, which uses additives in many of its products, have sponsored advertising campaigns to reassure the public that all additives are safe. Monsanto emphasized that natural foods are made up of chemicals and that "without chemicals, life itself would be impossible," so that we shouldn't worry about "man-made foods." General Foods' ads described the wondrous things that additives can do and explains that "our additives meet both Government standards and General Foods standards. And those are very exacting standards indeed."

To argue that all food additives have been, are, and will always be safe is as ridiculous as arguing that they are all dangerous. In fact, in the past half century, the federal government has banished more than twenty-five chemicals to the food additive cemetery, as discussed in Chapter VII. It is astonishing that with all these skeletons in their closets industry officials would continue to voice their shopworn homilies with such innocence and deny so vehemently that any chemicals currently in our food supply may be dangerous. Although people and water are made of chemicals, food additives can still be dangerous.

Another bit of twisted logic that defenders of processed foods use is that we shouldn't worry about food additives, because some dangerous chemicals occur naturally in fresh food. These people cite the arsenic present in one food or the aflatoxin in another. Sometimes, as in the case of arsenic, the amounts are so small that they are harmless. In other cases, as with aflatoxin, a cancer-promoting substance produced by microorganisms on moldy peanuts and corn, the risk is real . . . and should be decreased. In any case, the existence of unsafe natural chemicals does not excuse the use of unsafe additives. Our goal should be to maximize the safety of our entire food supply. You don't do that by allowing one risk to justify the presence of another. It makes no sense whatsoever to *intentionally* add unsafe chemicals to our food.

The general rule to follow on the safety of food additives is that there is no general rule. Some are safe, others are hazardous. Some are safe at low concentrations, but toxic at high concentrations. Some are perfectly safe for the general population, but deadly dangerous for sensitive individuals. Some are themselves safe, but make possible the fabrication of nonnutritious foods. Each chemical must be examined individually.

A few chemicals, preservatives in particular, may introduce into our foods a small hazard, but one worth tolerating because the chemicals also have health benefits. Big battles over sodium nitrite, a preservative, and the artificial sweetener, saccharin, revolved around this very question. Both chemicals promote cancer, but industry contended that their benefits outweighed their risks. Unfortunately, it proved impossible to accurately quantify either the benefits or the risks, so completely rational judgments are almost impossible. We will discuss the nitrite and saccharin cases in greater detail later in the book. The best remedy for situations in which beneficial additives introduce small hazards is to use the smallest quantities possible and then to switch to other additives or processes that are as effective but less hazardous.

Some additives introduce a hazard without offering any offsetting benefits. For many years, baby food companies used sodium nitrite in ham and bacon products. The chemical has a slight effect on the color and taste of food, but was of no value whatsoever to the baby. It did not act as a preservative, nor did it increase the nutritional value or palatability. Once parents learned that nitrite increases slightly the risk of cancer, they clamored for it to be removed from baby foods, but the unnecessary additive should not have been tolerated even before there was a question of safety. A substance has no business being in our food if it does not benefit the consumer. Incidentally, after suffering bad publicity for several years, the baby food companies finally relented and removed nitrite in the late 1970s.

A second additive in baby food was used to satisfy the parents' taste buds rather than the baby's health. The additive was monosodium glutamate (MSG), a flavor enhancer. Scientists had considered MSG innocuous, but then new research indicated that it posed a possible risk to infants. Manufacturers stopped using it only in the face of massive public pressure generated by scientists, legislators, and Ralph Nader. MSG should never have been in baby food.

A third example of unnecessary additives involves antioxidants. Synthetic chemicals, including BHA (butylated hydroxyanisole), BHT (butylated hydroxytoluene), and propyl gallate are added to some brands of vegetable oil and shortening to prevent them from going rancid. Each of these chemicals appears to pose a slight cancer risk. Some companies have discovered that improved manufacturing procedures eliminate the need for these additives, an indication that antioxidants are not necessary in oils and shortening.

Artificial colorings add nothing to food but hazard and a cosmetically improved appearance. Candies and breakfast cereals are routinely colored simply for the sake of variety. Not only do colorings add hazard without matching benefits, but sometimes consumers are not even told of their presence. Florida citrus growers sometimes treat oranges with a synthetic dye to cover up their natural splotchy green color. Sodium nitrite and sodium erythorbate contribute to the pink color of cured meats. Potatoes are sometimes dyed red. In all these cases, in spite of federal labeling laws, the consumer is almost never told that the food has been artificially colored. As discussed later, several colorings appear to promote cancer. In 1976, FDA Commissioner Alexander Schmidt admitted that the labeling law is being violated routinely but said his agency did not have the staff to enforce it.

In thinking about safety, it is extremely important to realize that if you eat a food containing an unsafe chemical (be it an additive, natural constituent, or contaminant), you generally are not risking certain and instant harm. Rather, the additive, perhaps in combination with other chemicals to which you are exposed, increases slightly your chance of harm either in the near or long term. In most cases, unsafe additives, such as those that have promoted cancer in laboratory animals, pose only a tiny risk to a particular individual, such as yourself. But, when that tiny risk is multiplied by the tens of millions of people who are consuming the additive, the risk to the population at large can be quite significant. For instance, the chance that a hypothetical chemical would cause a fatal cancer in a given individual might be one in a hundred thousand. Most people will not get worked up over such a slight risk, particularly when the death might come years or decades later. However, if one hundred million people consumed that chemical, one thousand people would be predicted to die. One thousand deaths is not an insignificant number, as everyone realizes whenever an airliner crashes or a flood devastates a town. That is why it is so important to have strong government agencies whose job it is to control substances that each and every individual should probably not be worrying about.

Most of the attention paid to food additives has focused on their safety. If they are safe, fine. If one is dangerous, get rid of it. This primary focus on safety has distracted attention from a more subtle problem with additives. Additives that are perfectly safe oftentimes enable the production of foods that are nutritional duds, foods like dessert topping, instant soups, gelatin desserts, soda pop, and hard candies. Where would these foods be without the plethora of artificial colorings, flavorings, preservatives, and sweeteners that prop up their otherwise shaky existence?

How Are Food Additives Tested?

Every few years the FDA, university scientists, or industrial testing labs discover that a supposedly safe substance is really hazardous. Red dye No. 2, Violet dye No. 1, agene, dulcin, butter yellow: these and other once accepted, now banished, food additives portend future scandals and worries. In Chapter VI we evaluate the safety of the more common additives. Let us now examine the tests that are—or should be—conducted to determine whether a food additive is safe.

A manufacturer who wants to introduce a new food additive bears the responsibility for conducting scientific tests to establish its safety. The FDA then evaluates the tests. The substance must be shown to be free from hazards before it may be used in foods. This process is of remarkably recent origin, having been incorporated into law only in 1958 (1960 for color additives). Prior to 1958 the situation was reversed: manufacturers could put anything they pleased into food; the FDA could ban a chemical only after it had proved that the chemical was dangerous. Millions of people would be consuming the additive while the FDA built its case.

The weakest part of the 1958 food additive law pertains to those chemicals that were already in our food when the law was passed. Such additives were accepted as being safe solely on the basis of their having been used in food for many years; scientific evidence of safety was not required. Colorings in use at the time the 1960 law was passed were supposed to be tested by 1963. However, in 1985—over two decades later—some of the tests were still dragging on.

Many of the chemicals that were used before 1958 have been legally classified "generally recognized as safe," or GRAS (pronounced "grass") for short. Little scientific evidence of safety was required for these additives to be considered GRAS. Most GRAS chemicals can be used in any food at any concentration. Manufacturers were authorized by the law to add new chemicals to the

GRAS list after 1958, but only if scientific tests showed that the chemicals were safe. The manufacturers themselves are allowed to decide what constitutes adequate scientific evidence. GRAS chemicals are controlled by the FDA only after they are in the food. If the FDA has reason to believe that a GRAS chemical may be dangerous, it can either order it out of the food supply or transfer it from the GRAS list to an "interim" list and require new tests.

As a result of the controversy over the artificial sweetener cyclamate, President Richard Nixon ordered the Food and Drug Administration to systematically evaluate the safety of all 415 GRAS additives. FDA appointed a committee of academic scientists to review the scientific studies on the GRAS compounds and make recommendations to FDA. FDA then decided whether to affirm the chemicals "safe," require additional tests, or ban them. In 1985—fifteen years after cyclamate—FDA was still reviewing the data for some of the chemicals. The more controversial—and potentially harmful—the chemical, the more slowly FDA moved. Delays of five years between the time of the scientific committee's recommendations and FDA's decisions have not been uncommon. The whole process has been so slow that new hazards have been discovered after a review was completed, but before FDA made its decision, thereby antiquating the initial recommendations. In at least one case, concerning the preservative sulfur dioxide, FDA never updated the seven-year-old GRAS review and made a fatal mistake by proposing to affirm sulfur dioxide as GRAS.

For chemicals that are not "generally recognized as safe," a manufacturer must conduct tests on animals and then petition FDA to permit the chemical in foods. The petitioner must state the composition of the additive, its function, the amount to be used in food, the types of foods in which it would be used, the testing procedures, and the results of the tests. FDA scientists evaluate the petition and, if the chemical appears safe, approve the additive and specify the conditions of safe use. The public has a brief period in which to object to FDA's decision, after which time food makers can use the new additive. Note that the FDA's role is usually limited to evaluating the manufacturer's data. The FDA does not ordinarily perform its own tests to verify the information that the petitioner has submitted.

As we have become more aware of the range of harmful effects a chemical may have, the FDA has required manufacturers to conduct more extensive tests. Prior to the 1950s, most toxicological studies involved only a few dozen animals, lasted several months, and could detect only out-and-out poisons. In the last thirty years, we have become concerned about subtle and long-range effects of chemicals, and the sophistication of testing has improved markedly. Scientists test more animals for longer periods of time and look for a wider variety of effects.

The most difficult effects to detect are those that show up only months or years after a person is exposed to a chemical. A food additive that had no immediately toxic effects, but that causes birth defects, cancer, or mutations, might escape detection indefinitely, because there is no simple way of associating the ingestion of a chemical in 1985 with the birth of a deformed child in 1986, the occurrence of liver cancer in 1999, or a case of hemophilia in 2052. Extensive testing on laboratory animals and microorganisms is the only practical means of weeding out dangerous food additives before they cause subtle or long-range damage in people. Even though laboratory animals are not physiologically or anatomically identical to humans, they are similar enough to permit fairly accurate predictions of the effects of a chemical on humans.

Testing usually begins with brief (one to six months) studies. Scientists examine animals' growth, blood, urine, and liver function. Once they know an animal's approximate tolerance to a chemical, they can select the most appropriate dose levels for the crucial lifetime feeding studies.

Feeding studies demonstrate the effects of a chemical on the animal; biochemical experiments reveal the effects of the animal on the chemical. By learning how an animal's body handles a chemical, one can frequently estimate a substance's toxicity. For instance, some chemicals, such as the thickening agents carboxymethylcellulose and karaya, are not absorbed by the body and are likely to be harmless when present in moderate amounts. Additives that are identical to chemicals occurring in the body, or that are converted to such chemicals in the digestive tract, are generally also safe. Some chemicals may themselves be harmless, but biochemical experiments can reveal that they are converted by bacteria living in the intestine or by liver enzymes into toxic agents. In other cases, potentially poisonous substances may be detoxified in the liver and then harmlessly excreted.

The way in which a chemical is administered to animals greatly influences the results and interpretation of studies. Ordinarily, scientists expose animals to a chemical by adding it to their food or water or by administering it through a stomach tube. The oral route is the most meaningful way of testing food additives, because additives enter the human body through the mouth. A stomach tube insures that the animal actually consumes the chemical, rather than scattering it around the cage. Administering the chemical by tube also increases the sensitivity of a test by exposing the animals to a sudden, high dosage of chemical. This type of exposure is similar to a person gulping down a can of soda pop or cup of coffee. When the chemical is mixed in with the food, the animal consumes it gradually throughout the day and is never exposed to a high concentration.

While feeding studies are generally the most informative, some information can be obtained by applying the additive to the skin or injecting it under the skin (subcutaneously), into a blood vessel (intravenously), or into the body cavity (intraperitoneally). Injecting a chemical with a syringe bypasses the animal's digestive enzymes, stomach acids, and intestinal bacteria, any of which may alter the substance under study, and also exposes the animal to sudden, exceedingly high levels of the agent. The results of this kind of experiment must be interpreted in light of metabolic studies that show whether the substance, when ingested, is absorbed into the bloodstream or is converted into a second substance by the digestive system. Otherwise, the conclusions drawn from injection studies are likely to be erroneous.

The most important test used to evaluate food additives is the chronic, or lifetime, feeding study. This test is designed to detect chemicals that cause cancer or are toxic when ingested over long periods of time. In a chronic feeding study, researchers feed animals a diet that contains ten times to one thousand or more times as much of the additive as a person might consume. These studies typically employ fifty animals of each sex of two species of rodents, usually mice and rats. As a control, an equal number of animals is fed identical food, except that the additive is left out. The animals are maintained on the diets for their entire lives, usually about two years. In the best tests, animals are first exposed to chemicals while they are still in their mothers' womb. Thus, an animal will be exposed from the very moment of conception, just as a person might be.

Technicians monitor the animals' weight, consumption of food, and blood composition. Special tests may be performed to measure the health of the liver, kidney, or other organs. After the animals die or are sacrificed, pathologists examine the major organs, first by eye and then microscopically, for evidence of tumors or other harm. The highest dosage that has no harmful effect is determined. FDA then sets a safe level for human exposure by applying a one hundredfold safety factor to the "highest no-observable-effect level." A chemical is unacceptable as a food additive if low dosages are harmful or if any amount causes cancer.

In interpreting the results of animal studies, it is crucial to keep one eye fixed on the chemical's effects and the other on the dosage levels used. Disregarding the quantity of chemical that causes a toxic effect all too commonly leads to groundless fears. Large enough doses of *any* chemical, even water, are injurious to animals and humans. Some substances upset the water balance, causing chronic diarrhea or increased production of urine; others taste so bad that animals would rather starve than eat their food; still others may overwork and damage the kidneys or liver. These effects do not arise when animals consume the small or moderate amounts that would likely be added to food. Thus, just because extremely high dosages of a chemical are harmful does not mean that normal dietary levels will be harmful and that the chemical should be prohibited as a food additive.

CANCER

Cancer, however, does *not* appear to be one of the effects that occur at high dosages, but not at low dosages. The scientific evidence strongly indicates that, if large amounts of a chemical cause tumors, we should assume that small amounts will also cause tumors, though less frequently. In 1979 all of the federal agencies that regulate cancer-causing chemicals agreed on this key principle.[1] The International Agency for Cancer Research came to the same conclusion. Despite this general agreement, however, it is conceivable that large dosages of some chemicals might disrupt an animal's metabolism to such an extent that only high dosages, but not low dosages, would cause cancer. If such chemicals are found, they would deserve to be regulated as exceptions to the general rule.

The 1958 food additive law recognized the importance of eliminating cancer-causing chemicals (carcinogens) from our food supply by banning any additive that "is found to induce cancer when ingested by man or animal." This section of the Food, Drug and Cosmetic Act is known as the "Delaney Amendment," in recognition of Representative James J. Delaney, Democrat of New York, whose efforts resulted in this and other consumer protection laws of the 1950s. Though relatively little was known about cancer when the amendment was passed, it has withstood well the tests of time. Cancer experts still generally support the basic assumption in the law: that if a chemical causes cancer in animals, it poses a threat to humans, also. In 1985 after much debate and soul-searching, the White House Office of Science and Technology Policy under President Reagan accepted this prudent philosophy.[2] While that assumption cannot be tested directly, it is known that almost all proven human carcinogens—there are several dozen such chemicals—also cause cancer in animals. Of course, exceptions may exist. For example, mice might have an enzyme that converts a harmless chemical into a carcinogen. Humans might lack such an enzyme and be immune to harm from that chemical.

Cancer tests that employ some method other than feeding (or stomach tube) must be interpreted cautiously. When a chemical is injected subcutaneously, local tumors (fibrosarcomas) often develop at the site of injection. Scientists argued for years over whether these tumors reflect a hazard to humans or are simply due to nonspecific physical irritation caused by repeated injections. Sometimes local tumors can be induced by implanting bits of inert plastic or by repeatedly injecting harmless chemicals under the skin. Many cancer specialists are not concerned abut tumors that arise only at the site of injection, but view with suspicion chemicals that cause tumors far from the point of injection—in the liver, lung, bladder, etc. Tannin, a substance in tea, and Citrus Red 2, the artificial coloring on some Florida oranges, are two substances that, when injected, cause tumors distant from the site of injection.

Lifetime animal studies designed to detect cancer-causing agents typically take three to four years to conduct and cost several hundred thousand dollars. These two factors stimulated scientists to seek quick, inexpensive tests that could identify cancer-causing chemicals. In the 1970s, Bruce Ames, a molecular biologist at the University of California at Berkeley, made the first real breakthrough. The "Ames test" takes just a few days and costs just a few hundred dollars.[3]

The Ames test measures a chemical's ability to cause mutations in bacteria. The researcher mixes the chemical with enzymes from a rat's liver. The enzymes convert the chemical to some of the metabolites that might form in the body. (Sometimes the basic chemical will be safe, but its metabolites harmful.) Bacteria are then exposed to the chemical mixture. The number of mutant bacteria that form is compared to the number of mutants that form in the absence of the chemical. The more mutants, the more mutagenic is the chemical. The ability to cause mutations correlates closely with the ability to cause cancer.

The Ames test and other similar microbiological tests are good, but not perfect indicators of carcinogenicity. Some cancer-causing chemicals do not cause mutations in bacterial tests. Other chemicals that do cause mutations in bacteria have not been identified in animal tests as being carcinogenic. Because the short-term tests are still not foolproof, food additives and other chemicals to which humans may be exposed still need to be subjected to the more expensive and lengthy animal tests before they can be considered safe.

Many chemical companies are now using the quick mutagenicity tests to routinely screen newly synthesized chemicals. The manufacturers can save enormous amounts of money by not developing chemicals that show up "positive" in the screening.

BIRTH DEFECTS

In 1962 the world was shocked by an epidemic in Europe of babies born with heartbreakingly deformed arms and legs. Medical detective work traced the cause of deformities in 4,000 babies to thalidomide, a sedative that the mothers had been taking during pregnancy.

The thalidomide disaster dramatized the possibility that supposedly safe chemicals in our increasingly synthetic environment may affect the development of an unborn baby. While such tragedies are rare, birth defects are common. According to the March of Dimes Birth Defects Foundation, every year 250,000 American babies are born with such defects as cleft palate, club foot, abnormal behavior, or open spine. Scientific experts agree that environmental factors, such as drugs, smoking, alcohol, pollutants, and additives, cause a sizable percentage of birth defects. Chemicals that cause birth defects are termed teratogens, from the Greek word meaning monster.

A person who is afflicted with a congenital defect must shoulder an unenviable burden through his or her entire life. And added to the human grief is the enormous monetary cost to the victim's family and to society in the form of doctor bills, hospital rooms, deprivation of earnings, and lack of contribution to the economy and our society. For serious birth defects, this dollar cost runs to hundreds of thousands of dollars per person. To minimize these costs it is essential that manufacturers of chemicals to which millions of people are exposed be required to test their products for their capacity to cause birth defects (teratogenicity).

In the 1960s, the FDA began asking manufacturers of proposed additives to conduct animal reproduction studies. These studies are usually integrated into lifetime feeding experiments. A good reproduction study spans four generations and reveals a chemical's effect on fertility, lactation, and the development of the embryo.

The multigeneration reproduction study is informative, but has important shortcomings. In the first place, rarely are progeny from more than twenty parent animals examined. This means that only relatively potent teratogens could be detected. Ideally, many more animals would be used in each study.

The second limitation of multigeneration studies follows from the way animals cope with foreign chemicals. Some chemicals stimulate an animal's liver to produce large amounts of detoxification enzymes, which are ordinarily present at low levels. These enzymes modify foreign substances to make them less toxic and more easily excreted. Thus, an animal exposed for a lengthy period to a potential teratogen may possess high levels of detoxification enzymes and dispose of it much more rapidly than would an animal encountering the chemical for the first time. For this reason, in some studies animals are fed a chemical for only brief periods, usually just one to three days, at different times during pregnancy. This method offers the best possibility of detecting a teratogen.

Most good reproduction studies take great pains to expose pregnant animals to only one chemical at a time. That keeps the experiment easy to interpret. However, such an experiment does not bear much resemblance to a pregnant woman's lifestyle. The average pregnant woman consumes dozens of food additives, may smoke cigarettes and drink alcohol, breathes scores of air pollutants, and may take a dozen different prescription and over-the-counter drugs. It should hardly surprise us, if some combination of all these chemicals multiplied the risk to the developing fetus . . . and one important recent study has found exactly that, a synergism between chemicals.

Doctors J. R. Ritter and J. G. Wilson of the Children's Hospital in Cincinnati exposed pregnant rats to caffeine and did not detect any malformations in the pups. Another chemical, acetazolamide, caused malformations in 21 percent of the offspring. When the pregnant rats were treated with caffeine and acetazolamide at the same time, 58 percent of the offspring suffered birth defects.[4] Other chemicals interacted with caffeine in the same way. This study proved that one chemical could greatly increase the teratogenicity of another.

A key problem with teratology studies is that scientists do not agree on how to interpret the results. For cancer studies, most experts agree that if large amounts of a chemical cause cancer in animals, a small amount would also cause cancer, but much less frequently. In other words, there is no "threshold" level below which a carcinogen is safe. This may or may not be the case for chemicals that cause birth defects. The reproductive process is so complicated and sensitive that huge amounts of otherwise safe chemicals could often cause birth defects or infertility. Thus, there may be threshold levels below which a chemical does not cause birth defects.

Also, cancer experts agree that a chemical that causes cancer in animals should be assumed to be a carcinogen in humans. By contrast, some birth defect experts question the relevance of animal studies to human beings. The lack of a consensus on how animal teratology studies relate to humans sometimes results in a "heads I win, tails you lose" situation for food and chemical companies. When animal studies indicate that large doses of a chemical do not cause birth defects, the manufacturer contends that the tests prove that the chemical is safe for humans. However, when large amounts of a chemical do cause birth defects in animals, industry scientists suddenly recognize weaknesses of the test: excessively high dosages were used, the animals may metabolize the chemical differently from humans, et cetera, et cetera. Hence, they argue, the chemical should not be considered harmful. The usual next step is to call for more animal studies, plus studies on human populations that have been exposed to the chemical, comparing the incidence of birth defects to a population that did not consume the chemical in question. In theory, such epidemiological studies would be informative. In practice, though they are usually prohibitively expensive, difficult to interpret because humans are exposed to so many chemicals, and inevitably unable to detect even a doubling or tripling in the rate of a birth defect, let alone a 1, 5, or 10 percent increase.

Though some scientists maintain that it is presumptuous to jump from animal reproduction studies to human risks, there does seem to be a close correlation. According to Dr. Vasilios Frankos, an FDA expert on developmental biology,

> FDA's review of the literature reveals a group of 38 compounds for which there are reports of birth defects in humans associated with intake of these compounds during pregnancy. Of these compounds, all except one have a positive study in at least one animal test species. Furthermore, over 80 percent of the compounds are positive in multiple species. The one exception is a compound that causes otologi-

cal [hearing] deficits in humans that would not normally be discovered in test animals at the time of caesarean section.[5]

In the late 1970s, federal officials were developing a uniform, governmentwide policy on interpreting animal reproduction studies, but this effort was torpedoed by the Reagan Administration. Nevertheless, the Food and Drug Administration did adopt a policy. According to FDA's Dr. Frankos, ". . . a thousandfold safety factor would be applied in those cases where there is evidence of serious developmental effects in two species." For minor or temporary birth defects, FDA would use its standard hundredfold safety factor.

MUTATIONS

It took the thalidomide episode to drive home the importance of examining the effects of food additives on reproduction. Some farsighted scientists are urging that we not wait for an analogous, and less easily detected, catastrophe to induce us to screen out food additives that affect our genes.

Biologists have known for decades that radiation or chemicals can cause changes—or mutations—in the genes of plants and animals. Genes in a woman's egg cells and in a man's sperm carry, in chemically encoded form, the instructions for the proper development of the next generation. Mutations in these genes may garble the precisely inscribed instructions and cause such "mistakes" as hemophilia, extra fingers, heightened need for certain nutrients, reduced intelligence, mongolism, and decreased resistance to disease. The mutations—and their effects—may persist from one generation to the next.

The importance of identifying mutagenic chemicals was cogently described by Dr. James F. Crow, chairman of the genetics department of the University of Wisconsin, in a National Institutes of Health genetic study section report entitled "Chemical Risk to Future Generations." Crow wrote:

> Special attention should be given to the danger of very low concentrations of highly mutagenic compounds that might be introduced into foodstuffs . . . Even though the compounds may not be demonstrably mutagenic to man at the concentrations used, the total number of deleterious mutations induced in the whole population over a prolonged period of time could nevertheless be substantial. Such increase in mutation rate probably could not be detected in a short period of time by any direct observations on human beings. Protection from such effects must depend on prior identification of mutagenicity.[6]

Geneticists developed practical tests for detecting chemical mutagens in the 1960s and 1970s. One of the first, the "dominant lethal" method, is quite simple. Male mice are fed or injected with large amounts of the suspected mutagen and then mated to untreated female mice. Two weeks after the mating, the researcher sacrifices the pregnant mice and counts the fetuses. If the chemical caused a high rate of mutations in the sperm cells, the average number of live fetuses per mother would be reduced. The major limitation of this technique is that only "dominant lethal" mutations—ones that kill the developing animals—can be detected.

A second way that scientists can identify mutagens is to treat animals with large doses of chemicals and then look under the microscope for damaged chromosomes. Bone marrow, spleen, and testes contain large numbers of dividing cells and are the tissues most likely to reflect genetic damage.

Mutation studies involving live animals are relatively expensive, time-consuming, and insensitive. They have been largely superseded by the Ames test, described earlier, which uses bacteria. Similar tests have been developed involving other microorganisms or cultured animal cells. These quick, inexpensive tests have made it possible to routinely screen all new chemicals for their ability to cause genetic mutations.

HOW GOOD ARE THE STUDIES?

Testing a proposed food additive for carcinogenic, teratogenic, and mutagenic effects and conducting metabolic studies is a major undertaking. But even after this great investment of time and money in what would appear to be a thorough investigation, an apparently safe additive could still cause trouble.

Food additives that cause only very occasional cancers, mutations, or birth defects would probably not be detected by current testing methods. In fact, the reason we are justified in being alarmed when an additive is found to cause cancer is that current methods are so coarse and insensitive. The primary weakness of feeding tests is that only a small number of animals are used. The results of these relatively small experiments are inevitably blurred by spontaneously occurring tumors or malformations, random variations, and the premature death of some of the animals. For instance, a typical reproduction study involves only twenty parent animals at each dosage level. A chemical would have to increase the incidence of malformations in the range of five to twelve times above normal before it could be positively identified as a teratogen.[7] In a typical long-term feeding study involving one hundred animals, at least about five to twenty animals would have to develop cancer before the chemical being tested could, with any confidence, be identified as a carcinogen. Using doses one hundred to one thousand times greater than amounts to which humans would be exposed compensates somewhat for the small number of animals, but the studies are still not all that sensitive. Even assuming that animals and humans are equally sensitive to a chemical, a "rigorous" experiment could detect only those carcinogens that cause more than about one cancer death in two thousand to twenty thousand persons. This means that a "safe" food additive could cause cancer in as many as ten thousand to one hundred thousand Americans.

It should be emphasized that feeding studies, which because of costs inevitably involve a limited number of animals, are as sensitive as they are only because massive amounts of chemical are fed to the animals. Even strong carcinogens might escape detection if a hundred rats were fed a chemical at the level at which it occurs in a human diet. Food industry officials sometimes argue that experiments in which huge doses of chemical-caused cancer are invalid because enormous amounts of *any* chemical will cause cancer. In fact, as discussed earlier, extremely high doses of most chemicals do *not* cause cancer. They may destroy the liver, or damage the heart, or cause continuous diarrhea, but they do not cause cancer.

In virtually all toxicologic studies only one or two species of animals are treated with the chemical. Yet we know that sensitivities to chemicals that cause birth defects and cancer vary greatly from one species to another, and it is impossible to know which species' reaction would be most similar to human's. The classical illustration of this problem is thalidomide, to which the human fetus is at least thirty to two hundred times as sensitive as rabbits, mice, rats, hamsters, and dogs.

In addition to the markedly different sensitivities of different species to a chemical, there are significant variations between strains of animals within a species. Animals used in experiments are not field mice or sewer rats recently captured in the wild, but rodents that have been highly inbred over many generations in the laboratory. Different strains of the same species may be extremely sensitive to or uniquely resistant to a specific carcinogen or teratogen. Usually only one strain of a species is used in a feeding study. In contrast, the entire extraordinarily diverse American population ingests food additives. Americans of African or European ancestry may react differently to an additive than a person of Asian descent. Moreover, subcultures within the United States —blacks, adolescents, vegetarians, suburbanites, etc.—have distinctive eating habits and lifestyles that may increase or decrease their sensitivity or exposure to a certain chemical.

Laboratory experiments are almost always conducted with well-fed, pampered animals, the kind that might be most resistant to the effects of marginally toxic chemicals. Humans, on the other hand, suffer infections and diseases and are frequently malnourished. Diabetes, alcoholism, hypertension, food allergies, and dozens of other problems could increase the toxicity of a chemical.

In one rare study conducted on malnourished animals, an emulsifier (polyoxyethylene-(40)-stearate) caused an abnormal increase in the number of stomach cells, which is often indicative of cancer, when rats were on a diet deficient in vitamin A but not when they ate a normal diet.[8]

In the mid-1960s, brewers used a chemical that everyone thought was safe to stabilize the foam in a glass of beer. Shortly thereafter, deaths due to congestive heart failure started occurring at an alarming rate in heavy drinkers. Doctors discovered that the normally harmless additive, cobalt sulfate, could be fatal to heavy drinkers. Food additives, including even those used in alcoholic beverages, are never tested on animals whose bodies are weakened by alcohol.

Sodium bisulfite is another additive that was long considered safe. Then, between 1976 and 1982, half a dozen studies were published proving that thousands of asthmatics were highly sensitive to the chemical. At least five deaths have been linked to this "safe" substance.

Dr. Tibor Balazs, a scientist in FDA's division of drug biology, has expressed concern about the effects of chemicals on subgroups of the population. He emphasizes "the importance of studying the toxicity of chemicals in conditions modeling those of human use."[9]

Another difference between laboratory conditions and real life is that typical toxicity tests measure the effects on animals of one food additive in an otherwise "pure" diet. Most Americans consume a rich assortment of synthetic antioxidants, thickening agents, emulsifiers, coal tar dyes, and preservatives, as well as drugs, air pollutants, water pollutants, and pesticides. The possibilities are endless for two otherwise harmless chemicals to interact and cause a problem. For instance, the preservatives BHA and BHT stimulate the liver to produce enzymes which may hasten the destruction and reduce the effectiveness of certain medicines.

Diethylpyrocarbonate (DEPC) was used as a preservative in beverages and thought to be safe, because it quickly broke down to carbon dioxide and water. However, in the early 1970s, scientists discovered that a tiny fraction of the DEPC reacted with ammonia to form urethane, a carcinogen. Additives are almost never tested for interactions with other chemicals.

Still another of the inadequacies of current testing procedures is that only a limited range of effects is monitored. Rarely studied are possible effects on the brain. A chemical that causes impaired eye-hand coordination, a slight reduction in memory, or hyperactivity would never be identified by current test procedures. Government and other scientists have developed special tests that can evaluate a chemical's effects on behavior, but the FDA does not require food additives to be so tested.

One of the biggest problems is that most testing of food additives is done by the manufacturers themselves. Companies either test chemicals in their own facilities or contract the work out to private testing laboratories whose financial solvency may depend upon delivering favorable results to its clients. One would not be surprised if companies used lax experimental protocols or overlooked an occasional tumor. At the subtle end of the spectrum, industry scientists might unthinkingly interpret ambiguous results in a way that absolves the chemical of any harmful effect. At the other end of the spectrum, are the horror stories about lying, cheating, greedy laboratories. In a brilliant summary of such practices, *Mother Jones* magazine (June and July 1982) described how Industrial Bio-Test Laboratories, physicians, and others withheld important data from the government, shredded incriminating records, underreported the number of tumors, and allowed dead animals to decompose instead of autopsying them. Other investigations have disclosed how animals that died in a study would be resuscitated in the records, how tests are designed so that they could not detect a problem, and how results presented in the body of a scientific paper would be ignored or distorted in the more widely read summaries and conclusions.

Concerned scientists and lawyers have suggested that testing frauds could be reduced by inserting a governmental intermediary between the company that developed a new chemical and the laboratory that tests it. This system would also enable testing laboratories to be truly independent and professional. Former Senator Gaylord Nelson proposed legislation in the 1970s to accomplish this, but it was derailed year after year, allegedly by drug industry lobbyists.

BRAVE NEW WORLD

So many additives have been found to be harmful over the years that scientists are working hard to develop fail-safe substitutes for questionable additives. Because most additives are harmless until they are absorbed into the bloodstream, some researchers are developing ways of preventing absorption. One way to accomplish this is to bond many individual, small molecules into one very large molecule that passes right through the stomach and intestine. In 1983 FDA approved an antioxidant called anoxomer that was synthesized on that principle. Another approach is to bind an additive, say a coloring or preservative, to a long, inert polymer. While the additive would serve its technical function in the food, it would be too big to get into the bloodstream. A third approach is being used by a small company that discovered a synthetic form of sugar that tastes sweet to the tongue, but, because of its molecular configuration, cannot be absorbed in the intestines. The synthetic sugar looks like the mirror image of real sugar, and is called "left-handed sugar."

Safe as they may appear, these new additives must still undergo safety testing. They could, for instance, harm the digestive system, with which they obviously come into contact, or prevent the absorption of nutrients.

Is The Government Guarding Your Health?

THE BUREAUCRACY

The United States has about the toughest food safety laws in the world, and American companies and government agencies have conducted more safety tests of food additives than anyone else. Nations around the world look to the U.S. Food and Drug Administration for leadership and guidance. The FDA has several thousand employees whose job it is to protect the public from unsafe food additives, drugs, and cosmetics. Yet, despite this huge investment by our society it seems that all too frequently a legislator or other party complains that the FDA is ignorant of or unconcerned about a dangerous chemical. Is FDA protecting us? Or is it asleep at the wheel?

Bad as some people claim FDA is, our nation surely enjoys a relatively clean and safe food supply. People are not frequently, or at least obviously, dying in the street from food additives or contaminants. And despite FDA's slowness (the letters F, D, and A could easily stand for Foot Dragging Agency), the agency eventually banned numerous chemicals over the years (see Chapter VII, Food Additive Cemetery).

FDA can ban additives most easily when the evidence that they are harmful is clear and conclusive. FDA's job would be pretty easy if a chemical were shown by three separate animal studies to increase by thirtyfold the incidence of cancer. In real life, though, the facts are rarely so clear-cut. The evidence is often incomplete and contradictory. One study might indicate no problem, while the other indicated a tiny increase in cancer risk. Reasonable arguments could be made both for banning the additive and for retesting it. Keeping the chemical until more tests were conducted would expose consumers to a slight, uncertain risk; banning it might throw hundreds of workers out of work. It's cases like these that make life difficult for FDA officials.

The importance and uniqueness of an additive influence the speed with which FDA moves. If just a few thousand pounds of the chemical are used each year, and several other chemicals could do the job equally well, FDA might encounter little commercial resistance to a ban. But if the chemical is widely used and not easily replaced, FDA will experience all the might of the food and chemical industries' political power. Such was the case with saccharin and sodium nitrite, the two big brouhahas of the 1970s. Those two chemicals are key ingredients in billions of pounds—and billions of dollars' worth—of foods. Without saccharin, diet sodas would not have existed (diet sodas now contain aspartame, an artificial sweetener first allowed in soft drinks in 1983). Without nitrite, hot dogs would look and taste strange. In both cases, product sales might have dropped sharply if the additives were banned. The processed meat and soda pop companies saw their very survival at stake. With their backs against the wall and their profits hanging in the balance, companies sought both to retain the use of those two additives and more importantly, to weaken the food safety laws to such an extent that FDA would never again pose a threat.

One of the big problems with FDA—and other federal regulatory agencies—is that the employees have no great incentives to find or act upon problems. In fact, most of the incentives run in the opposite direction. Let's say that a scientist thought he or she found a problem with an existing food additive (or drug or cosmetic). The first thing the scientist would have to do is persuade other agency employees . . . who, perhaps, had been involved in the original decision to declare the chemical safe.

Defending a minority opinion in the face of internal agency opposition, and, later, external corporate, congressional, and media pressures means work, a lot of work. It means psychological stress, time away from the spouse and kids, missed car pools, and, perhaps, a reputation as a troublemaker that might impede progress up the bureaucratic ladder. Who needs it?

If the big internal hurdle could be crossed, then the agency would tell the makers and users of the additive about the problem. The agency had better be well prepared, because the companies would have on hand a flock of scientists and attorneys to dispute every single point. If, after that encounter the agency still wanted to do something, it would have to invest large blocks of time in legal research and preparation of the appropriate documents. With meager resources, the decision to ban a chemical is not taken lightly. Afterward would come *Federal Register* announcements, comment periods, arguments about the quality of scientific research, and ultimately lawsuits, trials with expert witnesses, appeals, scrutiny by legislators and the media, and so on and on and on.

Fortunately for the public, not every troubleshooting government safety agency has its reward system organized in a way that discourages employees from finding problems. Police departments, for instance, place great value on investigating problems and solving cases. The problem-solvers are not vilified. Rather, they are publicly applauded and given medals and promotions. How outraged the public would be if police acted any differently, if detectives were patted on the back for not detecting.

The challenge to government leaders is to redesign the system of rewards and punishments so that regulatory scientists and officials would benefit personally by aggressively protecting the public's health. The benefits could be financial, such as a five-thousand-dollar bonus for identifying a dangerous chemical. Or the person could be honored by the President or FDA Commissioner at an awards ceremony, or given more technical assistance, or relieved of undesired duties. There are all kinds of ways of rearranging the carrots and sticks. Will it happen? Don't hold your breath, because all the forces that currently keep mouths sealed and rugs bulging with hidden problems would be at work to keep the bureaucracies maintaining their placid course. Major reforms would have to be ordered by the White House and would probably be triggered only by a major scandal.

Consumer advocate Ralph Nader has pinpointed another impediment to vigorous action by government officials: the "deferred bribe." If officials behave themselves during their years of government service, they have a good shot at getting juicy jobs in industry. Over the years numerous government officials, particularly the lawyers, have opted for the good life, taking with them expertise and information gained while on the public payroll.

Finally, numerous men and women have moved from industry into government: from food processing companies into FDA, or from the meat industry into the Department of Agriculture. While such people have an excellent understanding of industry practices, they usually bring with them a philosophy that has excessive respect for industry's interests. Appendix III of *Nutrition Scoreboard* lists some of the public officials who either came from or left for industries regulated by the FDA or the USDA. Citizens certainly have the right to ask whether the public interest is best served by those migratory patterns.

As numerous examples in this book and in your daily newspaper indicate, Food and Drug Administration officials have done an inadequate job of regulating food additives and food labeling. Congressional committees and Public Citizen Health Research Group have demonstrated that FDA has done just as poor a job when it comes to regulating drugs. We need nothing less than an inspiring FDA commissioner and a vigorous shake-up and shake-out of FDA's top layers of officials. The indecisive, spineless foot-draggers, the officials who search endlessly for every excuse to exonerate an arguably dangerous additive, those who are more touched by corporate lawyers than human suffering should all be invited to retire. The reluctant regulators should be replaced by men and women, from within or without the agency, who have demonstrated a zeal in promoting the public's health and who are capable of intelligent, decisive action. They should be aware that their top priority is protecting the public, not their job. What a tonic such changes would be for a cynical citizenry disgusted by years of governmental indifference and incompetence!

But we need more than good people. We also need a governmental structure in which they can function effectively. Traditionally, FDA was a science-based, relatively independent regulatory agency. But, in the past few years, FDA's wings have been clipped. Instead of analyzing the evidence and issuing a decision, FDA must now have its proposals approved by its parent agency, the Department of Health and Human Services. HHS, in turn, submits its verdict to the Office of Management and Budget, an arm of the White House. In just the past year, HHS or OMB blocked FDA's efforts to ban several cancer-promoting food dyes, ban or require better labeling of sulfites in drugs and foods, and halt the marketing of raw milk. In each case, it was politics, not science, that determined the outcome.

To be maximally effective, the Food and Drug Administration should be removed from the Department of Health and Human Services and set up as an independent agency. Commissioners should serve for fixed terms, of perhaps five years, rather than at the whim of the President. Even these steps would not guarantee a vigorous agency, but they would certainly improve the odds.

CHANGING THE LAW

America's basic food safety laws were revised most recently in 1958–60. While consumer groups, industry, and government have all proposed major changes during the past decade, Congress has retained the basic law. However, laws are flexible creatures and are constantly being reinterpreted by the courts and government agencies.

While the exact language of the food safety law has not changed for twenty-five years, the environment in which it has had to operate has changed dramatically. Animal tests are generally larger and more sensitive than they had been. This means that additives long thought safe may be found to be hazardous. Most important, scientists have developed exquisitely sensitive means of detecting minuscule amounts of chemicals. It is possible to detect certain chemicals at levels as low as one part in a trillion. An additive considered to be pure may actually be contaminated with a dangerous substance. Practically all foods, even those grown organically, are contaminated with low levels of toxic pesticides or other chemicals. These new developments have made the jobs of Food and Drug Administration officials increasingly difficult.

The most controversial and difficult to enforce portion of the food safety law is the Delaney Clause, which bans cancer-causing additives. The law specifically states:

> That no additive shall be deemed to be safe if it is found to induce cancer when ingested by man or animal, or if it is found, after tests which are appropriate for the evaluation of the safety of food additives, to induce cancer in man or animal . . .

The food and chemical industries have complained that this law should be repealed, because it prohibits many useful chemicals that have only a remote likelihood of causing cancer in humans. Industry spokespersons describe a grim scenario in which the government bans dozens of long-used chemicals as soon as one laboratory rat dies of cancer. They argue that strict enforcement of the Delaney Clause would ban hundreds of traditional foods that contain naturally occurring carcinogens. They also say that modern analytical methods are so sensitive that they can find very low levels of carcinogens in virtually any food or food additive.

In truth, the Delaney Clause is much more important as a philosophical statement than as a legal tool. The clause has actually been used to ban only a handful of food additives. To clear away one misconception immediately, industry's argument about banning natural foods is totally wrong, because the clause covers only *additives,* not *traditional foods.* In fact, the Delaney Clause does not even cover all food additives, but only those that were not sanctioned or approved by the FDA or USDA prior to the 1958 law. It is, unfortunately, virtually impossible to ban additives that were in use prior to 1958.

As you will find when you read about specific additives in the next chapter of *Eater's Digest,* the FDA enforces the law very loosely. One or two rats dying of cancer has never been enough to trigger Delaney. In most cases, a single study indicating cancer is not enough. FDA usually waits until one study is corroborated by a second or third study. Even then, chemicals are not banned abruptly. FDA usually appoints review committees and issues warning signals, allowing companies time to argue their case or switch to safer chemicals. All this takes years, and all the while people are consuming the suspect additive. Once an additive is approved, the whole legal structure favors industry, not consumers.

The courts and FDA have recently poked small loopholes into the Delaney Clause. The U.S. Court of Appeals ruled that even though Delaney bans cancer-causing chemicals, the amount of such a chemical in a food may be so small that it is not worth worrying about. The court decision was based on a case dealing with plastic bottles and applies only to substances that get into food accidentally, such as from packaging or chemicals used on processing machinery. While the court did not specify the exact number of molecules that would be tolerated, FDA has done a good job in not allowing every troublesome additive to sneak through this loophole.

In addition to carcinogenic packaging contaminants, FDA is giving the green light to certain other chemicals that might cause very small numbers of cancers. These chemicals include drugs added to animal feed and otherwise safe food additives that contain cancer-causing impurities. FDA allows the use of these substances if statisticians can establish that they pose a risk of less than one cancer death in a million people over their lifetime. This type of exception was inevitable in light of advances in analytical chemistry. Modern instruments can often detect impurities that constitute as little as one billionth of another chemical. With needle-in-a-haystack capabilities like that, it might be possible to find cancer-causing contaminants in practically everything.

When it enacted the Delaney Clause, Congress was certainly far more concerned about the safety of the food additives themselves than about the contaminants in our food or food additives. A weak carcinogen that constitutes one millionth of an additive that itself makes up just a ten millionth of our diet does not pose much of a threat to the public's health. Thus, through its new policies, FDA made sure it wasn't going to forbid useful chemicals that might seep into the food supply by way of drugs that farmers administer to livestock or that contain trivial levels of contaminants.

To implement these exceptions to Delaney, FDA statisticians calculate the degree of risk on the basis of animal experiments. These estimates are only rough approximations, because humans may be more or less sensitive than the animals tested and humans are exposed to dozens of hazardous chemicals unlike test animals exposed to only one. However, if done conservatively, as FDA has been doing them, risk assessments can indicate the approximate maximal risk an incidental additive poses to consumers. It would be very dangerous, though, if regulators gave a lot of weight to these rough estimates when regulating chemicals that were present in large quantity in food. The cost of an error could be great.

In June 1985, FDA assaulted Delaney head on. For the first time, the agency said that it would not ban a food additive (Red 3) that has been labeled a carcinogen by previous FDA officials and a federal cancer review committee. FDA Commissioner Frank Young maintained that during the time it would take to conduct and evaluate new studies the dye posed a negligible risk to consumers. Though the exact risk posed by Red 3 is unknown, it was crystal clear that the Reagan administration was effectively scuttling a law that was inconvenient to its business supporters. Whether the Administration succeeds will be decided in the courts over the next several years.

Perhaps the biggest crack in the barrier against dangerous food additives is FDA's lax interpretation of scientific studies. FDA usually moves excruciatingly slowly after learning that an additive may be harmful and sometimes bends over backward to accept a manufacturer's excuses as to why an additive should not be banned. The effects on the public's health of this practice are usually difficult to discern, because the effects of most chemicals would show up only years or decades later. An exception is sodium bisulfite, which has killed at least several persons, because of FDA's failure to act. If carcinogens expressed themselves as rapidly as bisulfite, FDA would be forced to act much more promptly.

Examples of FDA's slowness are legion:

- All food dyes were "provisionally" approved in 1960, pending further safety studies that were supposed to be completed in two and one-half years. In 1985 some of the dyes still had not been tested well enough to be permanently approved.

- In 1979 the committee reviewing "generally recognized as safe" (GRAS) additives advised FDA that the high levels of salt in food posed a health hazard and should be reduced. FDA asked companies to reduce sodium levels voluntarily, but did not initiate any regulatory actions that would achieve this.

- In 1977 the FDA proposed that the controversial preservative BHT be removed from the GRAS list and restricted to certain uses, pending further studies conducted by the manufacturers. Seven years later, that proposal was never finalized and the tests never conducted.

Besides being slow, FDA sometimes interprets studies in a way that endangers the public's health. Also, FDA has sometimes approved an additive or allowed the continued use of additives, even though few or no safety tests had been conducted. Consider these examples:

- Caffeine: even though it is generally acknowledged that caffeine poses a special risk to children, because of its druglike stimulatory effect on the brain, FDA continues to allow it in soda pop, the favorite drink of millions of children.

- Heptyl paraben: this preservative is specifically allowed in beer, but has never been tested on animals whose bodies were weakened by alcohol. (Twenty years ago a "safe" beer additive killed dozens of people, because it attacked alcohol-weakened hearts.)

- Methylene chloride: coffee processors began using this chemical to decaffeinate coffee, when trichloroethylene was found to cause cancer. FDA approved methylene chloride even though it had never undergone cancer studies and comes from the same chemical family (chlorinated hydrocarbons) as trichloroethylene and many other cancer-promoting agents.

- Blue 2: after the manufacturer reported to FDA that this dye caused an increased incidence of tumors in the brain and other organs of rats, FDA bent over backward to keep it in the food supply. FDA first appointed a special review committee, but this committee did not exonerate the dye, only saying that the evidence for brain tumors was "equivocal." FDA's own toxicologists and statisticians then conducted their own review and interpreted the data in ways that let Blue 2 off the hook.

At the same time that consumer groups were complaining about FDA's laxness, food companies were demanding that FDA be more lenient. The industry's prime target has been the anticancer Delaney Clause. The National Soft Drink Association and the American Meat Institute worked with Senator Orrin Hatch, a conservative Republican Senator from Utah, and drafted legislation that would have totally overhauled the food safety laws. This bill, submitted in 1981, would have replaced the flat-out ban on cancer-causing additives with a ban on only those additives that caused more than an "insignificant risk" of cancer. This change would have punched a giant loophole in the law, because nowhere was "insignificant risk" defined. It's one thing to tolerate a few errant molecules of a pesticide; it's quite another to allow large amounts of an additive that may cause hundreds or thousands of deaths a year. The legislation also would have accelerated the approval process of new additives, instituted several procedures that could extend the banning process for up to ten years, and required FDA to weigh purported health and economic benefits of an additive against its health risks. The latter measure—weighing risks against benefits—is an attractive one, but it is impossible to measure accurately either the risks or the benefits. The estimations depend largely on who is paying the statisticians and economists. As FDA toxicologist Robert Scheuplein has said, you can get "about any answer you want."[10]

The Hatch bill amounted to a "wish list" for industry and did absolutely nothing to make food safer for consumers. It was this very one-sidedness that doomed the bill. Consumer groups lobbied against the bills, and Senator Edward Kennedy and Congressman Henry Waxman blocked their passage in Congress.

Legislation never dies completely, though, and in 1983 Senator Hatch submitted a similar bill, but did not seem to be advocating it with much fervor. This bill also died in committee.

The food safety laws could use some revisions, though not necessarily of the type that Senator Hatch had in mind. The public would be significantly better protected if changes like the following were made:

- Additives in use prior to 1958 are now practically exempt from safety requirements. These "prior sanction" additives should be treated like any other additives. As a start, they should be subjected to safety reviews and retested when appropriate or banned.

- Once an additive has been approved, it is next to impossible to restrict or ban its use. Additives should be *licensed* for a period of ten years, rather than being approved permanently. At the end of the ten-year period, the license would be renewed if the testing of the additive met contemporary standards. If not, the chemical would be restricted or banned.

- Additives could conceivably impair intelligence, social skills, physical coordination, or other functions of the mind. Additives should be screened for effects on the central nervous system and on behavior.

- Additives should be tested in combination with other foods or chemicals with which they may interact in the diet. While every combination could not be tested, it would be feasible to test an additive both singly and in combination with a "cocktail" of caffeine, BHT, "the pill," aspirin, antihypertension medications, and other chemicals that are widely consumed. Additives should also be tested on animals whose bodies have been weakened by alcohol, diabetes, hypertension, and other relevant medical conditions.

- New additives should not be given permanent approval until their effects on humans have been evaluated. FDA's advisory committee on food additives (Select Committee on GRAS Substances, Federation of American Societies for Experimental Biology) has pointed out that with prospective additives being tested exclusively on animals, "no prediction of safety can be made with highest assurance unless accompanied with some confirmatory human experience." The committee recommended that temporary approval be followed by "a monitoring of any health complaints of consumers and appropriate epidemiological surveys with periodic reports to the FDA." The committee also suggested that lawmakers consider requiring carefully controlled human feeding studies before an additive is allowed into the food supply.[11]

These changes would address some of the real deficiencies in the current law. Needless to say, the companies that produce and use additives would lobby as strongly against legislation incorporating these changes as consumer groups lobbied against industry's bills.

While the legislative standoff continues, FDA will continue its plodding, reluctant regulation of additives. Consumer groups will continue to criticize FDA for allowing hazardous chemicals in our food. Industry will continue to complain that FDA is too slow in approving new additives and too quick in banning current additives. And scientists will continue to identify new risks associated with certain additives and from time to time dismiss old concerns. Meanwhile, the consumer is left in the grocery store wondering what is safe to eat and what is not. Therefore, let us now examine in detail the most commonly used additives, learn why they are used, and consider whether or not they are safe.

Notes

1. *Fed. Reg. 44,* 39858 (1979).
2. *Fed. Reg. 50,* 10371 (1985).
3. *Proc. Nat. Acad. Sci. (U.S.A.) 70,* 2281 (1973).
4. *Teratology 25,* 95 (1982).
5. "FDA Perspectives on the Use of Teratology Data in Human Risk Assessment," V. Frankos, speech, annual meeting of the Society of Toxicology, March 13, 1984.
6. *Scientist and Citizen 10,* 113 (June/July 1968).
7. *Fed. Reg. 49,* 46330 (1984).
8. *Fed. Proc. 25,* 137 (1966).
9. *Advances in Modern Toxicology,* ed. M. A. Mehlman, Hemisphere Publ., Washington, D.C. (1976), pp. 141–53.
10. *Food Chem. News,* p. 47 (April 29, 1985).
11. "Insights on Food Safety Evaluation," FASEB, Bethesda, Md. (Dec. 1982).

VI

A Close-up Look at Food Additives

The uses, abuses, and safety of the most widely used food additives are described in the following pages. Substances are listed in alphabetical order under their usual name. Some compounds, such as iodine and glutamic acid, are most frequently used as sodium, potassium, or calcium salts and are therefore listed as potassium iodide, monosodium glutamate, etc. Consult the index, if you have difficulty finding a certain additive.

Next to the heading for each additive is the word "Safe" or "Avoid" or a "?".

- "Safe" means that the additive has been reasonably well tested and appears to be safe for the general public. Nevertheless, a few individuals may be allergic to it, or large amounts may cause diarrhea or other transient problem.
- "Avoid" means that the additive has been very poorly tested or that some tests indicate a possible risk to the general population or a severe risk to sensitive individuals. As long as the government permits these additives, you should try to minimize your consumption of them.
- "?" means caution. Some additives so marked need to be better tested.

In other cases, many people consume too much of the additive, or some individuals may encounter a problem. Needless to say, these one-word summaries reflect a judgment that may emphasize a problem that clearly does not affect you or may downplay a problem that affects you very strongly, or that was rendered obsolete by new research. With but a stroke of your pen, you can adjust the author's views to conform to your own!

References to some of the more informative or recent resources are given for most additives. Abbreviations used in the references (except for scientific journals) are deciphered in the Bibliography. Additional articles may be located by referring to papers cited in these publications. The most recent scientific and medical papers can be found by using *Chemical Abstracts, Index Medicus,* and *Science Citation Index.* Actions taken by the Food and Drug Administration, as well as its trials and tribulations, are reported in the pages of the Washington *Post* and, even more exhaustively in *Food Chemical News,* an invaluable, weekly trade publication.

The cryptic numbers and letters at the end of many lists of references are a guide to the regulatory status of the additive. The combination beginning with 21 CFR, such as 21 CFR 74.203, refers to the official government listing of food additive regulations in Title 21 of the Code of Federal Regulations. Individual regulations list the foods in which the additive may be used and at what levels.

For explanations of scientific terms and food additive jargon, turn to the Glossary. The testing procedures referred to in the discussions of most additives were discussed in Chapter V and are summarized under *toxicity tests* in the Glossary.

Acesulfame-K   Approval Pending

The tremendous controversies over the safety of cyclamate, saccharin, and aspartame have spurred companies around the world to develop new, improved, noncaloric sweeteners. A German company, Hoechst, has developed acesulfame-K (also called acesulfame potassium; K is the chemical symbol for potassium), an inexpensive substance two hundred times sweeter than table sugar. Like saccharin, this chemical has a bitter aftertaste, so it must be used in combination with either sugar or aspartame to mask the bitterness.

Acesulfame-K has been subjected to more tests than practically any other food additive. It came through a battery of mutagenicity tests with flying colors. It also did not affect the action of various drugs. Nor did it cause cancer in mice. However, lung and mammary tumors occurred in two studies on rats. Though the manufacturer manipulates the data to downplay the significance of the tumors, it is dubious whether this chemical will ever be approved by the FDA. Another, unrelated question arose in a test on diabetic animals. Huge doses of the additive raised the animals' cholesterol levels by about 20 percent. Lower levels of the chemical were not, but should be, tested.

Despite the questions concerning cancer and cholesterol levels, the World Health Organization has given its stamp of approval to acesulfame-K. As of early 1985 the Food and Drug Administration had not approved acesulfame-K, though Great Britain allows it for all purposes and West Germany permits it as a tabletop sweetener.

Ref.: FAO(27); *Food Chem. News,* p. 34 (Nov. 5, 1984); FDA files.

Acetic Acid   Safe

Acetic acid is the substance that gives vinegar its sharp taste and odor. Manufacturers use it to preserve, flavor, or acidify foods.

Almost all of the billion pounds plus of acetic acid produced each year in the United States is produced chemically from alcohol and acetaldehyde. Much of this is used in manufacturing plastic; the food industry uses only a trivial amount.

Vinegar is produced by the bacterial fermentation of low-grade fruit and fruit by-products (apple cores, peels, etc.). Bacteria convert carbohydrate in the fruit first to alcohol and then to acetic acid.

Alcohol can also be converted to acetic acid by oxygen in air; acid produced in this way accounts for sour wine. Historical records show that mankind has been afflicted with this contretemps for at least five thousand years.

Ref.: ECT 8 386, *21* 254; *21* CFR 184.1005.

Acetone Peroxide   ?

Bakers have known for centuries that you cannot make good baked goods from freshly milled flour. Dough made from such flour lacks the strength and resilience needed to trap the gas bubbles that are produced by yeast, leavening, or whipping and that create fluffy, tender bread and cake. Until the twentieth century, bakers stored flour for months before using it, to let the oxygen in the air gradually condition the flour. However, at the same time the flour was aging, vermin would defile or devour part of it and another portion would spoil. To eliminate the costly and wasteful storage period, food chemists devised chemical methods that age flour almost instantaneously. Acetone peroxide is one of the newer of the chemical aging agents, but according to the American Institute of Baking it is rarely used. FDA estimates the total annual poundage consumed via food is 12,375 pounds. Like several other flour improvers, acetone peroxide bleaches the flour white in addition to aging it. This powerful oxidizing agent is a solid at room temperature and is used at levels of 5 to 120 parts per million (ppm), depending upon the flour.

Acetone peroxide has been tested on animals but not extensively. In one study, scientists fed four generations of rats bread or flour that had been treated with 450 ppm of this chemical. The treated food comprised 70 percent of the rats' diet. Pathologists did not detect tumors, birth defects, infertility, or tissue damage, but they did not examine the lungs or urinary bladder, two organs that frequently develop tumors. A lifetime feeding test involving at least one additional species, as well as careful tests for an ability to cause mutations and birth defects, must be conducted before we can consider acetone peroxide adequately tested.

Ref.: FAO (40A)-117; *Baker's Digest* 36 50 (1962); *Fd. Cos. Tox.* 5 309 (1967); *21* CFR 172.802.

Adipic Acid   Safe

Adipic acid is sometimes used as the acid in bottled drinks and throat lozenges. Because this additive has little tendency to pick up moisture, it may be used to supply tartness to powdered products, such as gelatin desserts and fruit-flavored drinks.

Adipic acid is occasionally added to edible oils to prevent them from going rancid. The acid's two negatively charged groups attract and trap positively charged metal ions, which may be present in the oil. Free metal ions promote chemical reactions that cause noxious odors and off-colors to develop.

Rats, and presumably humans, metabolize adipic acid without any difficulty. One small lifetime feeding study on rats indicated that moderate doses (1 percent of diet) are harmless.

Ref.: FAO(40A)-129; C&EN-117; CUFP-67; *21* CFR 184.1009.

Agar   Safe

Agar is a tasteless, odorless carbohydrate that is extracted from seaweed. Food manufacturers seldom use agar, but it is of great importance to microbiologists because it forms a stable gel that provides a good medium for growing cultures of microorganisms.

The natural source of agar is red algae, which grow off the coasts of Japan, Spain, and Southern California, ten to forty feet below the ocean's surface. The seaweed is harvested by hand by divers and then boiled in water. The boiling extracts the agar from the plant and when the water cools an agar gel forms. The gel is dried, and then the agar is ground to a powder. This is essentially the same purification scheme as was used in 1658 by the Japanese innkeeper who first discovered the gel-able constituent of seaweed.

The most important use of agar is as a solid support for growing bacteria. The idea of using agar in bacteriology was conceived in the nineteenth century by a German housewife. Her husband, a physician, had success with the technique and passed the idea along to Robert Koch, who proceeded to use it in

1882 to discover the bacterium that causes tuberculosis. Since that time agar gels have been standard equipment in microbiology laboratories.

Gels made from agar are tough and brittle compared to gels made of gelatin or carrageenan and do not "melt in the mouth," so they find little use in foods. However, agar is used in food at concentrations too low to form a gel. Its major use in the United States is in baking, where it prevents icings on cakes and cupcakes from drying out. It also serves as a stabilizer in ice cream, jam, and whipped cream.

Agar is nondigestible and swells greatly in water, suggesting another of its uses: as a bulk-type laxative.

Short- and long-term animal feeding studies on rats and mice, short-term animal experiments, and medicinal experience in humans all point to this seldom used additive's safety.

Ref.: FAO (35)-64; *ECT 17,* 763; *Fd. Chem. Toxicol. 21,* 305 (1983); *21* CFR 184.1115.

Alginates ?
(The ammonium, calcium, potassium, and sodium salts of alginic acid)

Alginic acid was first purified from brown algae in the late 1800s in England. In the seaweed, alginate constitutes an important part of the cell wall; as a food additive it acts as a thickening and stabilizing agent. The most important commercial source of algin is giant kelp, a seaweed that is "farmed" off the Southern California coast. Chemically, alginic acid consists of long polymers of mannuronic and guluronic acids.

Alginate solutions can be converted to gels by adding calcium. These chemically set gels are extremely stable, and while they do not possess that "melt in your mouth" texture, they help prevent jelly in pastries from oozing all over the oven. Industry also uses algin to help maintain the desired texture in ice cream, cheese, candy, pressure-dispensed whipped cream, yogurt, canned frosting, and other factory-made foods. Because alginate precipitates out of acidic foods, it cannot be used in salad dressings and soda pop.

The food that contains the most alginate is the cured, restructured pimiento ribbon used exclusively to stuff green olives. The red ribbon contains up to 6 percent sodium alginate.

Short-term feeding studies on animals have shown that alginate is not toxic. Alginate is not absorbed by the body, thus it probably does not cause cancer or birth defects, but until appropriate experiments are done, this chemical (and any impurities in it) cannot be pronounced safe. Like most other thickening agents, alginate binds a great deal of water in the gastro-intestinal tract and could inhibit the absorption of nutrients. This possibility deserves study.

In the early and middle 1960s Americans worried a great deal about radioactive fallout contaminating our food supply. Strontium 90 was particularly worrisome because it behaved much like calcium: it was present in milk and was deposited in bones and teeth. Scientists who were pessimistic—but perhaps realistic—enough to assume that radioactive fallout was going to be an unavoidable ingredient of modern life sought ways to minimize the hazard of fallout. Doctors working with alginate made the surprising discovery that the seaweed derivative had a much greater affinity for strontium than for other ions, including strontium's close relative calcium. When 1 percent algin was added to milk, the body's absorption of strontium was reduced by 75 percent while calcium absorption was decreased only 35 percent. Fortunately, the U.S.-Soviet ban on above-ground nuclear tests made further development of this discovery unnecessary.

Ref.: FAO (35)-68; FAO (46A)-135; *Can. Med. Asso. J. 99,* 986 (1968); "Kelco Algin" (Kelco Co., Chicago); *Fed. Reg. 47,* 29946, 47373 (July 9, 1982, October 26, 1982); *48* 52447 (November 18, 1983); *21* CFR 184.1011, 184.1133, 184.1187, 184.1610, 184.1724.

Alpha Tocopherol (Vitamin E)   Safe

Tocopherol is a vitamin, first discovered in 1923, that is abundant in wheat and rice germ and in vegetable oils. Americans' diets may be deficient in Vitamin E because little or none is present in white flour, enriched white bread, and enriched white rice. Because the biological effects of vitamin E are poorly understood, it is not known whether deficiencies actually exist and are causing adverse health consequences. Vegetable oil remains a good source of this vitamin, although approximately 25 percent is lost during typical commercial processing.

Both in nature and as a food additive, tocopherol acts as an antioxidant, preventing fats and oils from going rancid. It could replace many uses of BHA, BHT, and propyl gallate, three preservatives of questionable safety, but it is a bit more expensive, so is rarely used.

Occasional studies have indicated that vitamin E can alleviate the symptoms of heart disease, though other studies have found no benefit. Also, there are theoretical reasons to believe that this vitamin could slow the aging process. These glimmers of hope have led many people to consume huge amounts of vitamin E. Though the megadoses have not yet been proven to be beneficial (except for the treatment of rare diseases), at least they are relatively nontoxic, compared to two other fat-soluble vitamins, A and D.

Ref.: Am. J. Clin. Nutr. 17, 1 (1965); *Vitamin E Content of Foods and Feeds for Human and Animal Consumption,* Dicks, M. W., U. Wyoming, Laramie, Bulletin 435 (December 1965); *Agric. & Food Chem. 17,* 785 (1969); *Present Knowledge in Nutrition,* Nutr. Found. (1976); *Med. World News* p. 22 (May 2, 1977); *N. Engl. J. Med. 303,* 454 (1980); Recommended Dietary

Allowances, Nat. Acad. Sci. (1980); *New Engl. J. Med. 308*, 1063 (1983); *The Lancet i*, 225 (1983); *21* CFR 182.3890, 182.5890–182.5892, 184.1890.

Aluminum Compounds ?
(aluminum ammonium sulfate, aluminum potassium sulfate, aluminum sodium sulfate, aluminum sulfate, sodium aluminum phosphate, and other aluminum salts)

Aluminum is the third most abundant element on earth, so it is not surprising that many natural foods contain small amounts of this metal. Aluminum-containing food additives serve various functions in food. Sodium aluminum phosphate, a leavening agent, is the most widely used aluminum additive. It is attractive to bakers, because of its delayed action. It dissolves slowly in water, so if used in a cake mix, only 20 percent of the carbon dioxide gas is released during mixing, with the rest released during the actual baking. The same additive is used as an emulsifier in processed cheese. Consumers get moderate amounts of aluminum from additives, minuscule amounts of aluminum from cookware, and relatively huge amounts from certain antacids.

The human body absorbs only a small fraction of ingested aluminum, and most of this absorbed aluminum is excreted in the urine. Individuals with advanced kidney problems, however, do not excrete aluminum efficiently and should discuss with their doctors the desirability of avoiding aluminum-containing drugs and additives.

Aluminum additives have not been well tested for their potential to cause cancer. In 1975, Dr. Henry Schroeder, one of the pioneers of trace element nutrition and toxicology, published small studies on rats and mice. He found that male rats and both sexes of mice developed somewhat more tumors than expected. An FDA review committee used questionable reasoning to downplay the significance of the tumors. Considering the potential risk to the public, better studies should be conducted at once.

A variety of studies have linked aluminum to several forms of senility (Alzheimer's disease, parkinsonism dementia, dialysis encephalopathy). In regions of Japan, Guam, and New Guinea that are plagued with high incidences of senility, soil and drinking water have unusually high levels of aluminum. In a totally different line of research, numerous patients undergoing kidney dialysis displayed paranoia, delirium, confusion, and other symptoms, and soon died of brain damage. These patients had been consuming large amounts of aluminum-containing gels. Autopsies revealed concentrations of aluminum in their brains as much as tenfold higher than normal.

Aluminum, thought to be totally harmless until quite recently, may be contributing to mental deterioration, one of the saddest occurrences of old age. By far the greatest concern relates to aluminum-containing drugs. As more research is done, FDA may need to restrict the use of additives that contain aluminum, especially leavening agents, and provide guidelines for safely using aluminum cookware (such as not using it for salty, acidic, or alkaline foods).

Ref.: "Evaluation of the Health Aspects of Aluminum Compounds as Food Additives," Fed. Am. Soc. Exp. Biol. (1975); *J. Nutr. 105,* 421, 452 (1975); letter to FDA from Fed. Am. Soc. Exp. Biol. (Oct. 9, 1978); *Fd. Chem. Toxicol. 21,* 103 (1983); *21* CFR 182.1125–182.1131.

Ammoniated Glycyrrhizin ?

Licorice can be hazardous to your health. The medical literature describes twenty or thirty persons whose hearts began to fail when they ate several ounces of licorice candy a day for extended periods of time. One healthy fifty-three-year-old man developed congestive heart failure, hypertension, fatigue, edema, and headaches when he consumed twenty-four ounces of licorice in nine days. Symptoms disappear a week or two after the patients stopped eating licorice. The toxic agent in the candy is monoammonium glycyrrhizin, one of licorice's principal flavor components (0.5 percent).

Licorice is prepared from the roots of a small shrub that is cultivated in southern Europe and central Asia. Ammoniated glycyrrhizin is manufactured from root extracts. This chemical has a variety of physiological effects: it raises blood pressure, alleviates stomach ulcers, and reduces the toxicity of strychnine, carbolic acid, and diphtheria toxin. Food companies use it in licorice flavoring in beverages, candy, chewing gum, and baked goods. Glycyrrhizin is one of the sweetest natural substances known—one hundred times as sweet as sugar—so it is particularly useful when sweetness and licorice taste are both required.

Ammoniated glycyrrhizin is a fairly potent drug and should be tested for its ability to cause cancer, birth defects, and infertility. Its effect on children, who may consume enormous amounts of licorice, must be thoroughly investigated. As a minimal safety measure, packages of licorice candy should carry warnings against eating excessive amounts.

Ref.: J. Am. Med. Asso. 205, 492 (1968), *213,* 1343 (1970); *J. Pharm. Pharmacol. 15,* 500 (1963); *Chem. Abst. 63,* 1017c, 11933g. FASEB/SCOGS Report No. 28 (1977); *Fed. Reg. 48,* 54983 (Dec. 8, 1983); *21* CFR 184.1408.

Ammonium Compounds Safe
(Ammonium bicarbonate, ammonium carbonate, ammonium chloride, ammonium hydroxide, ammonium phosphate, ammonium sulfate, and other ammonium salts)

Salts of ammonium serve numerous purposes in food. Ammonium bicarbonate and ammonium hydroxide decrease the acidity. Ammonium chloride serves as a yeast food, providing needed nitrogen. Ammonium phosphate and ammonium sulfate are used as leavening agents.

Ammonium compounds are sources of ammonia, an important substance in the body. Much of the body's ammonia comes from amino acids. That ammonia is used in the synthesis of important nitrogen-containing compounds and to adjust the acidity of bodily fluids, with any excess converted to urea and excreted in the urine.

Few tests have been done to specifically test ammonium compounds as food additives, because ammonia is so widely available in natural forms. There is no reason to believe that these additives pose a risk, except for people with kidney or liver diseases.

Ref.: 21 CFR 182.1135–182.1141, 184.1143.

Amylases   Safe

Plant seeds contain rich reserves of nutrients that supply growing power until the plants can produce their own nutrients by photosynthesis. In cereal grains, energy is stored in the form of starch, which is broken down to sugar as the seeds germinate. The enzymes that convert starch to sugar are called amylases.

Plants contain two different kinds of amylases. Alpha-amylase attacks internal parts of starch molecules, creating new tips, while beta-amylase nibbles away at the tips. The large fragments of starch created by alpha-amylase are called dextrin. The small pieces generated by beta-amylase are called maltose, a close relative of sugar (sucrose). In addition to occurring in plant seeds, alpha-amylase is present in saliva, pancreatic juice, and microorganisms. Amylases, like all enzymes, are proteins and are safe.

Bakers add alpha-amylase to bread dough to supplement the small amount that the wheat flour naturally contains. The amylases convert a small fraction of the starch to sugar and dextrin as the oven's heat disrupts starch granules. The enzymatic action stops as the rising temperature in the oven destroys the enzymes. The sugar that the amylases produce serves as food for the fermenting yeast and also makes for better-tasting, better-toasting bread. The conversion of a portion of the starch to dextrin improves the dough's consistency and the bread's keeping quality.

Brewers use malt, which is simply germinated barley, to convert starch to sugars. Yeast then converts the sugar to alcohol. Malt is used instead of ungerminated grain because as a grain of wheat germinates, it develops huge quantities of alpha-amylase.

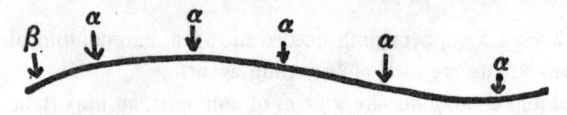

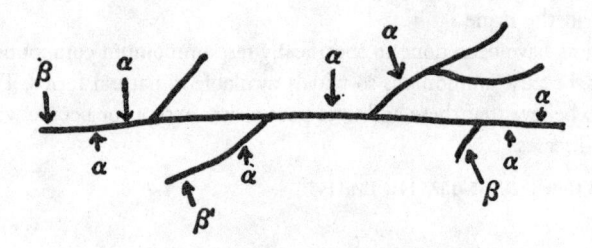

Amylase digestion of linear and branched starch molecules.

In another application amylases obtained from microorganisms are used to convert cornstarch to corn syrup or to dextrose.

Ref.: CRC-69-76.

Arabinogalactan (Larch gum) ?

Most natural compounds that manufacturers use to artificially thicken food are obtained from seaweed or from plants that grow in hot, arid climates. Larch gum is an exception. Producers obtain if from the Western Larch tree which is abundant in the northwestern United States. The gum can be collected by tapping trees, but more commonly it is extracted from wood chips because it is very soluble in water.

Like gum arabic, another very soluble gum, arabinogalactan forms thick solutions only at concentrations above 10 to 20 percent. Most other gums form thick solutions at concentrations of 1 percent or less. Only about one thousand pounds of arabinogalactan are used each year, primarily in dry soup mixes, gravies, and sauces.

Pure arabinogalactan is a carbohydrate consisting of galactose and arabinose in a ratio of six parts to one. Commercial preparations, however, contain significant amounts of tannic acid and other impurities.

As is true for most thickening agents obtained from natural sources, larch gum has been poorly tested. Small-scale, six-month studies on rats and dogs failed to reveal any toxic effects, but lifetime feeding, reproduction, and other tests need to be done before arabinogalactan can be certified safe. Nevertheless, the gum is probably harmless.

Ref.: TAPPI 46, 544 (1963); *Chem. Abst. 62,* 13759a, *66,* 77206, *70,* 106797; personal communication from FDA (summary of testing data); *Industrial Gums,* 2nd Ed., Ch. 18, editor: Whistler, R., Academic Press, N.Y. (1973); *21* CFR 172.610.

Artificial Coloring   Avoid

I. SYNTHETIC FOOD DYES

Natural foods contain pigments that do wonders for the attractiveness of a meal. Vegetables and fruits, especially, sparkle with almost every color in the rainbow. However, with the advent of factory-made foods, many of our meals would be drab affairs were it not for the generous use of food coloring. Imagine a meal with colorless cherry soda, gray frankfurters, colorless frozen lemon cream pies, pale raspberry sherbet, and off-white imitation pudding.

For thousands of years cooks have livened up their dishes with colorings derived from seeds, fruits, herbs, and even insects. While these natural products are still used as colorings, they have drawbacks such as fluctuations of supply and price, low coloring power, fading, and high cost. All of these difficulties were overcome—but not without the introduction of safety problems—when scientists discovered how to synthesize colored compounds from, of all things, coal.

Coal, when heated in the absence of air, is converted to coke (impure carbon), coal gas, and coal tar. The coal tar, a viscous black liquid, is a mixture of many organic compounds. In the 1800s, English and German chemists learned that they could produce intensely colored substances when they purified some of these compounds and reacted them with other chemicals. These synthetic substances are known as coal tar dyes and are used in great quantity by the food, fabric, and cosmetic industries. They are now produced from chemicals that are purer than coal tar, but they still contain many contaminants of questionable safety.

Americans are consuming food dyes at an increasingly rapid rate. According to the FDA, in 1940 251,000 pounds were certified* for use in foods, drugs, or cosmetics. In 1950 and 1961 the corresponding figures were 1,474,000 and 2,202,000 pounds. In 1971, slightly under 3.7 million pounds were certified by

---

* "Certified" means that a batch of coloring has been inspected and contains less than a certain level of impurities; certification does *not* mean that adequate toxicology studies have been conducted. Ingredient statements on labels that declare "U.S. certified food colors" are misleading, because they sound so authoritative and reassuring.

government inspectors. That figure jumped to 6,400,000 pounds in 1984.† On a per capita basis, food dye consumption has tripled since 1950 and risen 50 percent since 1971. This reflects the ever-increasing use of soda pop and other processed foods. Over 95 percent of these dyes are used in foods, particularly beverages, candy, ice cream, dessert powders, baked goods, and sausages. Levels used range from approximately ten parts to five hundred parts per million, the lower levels being used in liquid foods (beverages, gelatin desserts) and the higher levels in solid foods (breakfast cereals, snack foods).

Dyes frequently provide the only color in factory-made foods. In no case do they add to the nutritive value of the food. Rather, the presence of coloring in a food generally signals a deficiency or absence of natural and often nutritious ingredients whose colors the synthetic dyes seek to imitate.

A small, but good, example of how artificial colorings can be used to deceive consumers was furnished by the L. A. King Food Products Company, Denver, Colorado. *FDA Papers* (December 1970 and April 1971) reported that government inspectors caught that company adding two yellow food colorings (Yellow 5 and Yellow 6) to its Grandma's Fresh Frozen Egg Noodles to make the noodles look like they contained more egg than they did. Poor Grandma.

Manufacturers often use artificial coloring in candy, breakfast cereal, and pet food to create variety or eye appeal rather than to hide the absence of an ingredient or mimic a natural food. These rather frivolous uses of chemicals whose safety, as we shall see, is not of the highest repute are ill-considered and should be discontinued.

Processed food and chemical producers contend that dyes are important and that "legislation to ban food colorants would create a dilemma for our national nutrition program."‡ To arrive at this bizarre conclusion, industry spokespersons reason that food has to be attractive or people won't eat it. Many processed foods would go to waste, if they looked pale or ugly, and consumers might not get adequate nutrition. Someone ought to write to these food executives and remind them that foods like broccoli and brussels sprouts are still available in grocery stores.

At present seven synthetic dyes (Blues 1 and 2, Green 3, Reds 3 and 40, and Yellows 5 and 6) may be used in any food, and one, Citrus Red 2, is used only to color the skins of oranges. Orange B is allowed to color sausage casings, but is no longer manufactured.

People have been concerned about the possible toxicity of synthetic dyes ever since they were introduced in the late 1800s. These complex synthetic compounds were initially suspect because they are found nowhere in nature, and it

† These figures include both straight dyes and the dye portion of "lakes." Lakes are mixtures of the dyes with aluminum compounds and are used when insoluble colorings are needed, such as in certain candies, baked goods, and chewing gum.
‡ *Ref.:* Institute of Food Technologists' Expert Panel on Food Safety and Nutrition, *Food Tech.* p. 77 (July 1980).

was not clear how humans would react to them. In many cases, intuition has been backed up by scientific experiments, which showed that some dyes promote cancer. Repeatedly, colors approved for use in food have been shown to be toxic or carcinogenic and have been banned. The history of approved dyes reads like the guest register in a hotel for transients (see Table 2, p. 361–62).

In view of the frequent hazards associated with food dyes, one might assume that the dyes would have been thoroughly tested before being permitted in food. Such was not the case. The 1960 food coloring law states that new coloring agents must be proven safe *before* they may be used in food. Prior to 1960, a coloring could be added to foods until government proved that it was dangerous. For color additives already in use at the time the 1960 law was passed, provisional approval was granted for a period of two and a half years (until January 1963) to allow companies to complete any necessary safety tests. Then, FDA was to make a final determination as to whether the dyes should continue to be allowed in foods. The law included a clause that permitted the FDA to extend the two-and-a-half-year deadline for an indefinite period. And this is exactly what happened for many of the dyes in use in 1960: FDA extended the deadline more than a dozen times.

In 1977, Public Citizen Health Research Group (HRG) sued the FDA for violating the intent of the law. The government won this suit and kept on postponing decisions . . . as many as a total of twenty-seven times for several of the dyes. As the postponements tumbled forth, HRG told FDA, "The Reagan administration is making a mockery out of its alleged cancer reduction goals and is completely demoralizing dozens of FDA employees who know these dyes are too dangerous for continuous use by the public." Even a top FDA official, Sanford Miller, director of FDA's foods division, advised the commissioner, "We have already extended the provisional list so many times that we are in danger of losing both a lawsuit and our credibility as a regulatory agency." FDA's desire to ban several food and cosmetic dyes, including Red 3, was being stymied by FDA's parent, the Department of Health and Human Services, because of industry pressures.*

In June 1985 FDA rejected HRG's most recent petition to ban dyes that had been on the provisional list since 1960. This time, not only did FDA Commissioner Frank Young extend the deadlines for Red 3, Yellow 6, and several dyes not used in foods, but he became the first FDA commissioner to contend that the Delaney Clause did not apply to additives that cause just occasional tumors. In a letter to HRG director Dr. Sidney Wolfe, Young wrote:

> Yet, if the risk associated with a color is essentially negligible, there is no gain to the public [if the color is banned] . . .

* *Hearing*, House Committee on Government Operations, Subcommittee on Inter-Governmental Relations and Human Resources (Oct. 5, 1984).

Not only is this reasoning directly contrary to the law, but since "negligible" is nowhere defined, a risk that Commissioner Young or the food dye industry considered negligible might be completely unacceptable to a parent. FDA's decision marked the most serious assault yet on the Delaney Clause. Whether or not it is ultimately retained will depend first on the courts, then on Congress.

Most of the recent concern about food dyes has focused on their potential for causing cancer, but in the early 1970s a California allergist, Dr. Ben Feingold, startled the nation by claiming that dyes and other food additives were responsible for about half of all hyperactivity in children. The idea that additives might affect behavior was a shock not just to the public, but to food processors as well. Feingold was a tireless salesman for his theory. He published a book, *Why Your Child Is Hyperactive* (Random House, New York, 1975), appeared on countless talk shows, and organized parents of hyperactive children into a Feingold Association, which has dozens of local chapters. Thousands of parents swear by the Feingold diet and carefully choose foods that are free of dyes, certain preservatives, and sugar (not a bad diet for everyone!).

Government and industry (Nutrition Foundation) both sponsored studies to evaluate (and, they hoped, debunk) Feingold's hypothesis. Most of the tests involved feeding children dye hidden in capsules or foods and then having parents, teachers, and researchers evaluate their behavior. Critics of the Feingold diet contended that the studies showed that few or no children were affected by the dyes. Feingold and his supporters, however, said that most of the tests were inconclusive, because too little dye was used or because the dye was not mixed with other chemicals that a child might consume. One study, conducted by Bernard Weiss and Sheldon Margen at the University of California, Berkeley, was especially interesting. This study tested children whose parents said they were hyperactive.[†] Most of the participants did not appear to be affected by the dye. But one little girl was clearly affected. This child's sensitivity proved that additives could affect behavior, even if the problem is not as widespread as Feingold claimed.[‡]

Though Feingold did not convince the medical community that additives were a major cause of hyperactivity, he did accomplish two important things: everyone is now aware of the possibility that additives can affect behavior, and many companies voluntarily reduced their use of colorings and preservatives.

The listing of dyes on food labels is as inadequate as the testing some of the chemicals have undergone. Coloring in butter, cheese, and ice cream need not be specified at all, due to an exemption in the 1938 labeling law won by the dairy industry. In other foods, except for Yellow 5, colorings are never identi-

[†] *Science 207*, 1487 (1980).
[‡] *Ref.:* "Defined Diets and Childhood Hyperactivity," NIH Consensus Development Conference Summary *4* (3) (1982).

fied specifically (Blue 1, Green 3), but only as "artificial coloring." This is a great inconvenience to persons—such as sufferers of allergies or people who believe that a dye is poorly tested or dangerous—who want to avoid certain colorings. Because of the vague labeling, a person who is allergic to one food coloring may have to avoid all foods containing any artificial coloring. Allergists (and their patients) have urged that all food additives including colorings be specifically identified on all food products. Dr. F. H. Chafee, a physician at the Rhode Island Hospital in Providence, has pleaded for complete labeling:

> It is difficult for the average physician, and nigh impossible for the patient, to obtain this information. It would be far easier for the physician, let alone the patient sensitive to these chemicals, if the FDA were to require listing of the dyes on the package . . . Required listing of these dyes on drug and food packages might be lifesaving.

Congress has considered legislation that would require food dyes to be identified on labels, but food industry lobbying prevented passage.

Let us now examine each of the food dyes in more detail.

Blue 1 (Brilliant Blue FCF)   Avoid

This synthetic food coloring is used primarily in beverages, candy, baked goods, as well as a variety of other blue-tinted foods. The FDA certified 260,417 pounds in 1984.

Blue 1 was the subject of several small studies in the 1950s and 1960s. The dye is poorly absorbed in the intestinal tract and was long thought to be harmless. However, as larger studies were done in the past decade, some real questions arose. In one study, the dye appeared to increase the incidence of kidney tumors in male mice. The largest study on rats, conducted for the Certified Color Manufacturers' Association, indicated that the dye promoted breast tumors. But the sponsors reexamined their data and discovered two tumor-free rats that were inadvertently forgotten. When these animals were included in the analysis, the presence of tumors was no longer statistically significant. Industry, therefore, claims that the dye is safe. Until additional, more sensitive studies are done, a cloud of doubt will hang over Blue 1.

One study on rats indicated that the dye did not interfere with reproduction, but at least one other species should also be tested.

Ref.: WHO, *IARC Monographs 16,* 171 (1978); *Food Chem. News,* p. 20 (Dec. 14, 1981); *21* CFR 74.101.

Blue 2 (Indigotine)   Avoid

When the 1960 food coloring law went into effect, Blue 2, like other dyes, was only "provisionally" approved. This meant that the dye industry had to conduct additional tests. Twenty years (!) later, in 1981, the tests were finally completed. Not surprisingly, considering that so many other food dyes have proven unsafe, the tests indicated problems.

Bio-Dynamics Inc., which conducted the tests, reported that large amounts of Blue 2 increased the incidence of malignant brain gliomas, mammary cancers, and urinary bladder tumors, all in male rats. Female rats and both sexes of mice were apparently unaffected.

Dr. Samuel Epstein, a University of Illinois (Chicago) cancer expert who has long advocated tighter controls over cancer-causing agents, examined the animal data and concluded that they "unequivocally demonstrate that FD&C Blue 2 is carcinogenic." In September 1982, Public Citizen Health Research Group asked FDA to "ban this useless but dangerous dye immediately."

Ronald W. Moch, an FDA pathologist, also examined the data and in July 1982 wrote a cautious memo indicating his concern:

> "Although it is not possible for us to state categorically that FD&C Blue No. 2 is a brain carcinogen . . . the possibility cannot be excluded . . ."

Moch was dubious about the urinary bladder tumors and concluded that the dye did not cause breast tumors.

The FDA convened a Board of Scientific Counselors to review the data. The Board concurred with FDA that the dye did not cause mammary or urinary bladder tumors, but concluded that the data on brain tumors were equivocal. The FDA, apparently determined to exonerate this dye, took it upon itself to analyze additional tissue samples. After this was done, FDA officials said that the brain tumors were probably a statistical fluke and not caused by Blue 2. FDA then proposed that the dye be permanently approved.

Health Research Group, with its customary perseverance, contended that FDA's approval was illegal and continued to press for a ban. HRG argued that the law requires industry to prove that a color is safe before it can be permanently approved. The apparent increase in brain tumors, even if only equivocal, certainly did not achieve the high standard set by the law. HRG also maintained that the cancer study was irreparably flawed, because the test animals were not fed high enough levels of dye. FDA held a judicial-like hearing, with HRG on one side and FDA and its industry allies on the other. FDA's administrative law judge, Daniel Davidson, ruled that "Blue No. 2 has been shown to be safe to a reasonable certainty," and endorsed FDA's decision to approve the dye. In March 1985 HRG's attorneys William Schultz and Katherine Meyer appealed the judge's decision. Assuming that the FDA commissioner rejects the appeal, HRG may probably then go to court.

The FDA may consider the evidence about Blue 2 too weak to support a ban, but this does not mean that you should not try to avoid Blue 2. The dye tints candy, beverages, and baked goods, as well as such vital products as pet foods and mouthwashes. Approximately 101,000 pounds of this dye were approved for use in 1984.

Ref.: Health Research Group letter to FDA, Sept. 23, 1982; *Fed. Reg. 47,* 49637 (Nov. 2, 1982), *48,* 5252 (Feb. 4, 1983); unpublished studies in FDA files; FDA Hearing, Docket No. 83N-0009; *21* CFR 74.102.

Citus Red 2 — Avoid

Florida citrus growers use Citrus Red 2 the dye, mainly from October through December, to cover up a green or yellow color on oranges, tangelos, and temple oranges. Occasionally, Valencia oranges, which mature in the late spring, are also colored. In 1980–81, the Florida Department of Agriculture reported that 45 percent of fresh oranges, tangelos, and temple oranges were "color added." Many Florida growers fear that if they did not use the dye they would lose sales to California oranges, which have a natural, uniformly orange color, thanks to cool nights. An orange may contain dye at levels up to two parts per million. The dye is almost entirely on the outside of the fruit. No more than a few thousand pounds of Citrus Red 2 are used annually.

Feeding studies on mice and rats have indicated that large amounts of dye promote bladder cancer. The FAO/WHO Expert Committee issued the following warning at its 1969 meeting:

> Citrus Red 2 has been shown to have carcinogenic activity and the toxicological data available were inadequate to allow the determination of a safe limit, the Committee therefore recommends that it should not be used as a food color.

The International Agency for Research on Cancer has concluded that "Citrus Red 2 is carcinogenic in rats and mice." Consumers incur a minuscule risk if they eat or suck the peel of treated oranges or use the peel in marmalade. Unfortunately, oranges are no longer individually stamped "color added" so it is difficult to identify treated oranges. When oranges are not stamped, supermarkets are supposed to post signs saying "artificially colored." FDA administrators in Washington admit that grocers from one end of the country to the other are ignoring FDA's regulations, but plead that they have too little manpower to stop this minor infraction. Workers who produce Citrus Red 2 and who dye the oranges may ingest or inhale relatively large amounts of the chemical. They would be exposed to a proportionately greater hazard than the average consumer.

The Food and Drug Administration should ban this suspicious chemical or, at the very least, enforce the law requiring "color added" fruit to be clearly labeled.

Ref.: FAO (46A)-30; *J. Pharm. Exp. Ther. 134,* 100 (1961); *Proc. Univ. Otago Med. Sch. 43,* 31 (1965); *Fd. Cos. Tox. 4,* 455, 493, (1966); *Br. J. Cancer 22,* 825 (1968); *New Zealand Med. J. 73,* 74 (1971); *IARC 8,* 101 (1975); letter from FDA Commissioner A. Schmidt to CSPI (June 25, 1976); *21* CFR 74.302.

Green 3 (Fast Green FCF)   Avoid

Green 3 is one of the least used food colorings and provides an example of how studies that everyone hoped would provide unequivocal results oftentimes yield findings that are open to different interpretations.

In 1981, after years of procrastinating, industry finally completed a thorough test of Green 3. The initial results did not look good. Dr. Mark Nicolich, the statistician who analyzed the study sponsored by the Certified Color Manufacturers' Association, reported that "there is statistical evidence that the high dose of the test material increases the occurrence of certain types of tumors in rats." The tumors occurred in the urinary bladder, liver, testes, and thyroid of males. No increase occurred in mice.

The dye manufacturers, concerned about the apparent ability of Green 3 to promote cancer, hired a consultant to review the data. He concluded that certain tissues had been erroneously classified as being cancerous. The FDA then examined both the data and the original microscope slides. FDA concluded that industry had overestimated the risk associated with the dye by interpreting bladder tissue samples incorrectly and using incorrect statistical tests on the liver and thyroid results. After FDA's reanalysis, increases in tumor rates changed from being statistically significant to only borderline significance. With regard to the testicular tumors, FDA concluded that the doubling in the tumor rate between animals fed 5 percent dye and the controls was due to a freakishly low rate of tumors in the controls. So, in November 1982, FDA gave its official blessing to Green 3.

The test results on Green 3 do not provide great assurance of safety, but neither are they clearly damning. I think there is enough smoke that there just might be a fire, and I recommend avoiding the dye. Because this and most other dyes are not listed specifically on labels, the only way to be sure of avoiding Green 3 is to avoid all artificially colored foods. Considering the problems related to other dyes, this is a sensible practice even if Green 3 turns out to be safe.

Only 3,600 pounds of Green 3, which actually has an aqua blue hue, were certified by FDA for use in foods in 1984. It is used in candy, beverages, dessert powders, and ice cream.

Ref.: Fd. Chem. News, Nov. 23, 1981, p. 9; *Fed. Reg. 47,* 52140 (Nov. 19, 1982), *48,* 6329 (Feb. 11, 1983); *21* CFR 74.203.

Orange B   Not Used

Meatpackers in the southeastern United States sometimes coated the outside of hot dogs with a red coloring. One food coloring, Orange B, was used solely for that purpose. Each year, ten to twenty tons of the dye would brighten up the products that Ralph Nader dubbed "fatfurters."

Orange B had never been well tested. For instance, in studies conducted by Dr. John Doull at the University of Chicago, tissues from fewer than 13 percent of the animals tested were examined microscopically. In February 1976, the Center for Science in the Public Interest asked FDA to outlaw the coloring, unless better tests were done. CSPI pointed out that one metabolite of Orange B is identical to a metabolite of Red 2, which FDA had banned because it increased the risk of cancer. A second metabolite was identical to a metabolite of Yellow 5, which can cause allergic reactions.

In January 1978, Stange Co., the one producer of Orange B, told FDA that the dye was contaminated with tiny amounts of beta-naphthylamine, a known carcinogen. In April, Stange told its customers that rather than producing a purer product, it was ceasing production.

FDA has proposed a ban on Orange B, but has never finalized it, so another company could produce and market it. Needless to say, FDA should complete its action and get rid of the poorly tested, contaminated dye once and for all.

Ref.: J. Pharm. Exp. Ther. 116, 26 (1956); *Food Chem. News,* p. 21 (Oct. 9, 1978); *21* CFR 74.250.

Red 3 (Erythrosine)   Avoid

FDA officials agree that Red 3 dye causes cancer, but, because of political pressures, have not banned it.

In 1982 the food coloring industry's own tests indicated that Red 3 caused thyroid tumors in male rats. While FDA planned to allow the dye's "provisional" approval to expire, companies commenced a battle to save the dye. They said that maybe a contaminant and not the dye itself was the problem, but eventually admitted that this could not be proven. Then they maintained that the dye was too weak a carcinogen to worry about, but FDA scientists dismissed their evidence as shoddy. Next the companies suggested that the tumors were caused by hormonal imbalances caused by huge doses of Red 3, but would not occur at low doses. Amid these industry pleas, an FDA attorney held that the dye would have to be banned or HHS would risk "a lawsuit that the agency almost certainly will lose."

Industry officials leapfrogged their bureaucratic nemeses by going to higher-ups in HHS and the White House. They got the delays they wanted. First, HHS gave the dye a reprieve for the "sole purpose" of allowing the National Toxicology Program (NTP), a government agency that specializes in evaluating cancer tests, to conduct a special review. In short order, the NTP found "convincing evidence" that the dye causes cancer in animals. In November 1983 FDA itself officially concluded that Red 3 is a carcinogen.

But, as it is wont to do when profits are jeopardized, industry maintained its vigorous fight, with assistance from its White House allies whose sympathy for business interests outweighed any concerns for the public health or legislative mandates. They called for more reviews and more delays. In March 1984 the acting commissioner of FDA, Mark Novitch, urged HHS to ban the dye, saying:

> The agency should not knowingly allow continued exposure (at high levels in the case of FD&C Red No. 3) of the public to a provisionally listed color additive that has clearly been shown to induce cancer while questions of mechanism of action are explored . . . [T]he credibility of the agency and the Department would suffer if decisions are not made soon . . .

After still more delays, in November 1984 Sanford Miller, director of FDA's food division, wrote to FDA Commissioner Frank Young:

> In our judgment we have already extended the provisional list so many times for such tenuous reasons that we are in danger of losing both a lawsuit and our credibility as a regulatory agency.

Rarely has it been more self-evident that calls for more scientific tests and reviews reflect not a desire to gain crucial information, but simply a ruse to allow companies to profit while unwitting consumers suffer an increased risk of cancer.

In October 1984 a subcommittee of the House Committee on Government Operations conducted a detailed investigation into why FDA was not banning cancer-causing dyes. In its official report, the committee, whose investigation was directed by New York Representative Ted Weiss, concluded that Commissioner Young "completely misunderstands his and the Department's responsibilities under the law." The committee held that the effect of HHS's repeated demands for unnecessary reviews was "to subvert, if not completely paralyze, enforcement of the Nation's public health and safety laws." The legislators concluded unanimously that the Department of Health and Human Services had violated federal law by refusing to ban Red 3 and five other colorings. (Republican legislators added, though, that the law should be weakened.)

Ohio Congressman Edward Feighan introduced legislation to ban Red 3 and other apparently carcinogenic dyes. On the other hand, the Department of Agriculture, eight U.S. senators, and several representatives were lobbying for the continued use of the dyes. These parties' interest was spurred by cherry growers and the canned fruit cocktail industry. Red 3 is what gives those fruit cocktail cherries their color; other red colorings "bleed" onto other fruits (horrors!). Red 3 is also used to color pistachio. The dye's original purpose was to mask the blemishes in Iranian pistachios. Now, however, with California growers providing higher quality pistachios, the dye serves no purpose other than to meet consumers' expectations that pistachio nuts look like the dyed Iranian nuts.

In June 1985 FDA granted industry yet one more year—and possibly five additional years after that—to try to exonerate Red 3 of carcinogenicity or other form of toxicity. FDA officials (other than Commissioner Young) were reported to be totally demoralized over their inability to ban a chemical that is an acknowledged carcinogen. As one observer put it, FDA officials feel that if they can't ban Red 3, they can't do anything.

As much as any other food additive controversy, the battle of Red 3 demonstrates how government has turned the law on its head: instead of outlawing the dye until it is proven safe, the Reagan administration is insuring that consumers will be ingesting the probable carcinogen for years to come.

Even before Red 3 was found to be a carcinogen, scientists were concerned about it for other reasons. In August 1979 the official newsletter of the National Institutes of Health was headlined "Red Dye No. 3 May Affect Brain, Research Shows." The studies suggested that the dye might enter brain tissue and interfere with the uptake of dopamine, a neurotransmitter. If this phenomenon occurs in humans—and that is a big if—the dye could be responsible for learning disabilities in some children.

Scientists at FDA have expressed concern about this dye's iodine content. Many years ago iodine *deficiency* was a problem in certain regions of the United States. But now salt is iodized, many processed foods contain iodized salt, iodine-containing sterilants are used in milk handling, and people in iodine-poor regions are not dependent on locally grown foods. We are getting plenty of iodine and *iodine excess* may be a bigger problem than iodine deficiency. Too much iodine can cause goiter and other thyroid problems. It is unlikely, though, that Red 3 is the primary culprit. Even though iodine accounts for 58 percent of the dye's weight, less than 5 percent is absorbed by the body, according to FDA nutritionist John Vanderveen.

The controversy surrounding Red 3 has spurred smart food manufacturers to switch from Red 3 to other dyes. In 1984 FDA certified only 211,000 pounds of the dye, down from 464,000 pounds the previous year.

Ref.: J. Pharm. Exp. Ther. 137, 141 (1962); *Tox. Appl. Pharm. 17,* 300 (1970); *J. Am. Med. Asso. 242,* 453 (1979); "NIH Record" (Aug. 21, 1979); *Science 207,* 535 (1980); *Food Chem. News* p. 3 (Oct. 11, 1982), p. 50 (Oct. 31, 1983), p. 40 (Feb. 27, 1984), p. 40 (Jan. 14, 1985); *Eleventh Report,* House Committee on Government Operations (June 3, 1985); *The New York Times,* p. C1 (Feb. 13, 1985); *21* CFR 74.303.

Red 40 (Allura Red AC)   ?

If you ever eat artificially colored red, orange, brown, or purple foods, the chances are you consume Red 40. Though it was originally conceived of as a possible replacement for Red 4, which was used only in maraschino cherries, Red 40 proved popular with many food processors. Then, in the early 1970s when Red dyes 2 and 4 were first the subject of controversy and then banned in 1976, Red 40 became the most widely used dye in our food supply. In 1984 Americans consumed about 2.6 million pounds of the dye in candies, cherries, ice cream, soft drinks, baked goods, desserts, and other foods.

Red 40, itself, has been the subject of a controversy, which provides insight into how additives are regulated and into limitations of animal tests.

FDA approved Red 40 in 1971 on the basis of tests that were quite good in one regard, but inexcusably deficient in another. Red 40 was one of the first additives tested for effects on animal reproduction before being used in food. No problems were found. The dye was also tested for cancer-causing properties in rats. Again, no problems were found. However, it was not tested on mice, despite guidelines stipulating that food additives should be tested in at least two species—usually mice and rats. FDA figured that because only a few thousand pounds a year of the dye were going to be used in just a couple of foods, more stringent tests were not necessary.

In early 1976 enormous amounts of the dye were being consumed. Because the original tests had been so inadequate and geared to a rarely used additive, the Center for Science in the Public Interest petitioned FDA on February 25, 1976, to revoke approval of the dye. Unbeknownst to us, on the very day we wrote to FDA, Allied Chemical, which produced the dye, told FDA that at the ten-month mark of a new two-year study, it looked like the dye was causing cancer in mice. Seeing the results, Dr. Adrian Gross, a top FDA pathologist (now working at the Environmental Protection Agency), said Red 40 had "all the properties of a known carcinogen." Allied had undertaken the new study because the British and Canadian governments would not approve the dye without additional tests.

Needless to say, Allied's call sent FDA officials into a tizzy. FDA ordered Hazleton Laboratories, which was conducting the mouse study, to sacrifice and examine an additional group of animals. This turned out to be a big mistake, because little could have been learned from this "interim sacrifice," but the action reduced the total number of animals exposed to the dye for two years and greatly weakened the ultimate strength of the study. Gross called the sacrifice "unwise, unnecessary, and inept." At this point in the study, the dye seemed to be increasing the number of tumors in lymph glands. In May 1976 FDA informed Coca-Cola Export Corp. that ". . . the lymphomas appeared to be related to the ingestion of the color." If the dye was causing the tumors, it would have to be banned.

As the study proceeded, though, the animals not consuming the dye (the controls) developed lymphomas. At the end of the two-year study, both the controls and the experimentals had about the same number of tumors. The argument boiled down to whether the dye caused tumors to develop earlier than they otherwise would have. Early development of tumors is considered a sign of carcinogenicity.

Once tumors started showing up in the mice, FDA asked Allied to sponsor a second mouse study, using more animals and more care. Whatever the final interpretation of the first study, conducting the second one insured that a final decision would not be made for at least three years, during which time millions of people would be consuming the dye.

FDA's Dr. Gross, who was viewed within the agency as a consumer-oriented extremist, argued that in the first mouse study the dye was accelerating tumor formation. Other FDAers said "no problem." To resolve the dispute, FDA convened a working group of government toxicologists, statisticians, and cancer experts. FDA also sought the advice of several leading nongovernment statisticians, who reviewed and analyzed both studies. The statisticians acknowledged the ambiguity of the results of the first mouse study. In the end, though, they generally agreed that the evidence was not adequate to prove that the dye caused tumors to form earlier than in unexposed animals. Deciding whether the dye promoted cancer was a close call that ultimately boiled down to statistical analyses of almost unprecedented complexity.

The second study seemed to go without a hitch—until the results were analyzed. There were two ostensibly identical groups of control animals. These groups should have had approximately equal numbers of spontaneous tumors. In fact, though, they had very different numbers of tumors. Furthermore, among animals exposed to the dye, the largest number of tumors occurred in the low dosage group, and smallest number of tumors occurred in the high dosage group. Whether this effect was real, a statistical fluke, or a reflection of a snafu at Hazleton Labs was anyone's guess. Also, according to two Harvard statisticians who were acting as consultants for FDA, there was again an indication that the dye was causing tumors to form earlier than they otherwise would have.

FDA ended up explaining away the discrepancy between the two control groups by citing careless laboratory methods. Normally the animals' cages are rotated from one position to another. In the Red 40 study, however, the cages stayed in the same spot for two years. FDA suggested that perhaps being closer to the ceiling, as one group of controls was, might increase the cancer risk, because of exposure to the fluorescent lights or some other unknown factor.

After five years of debate, in October 1981, FDA officially cleared Red 40. FDA acknowledged that there was evidence of a problem, but that the evidence was not always "consistent" and that there was "no substantial question of safety."

Once an additive is allowed, the law can be interpreted to require the government to have very clear and consistent evidence of harm before banning it. The evidence on Red 40 was clearly mixed, and perhaps in an ideal world it would not be used. Until this utopia arrives, those concerned about this dye will have to make a personal effort to banish it from their little corner of the world.

Ref.: FDA files; *Fed. Reg. 46,* 51037 (Oct. 16, 1981); *21* CFR 74.340.

Yellow 5 (Tartrazine)   Aspirin-sensitive people: Avoid

After Red 40, Yellow 5 is the most widely used artificial coloring in processed foods. About 1.6 million pounds of this chemical were approved for use in 1984.

While Yellow 5 is not suspected of causing cancer or birth defects (though it does belong to the suspicious family of chemicals called azo dyes), it does cause allergic reactions in some people. Asthma, hives, and a runny or stuffy nose are the most common reactions, though occasional, more severe reactions have also been reported. For some reason, most of those who have been found to be sensitive to the dye are also sensitive to aspirin. The Food and Drug Administration has estimated that between 47,000 and 94,000 people are sensitive to the dye.

The first evidence that tartrazine causes allergic reactions was published in 1959 by Dr. Stephen Lockey, a Pennsylvania allergist who has long been concerned about additives in foods and drugs. The evidence began piling higher through the 1960s and early 1970s. Only in July 1981, did FDA require that ingredient listings disclose the presence of Yellow 5, instead of just stating "artificial coloring," so that sensitive people could avoid the dye. Meanwhile, many consumers are wondering why *each* of the synthetic food dyes should not be listed on the label. And other consumers wonder why Yellow 5, which adds nothing to the nutritional value of a food, is not banned completely, as it is in Sweden and Norway. Colorings obtained from turmeric and annatto can be used in place of Yellow 5.

Ref.: FAO (38B)-88; *Tox. Appl. Pharm.*, 6, 621 (1964); *Fd. Cos. Tox.* 7, 287 (1969); *Fed. Reg.* 42, 6835 (1977), 44 37212 (1979); 21 CFR 74.705.

Yellow 6 (Sunset Yellow FCF)   Avoid

Yellow 6 is the third most widely used dye. It has more of an orange tint, compared to the true yellow of Yellow 5.

Government and industry sponsored lifetime feeding studies in the late 1970s and early 1980s, respectively, because the dye is so widely used and because earlier studies were considered "less than adequate," though they did not indicate any problems. Furthermore, Yellow 6 belongs to the "azo" family of dyes, several of which have proven harmful.

The government studies on rats and mice gave Yellow 6 coloring a clean bill of health, except for one small indication of liver cancers in the mice. The scientists who reviewed the study concluded that the apparent increase in liver cancer was more likely a random statistical fluke than an effect of the dye. They noted that the strain of mouse used frequently developed liver tumors spontaneously.

The industry-sponsored study, still being analyzed in 1985, suggested a problem in female rats. According to an FDA memo, agency scientists had a "concern over the occurrence of kidney tumors in the female groups . . ." Tumors were also showing up in adrenal glands. The tumors could be due to the dye itself or to the half-dozen carcinogenic contaminants that FDA has acknowledged are present in commercial batches of the dye.

More than 1.5 million pounds of Yellow 6 dye were certified for use in 1984. Most of the billions of pounds of foods in which the dye was used possessed relatively little in the way of nutritional worth.

Ref.: National Toxicology Program, Technical Report Series No. 208 (U.S. National Institutes of Health), May, 1981; *Food Chem. News,* p. 3 (May 28, 1984), p. 21 (July 2, 1984), p. 19 (Oct. 1, 1984); *Eleventh Report,* p. 6, House Comm. on Gov. Operations (June 3, 1985); 21 CFR 81.10.

II. NATURAL FOOD COLORINGS   ?

Artificial colorings derived from plants, insects, and minerals were used in food long before coal tar dyes were developed. Currently they account for only about 5 percent of the artificial food coloring used in the United States. Table 1 (pages 235–36) lists the natural food colorings currently approved by the FDA.

Most of the natural colorings have not undergone detailed chemical analysis or biological testing. The extracts of herbs (turmeric, annatto, tagetes, and others) and substances processed at high temperatures (caramel, toasted cottonseed flour) should have the highest priority for testing. As an example of the minimal testing these colorings have undergone, the only test on carmine, a complex organic molecule that comprises 10 percent of cochineal extract (made from a colorful insect), is an old three-month study on rats. Such a study says little about the chemical's safety. About 2,000 pounds of cochineal extract are used annually, according to FDA data. Canthaxanthin, a 64-pound-per-year coloring, is just as poorly tested. Annatto, which is widely used in butter and cheese (630,000 pounds per year), has never been studied for longer than one year. There is no evidence to suggest that any of these substances is harmful, but the mere fact that they were obtained from a natural source should not exempt them from safety tests.

Sodium nitrite and nitrate, which contribute to the red or pink color of bacon, ham, hot dogs, and luncheon meat, are considered preservatives, not artificial colorings. These chemicals are described in separate entries in this book.

The one coloring that you should not worry about—except whether you get enough of it—is beta-carotene, which is discussed in a separate entry. The body converts beta-carotene to vitamin A. Beta-carotene serves as a coloring and nutrient in margarine and other foods.

Ref.: Food Eng., May 1977, p. 66.

Artificial Flavoring   ?

Flavorings comprise one of the most important classes of food additives, because they are able to replace, or mask the absence of, expensive natural products and to improve the taste of manufactured foods. A measure of their importance and variety is the fact that about 1,500 chemicals—two thirds of all food additives used in the United States are natural or synthetic flavorings. Despite this large number, the average person consumes only an ounce or less of artificial flavorings over the course of a year.

If you notice that a food contains "artificial flavoring," you can generally assume that the food contains little or none of the ingredient that would normally supply the flavor. For instance, some brands of strawberry yogurt derive their flavor from real strawberries, while others are based on artificial strawberry flavoring. The peach ice cream that you make at home contains peaches; most commercial peach ice cream contains imitation peach flavoring. Substituting artificial flavorings for traditional sources of flavor does permit lower prices or higher profits, but many consumers believe that it also constitutes adulteration.

Natural flavors are produced by the combined effect of tens or even hundreds of different chemicals, although frequently the taste of one or two

TABLE 1. Food Colorings (other than coal tar dyes)*

Substance	Source	Color	Restrictions on Use
dried algal meal	algae (*Spongiococcum*)	yellow	in chicken feed to enhance the yellow color of skin and eggs
beta-apo-8'-carotenal	synthetic (or plants)‡	yellow to red	15 milligrams per pound
caramel †	heated carbohydrate	dark brown	—
beta-carotene † (provitamin A)	synthetic (or plants)‡	yellow	—
annatto extract	seeds from annatto, a tropical tree	yellowish red	—
tagetes (Aztec marigold) meal	*Tagetes* flower petals	yellow	in chicken feed to enhance the yellow color of skin and eggs
paprika (oleoresin)	ground dried pod of *Capsicum*, a sweet pepper	reddish orange	—
turmeric (oleoresin)	ground rhizome of *Curcuma*, an East Indian herb	yellow	—
saffron	dried stigma of *Crocus* plant	deep orange	—
fruit juice			—
vegetable juice			—
toasted partially defatted cooked cottonseed flour	cottonseed	brown	—

(continued)

TABLE 1. Food Colorings (other than coal tar dyes)* *(continued)*

Substance	Source	Color	Restrictions on Use
titanium dioxide †	synthetic	white	up to 1 percent in food
cochineal extract (carmine)	dried body of cochineal insect	red	—
grape skin extract	grape	purple red	coloring of beverages
grape color extract	Concord grape	purple red	for use in nonbeverage foods
ultramarine blue	synthetic $Na_7Al_6Si_6O_{24}S_3$	blue	coloring salt for animal feed (up to 0.5 percent)
ferrous gluconate †	synthetic	develops black color	coloring of ripe (black) olives
dehydrated beets	beets	dark red	—
corn endosperm oil	yellow corn grain	reddish brown	in chicken feed to enhance the yellow color of skin and eggs
riboflavin † (vitamin B_2)	synthetic (or natural) ‡	yellow	—
carrot oil	carrots	orange	—
iron oxide	synthetic	reddish brown	dog and cat food (up to 0.25 percent)
canthaxanthin	synthetic (or natural) ‡	orange to red	30 milligrams per pound

*See 21 Code of Federal Regulations.
†See separate entry in this book.
‡Occurs naturally, but the synthetic chemical is more economical.

chemicals predominates. Once the basic composition of a natural flavor is determined, scientists can construct a realistic artificial flavoring. The major components may be isolated from a natural source or may be synthesized chemically; in addition, chemicals not present in the natural flavoring may be used.

The job of creating realistic flavors out of purified chemicals is that of taste specialists. These persons, with their highly educated taste buds, prepare and evaluate the tastes of different mixtures and proportions of chemicals. The complexity of their job is reflected in the complexity of flavor recipes. A typical artificial cherry flavoring, for example, is not a single chemical as many persons might assume, but a mixture of thirteen chemicals:

Merory imitation cherry flavor MF 83*
- 1.75 eugenol
- 4.50 cinnamic aldehyde
- 6.25 anisyl acetate
- 9.25 anisic aldehyde
- 12.50 ethyl oenanthate
- 15.50 benzyl acetate
- 25. vanillin
- 25. aldehyde C_{16} (strawberry aldehyde)
- 37.25 ethyl butyrate
- 50. amyl butyrate
- 125. tolyl aldehyde
- 558. benzaldehyde (primary flavor)
- 130. alcohol-95% (solvent)
- 1000.

The Food, Drug and Cosmetic Act allows spices and flavorings in a food to be listed on the label under a general term instead of their specific names.

The government regulates flavorings more leniently than most other food additives, because relatively small amounts are used (usually less than 0.03 percent of a food) and almost all occur naturally. That a chemical is used very sparingly in food, reduces but of course does not eliminate its potential hazard; that a chemical occurs naturally, suggests safety but does not guarantee it. Safrole, for instance, occurs in sassafras and was used in root beer flavoring until 1960 when scientists found that it causes cancer of the liver. A second natural flavoring, oil of calamus, was discovered in 1967 to cause intestinal tumors.

* *Food Flavorings*, Merory, J., AVI Publishing Co., Westport, Conn. (1968). Amounts of ingredients are expressed in parts per thousand.

More recently, additional flavorings have drawn suspicion, and the more flavorings that are subjected to rigorous studies, the more problems will be found.

- In May 1982, FDA proposed banning cinnamyl anthranilate, a synthetic chemical in grape or cherry products. It caused liver cancer in mice and kidney and pancreas cancer in rats. Only a few hundred pounds were used annually. Though the ban has not been finalized, the flavoring is no longer used.

- Benzyl acetate occurs in some flowers and is also manufactured. It is used as an artificial flavoring in chewing gum, puddings, candy, and other foods. In a 1982 study sponsored by the National Toxicology Program, benzyl acetate caused cancer of the pancreas in rats and liver tumors in mice.

- In February 1983, the National Toxicology Program reported that allyl isothiocyanate caused cancer in male rats. It occurs naturally in oil of mustard and is used as a flavoring in a variety of processed foods.

The food additive law allows companies or trade associations to declare that a chemical is "generally recognized as safe" (GRAS) and to use it in foods without further ado. Flavorings, while not actually on the GRAS list, are handled similarly. Thus, manufacturers can synthesize a new flavoring, proclaim it safe on the basis of minimal or no testing, and add it to our food without obtaining specific permission from the FDA. Ordinarily, the public is safeguarded from dangerous GRAS compounds, because GRAS compounds, like other food additives, must be declared on most food labels. If FDA inspectors discover what they believe to be an unsafe chemical in food, the FDA can challenge the food manufacturer. But this safeguard does not work for flavorings, because they are not identified specifically on the label. A company could call arsenic an "artificial flavoring" and add it to a food without the FDA or the American public ever finding out (except the hard way). The public's only insurance against dangerous flavorings is that the flavor industry periodically informs the FDA of new substances that they are using in foods.

Most of the hundreds of flavorings—natural or synthetic—have not been tested for their capacity to cause cancer, birth defects, or mutations. The FDA with the assistance of industry and academic scientists should identify the flavorings that are used in the greatest quantity or, as judged from their chemical structure, might pose a problem. Once the priorities are established, the manufacturers of these chemicals—with financial assistance from those segments of the processed food industry that use artificial flavorings—should be required to conduct detailed toxicologic studies. In this way, over a period of years, we should be able to establish the safety of these ill-tested food additives.

Ref.: Residue Reviews 24, 7 (1968); "Criteria for Evaluation of the Health Aspects of Using Flavoring Substances as Food Ingredients," Fed. Am. Soc. Exp. Biol. (1976); *Fed. Reg.* 47, 22545 (1982), *48,* 4557 (1983); Nat. Toxicol. Program "Technical Report No. 250" (1982); seemingly endless lists of artificial and natural flavorings and spices appear in *21* CFR 172.510, 172.515, 182.10–182.60.

Ascorbic Acid (vitamin C)   Safe

One difference between man and most other animals is that the human body cannot synthesize ascorbic acid. The only other animals that have the same genetic defect are the primates, guinea pig, bulbul bird, and Indian fruit-eating bat. For these species ascorbic acid is a vitamin (vitamin C). They must obtain this vital nutrient from their diets.

Persons whose diets are seriously deficient in vitamin C suffer from scurvy. The symptoms of mild scurvy are muscular weakness, poor teeth, and bleeding gums. Severe and prolonged deficiencies of vitamin C cause fever, degeneration of muscles, hemorrhaging of internal organs, and painful joints. Some of these symptoms are obviously related to ascorbic acid's role in the synthesis of connective tissue (collagen). Biochemists are searching for additional, perhaps more subtle, functions of the vitamin.

Food manufacturers use ascorbic acid, most of which is produced synthetically, in several ways. First and foremost it serves as a vitamin supplement in beverages, potato flakes, and breakfast foods.

Ascorbic acid is the only food additive that is used both as an antioxidant to prevent the oxidation of food and as an oxidant to promote the oxidation of food. It operates as an antioxidant to increase the shelf life of food in one of two ways. First, it reacts readily with oxygen. As a result of the reaction, the ascorbic acid loses its nutritive value, but the oxygen is prevented from affecting the taste or appearance of the food. The second way ascorbic acid is used as an antioxidant is in conjunction with BHA, BHT, and propyl gallate, three of the most effective "primary" antioxidants. Ascorbic acid regenerates these antioxidants following the chemical changes they undergo when they stop fat from going rancid. The ascorbic acid added to bologna and other processed meats acts as an antioxidant and also inhibits the formation of cancer-causing nitrosamines.

Bakers use ascorbic acid as an oxidant to improve the properties of dough. Flour contains two enzymes that enable ascorbic acid to affect dough. One enzyme reacts ascorbic acid with oxygen, converting it to dehydroascorbic acid. A second enzyme reacts the dehydroascorbic acid with protein in the dough. This second reaction regenerates ascorbic acid and affects the dough in such a way that it kneads more easily and forms a lighter loaf with a finer texture. The ascorbic acid is entirely destroyed in baking and does not contribute to the nutritive value of the bread. Ascorbic acid is used more widely in Europe than in the United States because of differences in the wheats.

For further discussion of this remarkable chemical, please turn to page 97, in the *Nutrition Scoreboard* section.

Ref.: Fed. Reg. 48, 1735 (Jan. 14, 1983); *21* CFR 182.3013, 182.3189, 182.3731, 182.5013.

Ascorbyl Palmitate   Safe

Ascorbyl palmitate is formed by combining ascorbic acid (vitamin C) with palmitic acid (derived from fat). The raison d'être of ascorbyl palmitate is interesting. Ascorbic acid is a good antioxidant but is not soluble in fats. Palmitic acid, on the other hand, is readily soluble in fats and oils. A clever chemist hit upon the idea of chemically combining ascorbic and palmitic acids, thereby creating a fat-soluble antioxidant.

This additive functions as an antioxidant in shortening in the same fashion as ascorbic acid: it readily reacts with oxygen, preventing the latter from reacting with unsaturated fats and causing rancidity. Ascorbyl palmitate also serves as a source of vitamin C in vitamin pills and fortified foods.

Several studies indicate that ascorbyl palmitate is totally metabolized. The ascorbic acid portion of the molecule is available as vitamin C, and the palmitate portion is converted to energy or fat. In the early 1940s, FDA conducted a lifetime feeding study on rats and concluded that this compound is safe.

Ref.: FAO (31)-25; FAO (46A)-149; *Arch. Biochem. 12,* 375 (1947); *Chem. Abst. 65,* 15843h; *68,* 66889; *Science 113,* 628 (1951); *Fed. Reg. 48,* 1735 (Jan. 14, 1983); *21* CFR 182.3149.

Aspartame   Sensitive individuals; Pregnant women: Avoid
                                                         Others: ?

The history of artificial sweeteners is a grim one:

- dulcin: banned in 1950, because it caused liver cancer;
- cyclamate: banned in 1970, because it appeared to promote cancer and mutations;
- saccharin: ban proposed in 1977, because it increased the risk of bladder cancer.

Despite this depressing record, people still clamor for an artificial sweetener. Overweight people think that the calories saved by not eating sugar will be reflected in slimmer waistlines. Diabetics who need to avoid refined sugar want to satisfy their sweet tooth. And anyone concerned about tooth decay can protect their teeth by avoiding sugar. Because of this huge market for a sugar substitute, manufacturers have been identifying and testing a wide range of supersweet chemicals, both synthetic and natural.

The latest artificial sweetener to move into the spotlight is aspartame, which is marketed under the names Equal and NutraSweet and is about 180 times sweeter than sugar. Thus, a tiny amount can replace a very large quantity of sugar. Aspartame has one tenth the number of calories as an amount of sugar with equal sweetening power.

Like saccharin and many other chemicals, aspartame's sweetness was discovered serendipitously, in this case by a Searle drug company scientist in 1965. Aspartame is synthesized from two amino acids that occur naturally in food, phenylalanine and aspartic acid, and methanol (wood alcohol). Aspartame itself does not occur in nature.

FDA first approved aspartame on July 24, 1981, for use as a tabletop sweetener (the little packets) and in breakfast cereals, powdered beverage mixes, and other dry packaged foods. Two years later, FDA approved the use of aspartame in soft drinks, by far the biggest and most lucrative market for the additive. Aspartame cannot be used in foods that are baked or otherwise heated, because it loses its sweetness as it gradually breaks down to form diketopiperazine (DKP) or to form the amino acids of which it is composed. However, it can be added shortly before such foods are finished cooking. Packages of the artificial sweetener bear notices advising, "Not to be used in cooking or baking."

At first glance aspartame, which is advertised as "the good stuff," might appear as harmless as any other source of amino acids—such as meat, eggs, or beans—but aspartame has been the focus of a vigorous controversy going back to 1973, when Searle first petitioned FDA to permit its use. A basic difference between aspartame and food sources of amino acids is that when we eat meat or beans the protein is digested slowly, the amino acids are released gradually, and small amounts of a wide variety of amino acids are present. But when we eat aspartame, our body is exposed to a quick burst of just two amino acids.

One undisputed problem relates to the phenylalanine portion of the sweetener. One out of 20,000 babies has the genetic disease called phenylketonuria (PKU) and cannot metabolize this amino acid. Phenylalanine rises to toxic levels and causes mental retardation. All newborn babies are tested for PKU, and sufferers are put on a special diet without phenylalanine. These babies also have to be protected from aspartame. FDA requires that all packaged foods containing aspartame bear a notice saying: "PHENYLKETONURICS: CONTAINS PHENYLALANINE." Foods served at restaurants and cafeterias are not covered by this requirement.

A more subtle question concerns people who do not have PKU themselves, but unknowingly carry the genetic trait (about 1 percent of the population). A woman who carried the PKU gene could give birth to a baby with the disease. Some scientists warn that if such women consumed large quantities of aspartame or other sources of phenylalanine during pregnancy, their babies might be born mentally retarded. FDA scientists, however, disagree. According to then FDA Commissioner Arthur Hayes, "aspartame appears to present no greater hazard than common protein-rich foods considered essential for proper nutrition." This contention is hotly disputed, though, especially in light of the proliferation of aspartame-containing foods. In July 1984, the American Academy of Pediatrics' Committee on Genetics and Environmental Hazards expressed concern about aspartame consumption among young children and pregnant women. The committee concluded that "insufficient information is available to indicate whether high, but nonabuse level, intake by certain individuals is likely to cause harm."

The controversy over aspartame's safety is much broader than the PKU issue. The debate was initially sparked in 1974 by Washington attorney James S. Turner and Dr. John Olney, a Washington University scientist. Olney had previously shown that MSG (monosodium glutamate, a common flavor enhancer), might cause brain damage in babies. Olney's studies helped force MSG out of baby foods. Aspartame contains aspartic acid, which is chemically quite similar to glutamate. Olney charged that aspartame, along with glutamate and aspartic acid from traditional foods, could gang up to cause brain lesions. He didn't have proof of this, but he and Turner felt that the evidence was sufficiently suggestive that aspartame could not be considered proven safe.

Before FDA ruled on Olney and Turner's charge, the agency itself became suspicious of the quality of Searle's animal experiments on many different chemicals. As writer Judith Randal related in a major story about aspartame in the Washington *Post*, an FDA task force reported that "Searle made a number of deliberate decisions which seemingly were calculated to minimize the chances of discovering toxicity and, or, to allay FDA concern." FDA found major flaws in many of Searle's studies, including some on aspartame. Then FDA Commissioner Alexander Schmidt refused to approve the sweetener and later told Randal that "Searle has been running a cruddy operation."

In addition to doctoring records, a Searle official sought to increase aspartame's chances of approval by inculcating in FDA officials a "subconscious spirit of participation" in the Searle studies. In January 1977, FDA General Counsel Richard Merrill wrote, "The FDA must receive the truth, not psychological warfare." That statement was part of a thirty-three-page letter to the Justice Department, in which Merrill requested a grand jury investigation into Searle's alleged violations of the law. The Justice Department denied the request, and, as grand jury rules dictate, never provided a public explanation.

With a grand jury ruled out, the next step in the aspartame saga was a review of fifteen out of eighty of Searle's studies. This review, conducted by a consulting firm called Universities Associated for Research and Education in Pathology (UAREP), was supposed to answer all the questions, but it was so narrowly focused that it proved of little value. It reviewed the pathology, but not the design, supervision, and conduct of the studies.

Turner blasted the UAREP review and persuaded FDA to appoint a precedent-setting public board of inquiry to examine the whole range of complaints about aspartame. The board of three scientists—chosen jointly by FDA, Turner, and Searle—was established in 1979. Ultimately, to the dismay of Turner and others, this committee, too, focused only on a limited number of issues, including Olney's charge about brain damage and another charge that aspartame caused brain tumors in laboratory animals. The board concluded in September 1980, that aspartame did not increase the risk of mental retardation or noncancerous brain lesions. Olney held his ground, however, arguing that the industry-sponsored studies were deficient and urging that new, independent tests be conducted. FDA sided with the board.

The cancer question arose from a feeding study in which aspartame was fed to rats. Ordinarily, brain tumors occur very rarely in laboratory rats. The board said that "aspartame, at least when administered in the huge quantities employed in these studies, may contribute to the development of brain tumors" and urged that the tumor tests be repeated. Because of the possibility that aspartame caused brain tumors, the board said that aspartame should not be allowed in our food supply until further tests confirmed or refuted the study linking the sweetener to brain tumors.

FDA rejected the board of inquiry's conclusion concerning brain tumors, saying that the apparent increase in brain tumors was a statistical fluke. FDA said that the number of tumors occurring in the control (untreated) rats was uncharacteristically low and presented National Cancer Institute evidence in support of this notion. (Comparing the incidence of tumors in test animals to "historical" controls, rather than to the control animals used in the current study, is a potentially mischievous practice that can be very misleading if not done carefully and interpreted cautiously.) Also, a new rat study, completed after the board's review, was conducted by Ajinomoto, a Japanese marketer of aspartame. FDA said that this study did not show any evidence of harm. However, the new study was done on a different strain of rat and could not confirm or disprove the previous study.

In June 1985, a former high-ranking FDA toxicologist, Dr. Adrian Gross, charged that the research "has established beyond any reasonable doubt that aspartame is capable of inducing brain tumors in experimental animals." Yet another controversy centers on DKP, the breakdown product of aspartame.

One study indicated that DKP did not cause cancer. However, there was evidence that the DKP was not mixed in well with the rest of the rats' food. Thus, the rats may have eaten much less of the chemical than was intended. FDA's own scientists criticized the study sharply, but later FDA said that this was one loose end that would just have to be left dangling. FDA could have demanded that this and other dubious studies be repeated. Attorney Turner pointed out that Searle and FDA could have saved themselves a lot of grief—and the public a lot of worry—if they had only repeated the flawed studies years ago.

And so it was that after eight years of debate FDA approved aspartame, first for use in dry foods, then soft drinks. Days before FDA was going to approve aspartame for soft drinks, Richard Wurtman, a respected neuroendocrinologist at MIT, wrote a letter of objection. He acknowledged that small amounts of aspartame were safe—he even said he used the sweetener himself—but expressed concern about large amounts. He was particularly concerned that allowing aspartame in soft drinks would lead to excessive consumption by children. Wurtman told FDA that studies he had just completed raised the possibility that aspartame would alter levels of brain chemicals (neurotransmitters) and cause behavioral changes. His studies on rats suggested that aspartame could reduce levels of serotonin in the brain, especially when the artificial sweetener was consumed with carbohydrate-containing foods, such as potato chips or a cupcake. The FDA acknowledged a theoretical possibility of a problem, but said that without more evidence, it could not accept Wurtman's argument.

Food sciences professor Woodrow Monte, of Arizona State University, raised another objection. He pointed out that as aspartame is metabolized, methanol, a poorly tested, toxic chemical, is released. Monte said that methanol might cause visual and nervous system problems. FDA rejected this contention, too, saying the amounts of methanol were trivial, and then gave aspartame its stamp of approval.

Several months after FDA approved aspartame in soft drinks, news media ran major stories about possible dangers of the additive, and hundreds of consumers wrote to Wurtman, FDA, Monte, and others. These consumers complained of such symptoms as dizziness, headaches, epileptic-like seizures, and menstrual problems. One Yale physician told me that after drinking a can of Diet Coke her "head felt like it was coming unscrewed." She had never experienced that sensation prior to drinking Diet Coke, and it never recurred once she stopped drinking Diet Coke.

FDA and Searle continued to defend aspartame's safety, but FDA asked the Centers for Disease Control (CDC) to evaluate the consumer complaints. It was quite possible that even though the problems being reported had not been detected in any of the past studies, a small fraction of consumers was indeed experiencing serious problems. CDC's inquiry was doomed to be inconclusive, because CDC used questionnaires rather than clinical experiments to investigate the complaints. It would have been so easy to invite individuals who believed they were sensitive to volunteer for a controlled experiment. The individuals would be given either small amounts of aspartame or a placebo and then monitored for several hours. Such a study could have determined once and for all whether aspartame caused these immediate reactions. CDC concluded that:

> Although it may be that certain individuals have an unusual sensitivity to the product, these data do not provide evidence for the existence of serious, widespread, adverse health consequences attendant to the use of aspartame.

FDA said that it supported the CDC findings and believed that "clinical studies may be useful" in resolving concerns about aspartame. Searle has undertaken such studies.

In early 1984, Turner and the Community Nutrition Institute (CNI), a nonprofit citizens' group, filed a law suit against FDA, hoping to force the agency to hold a comprehensive, public hearing that would at long last examine all the still-disputed issues. As of July 1985, the case was still wending its way through the courts.

As summer 1984 approached, the aspartame controversy heated up when Common Cause published an exposé that found "such serious deficiencies in the Food and Drug Administration's process of approving aspartame that we are calling on Congress to begin its own investigation of this approval process immediately."

Aspartame's critics predicted that heavy soft drink consumption during the hot summer months would lead to an enormous number of new consumer complaints. However, those complaints never materialized. The relative silence provided some reassurance that aspartame was not causing many—or any—adverse reactions. In Canada, where aspartame had been used since 1981, the Common Cause report acknowledged that few people had ever complained to health officials.

The aspartame controversy continued into 1985. Dr. Keith Connors, of Children's Hospital in Washington, D.C., has been investigating the behavioral effects of various sweeteners. In February 1985, the New York *Times* reported that Dr. Connors "has studied two young children who suffer extreme agitation following doses of aspartame equivalent to the amount found in a six-ounce serving of Kool-Aid sweetened with NutraSweet. One of the children becomes so agitated he has to be restrained." The article also quoted a Searle executive who acknowledged that "a few people may be allergic or sensitive to it."

Aspartame poses difficult questions for government policy makers. Clearly, not all of the questions have been answered, and even FDA acknowledges that aspartame introduces some small risks. Ideally, more tests would have been conducted to replace the many flawed and disputed tests *before* the chemical was approved. As FDA Commissioner Hayes told *Science* magazine, "In the best of all possible worlds Searle would have conducted additional tests of its own. I wish they had, sure. On the other hand, I didn't feel there was justification for saying, okay, let's wait a few years." In the absence of commercial pressures, FDA probably would have demanded such tests. But such pressures do exist, and now millions of consumers are participating, unwittingly, in a giant new experiment.

The reason for Searle's desire to speed aspartame to market and keep it there is obvious when you examine recent sales records and future sales prospects. Sales of aspartame, according to *The Wall Street Journal,* would total $600 million in 1984—half of Searle's total sales—and $1 billion in 1985. The market for tabletop sweeteners doubled since aspartame was introduced. A beverage industry trade journal predicted that in 1990 diet sodas would account for half of all soda sales, twice the current level. Searle's future is rosy, indeed, unless a judge forces its golden goose off the market or a scientist proves conclusively that the chemical is indeed dangerous.

Until further studies are conducted, aspartame should be considered of questionable safety for most people, and risky to certain individuals. If you believe you have experienced a problem after consuming the sweetener, you should simply avoid it. If you have not noticed any problem, modest amounts —up to a few servings a day—should not pose a significant risk. But, just to be on the safe side until the uncertainties are resolved, no one should be consuming five or ten aspartame packets or aspartame-sweetened sodas a day. Pregnant women and infants should avoid aspartame. Safety aside, aspartame probably isn't much of a weight-loss aid. Most people who save a few calories by drinking a diet beverage will probably make up those calories by eating a few more bites of some other foods.

Ref.: Fed. Reg. 46, 38285 (July 24, 1981), *49,* 6672 (Feb. 22, 1984); Science *213,* 986 (1981); *Toxicol. 21,* 91 (1981); *New Engl. J. Med. 306,* 173 (1982); Washington *Post,* p. B1 (April 15, 1984); *Am. J. Clin. Nutr. 40,* 1 (1984); *Common Cause Magazine,* p. 25 (July/August, 1984); *The Wall Street Journal,* p. 1 (Sept. 18, 1984); "Evaluation of Consumer Complaints Related to Aspartame Use," Centers for Disease Control (Nov. 1, 1984); The New York *Times,* p. C1 (Feb. 5, 1985); Hearing, Senate Committee on Labor and Human Resources (April 2, 1985); *21* CFR 172.804.

Azodicarbonamide   Safe

Azodicarbonamide is one of the most effective dough conditioning agents employed by the baking industry. Dough conditioners such as this have replaced long months of storage as the standard way of aging flour. Natural and chemical aging have identical chemical effects on flour; both produce more manageable dough and lighter, more voluminous loaves of bread.

Azodicarbonamide is as effective as chlorine dioxide—another leading bleaching/maturing agent—but it is also a powder and easier and cheaper to use than the gaseous chlorine compound. It is used at concentrations of 2 to 45 parts per million.

Azodicarbonamide does not bleach flour. Therefore, a baker who wishes bleached as well as artificially aged flour must use this chemical in conjunction with a bleach, such as benzoyl peroxide.

When azodicarbonamide reacts with dough, the additive is rapidly and completely converted to a second compound, biurea. In the same chemical reaction, the protein (gluten) of flour is oxidized, accounting for the change in the dough's properties. (When flour oxidizes, cysteine residues in protein react with one another to form disulfide bonds.)

Biurea has a reputation for being inert and insoluble. Digestive enzymes do not affect it and most of it is eliminated in the feces. The 10 percent that the body does absorb is excreted in the urine. When scientists fed massive amounts of azodicarbonamide or biurea to rats and dogs for two years, no adverse effect on appearance, survival, growth, organ weight, or pathology was noted. Rat reproduction and lactation were not affected in a study that spanned three generations of rats.

The nutritive value of vitamins and amino acids in bread is not affected by azodicarbonamide or biurea. By all accounts, then, this food additive appears to be safe.

Ref.: FAO (40A)-104; *Baker's Digest 37,* 69 (1963); *Cereal Chem. 40,* 539 (1963); *Tox. Appl. Pharm. 7,* 445 (1965); Am. Inst. of Baking Bulletin #127 (February 1967); *21* CFR 172.806.

Benzoyl Peroxide   Safe

Benzoyl peroxide has been an important flour bleach since 1917. Because this chemical bleaches but does not "age" flour, bakers use it in conjunction with "aging" agents (azodicarbonamide, iodate, bromate). Fifty parts per million peroxide (usually mixed with twice as much cornstarch) is sufficient for most flours.

Benzoyl peroxide is a powder that bleaches flour within twenty-four hours. As the bleach does its work, most of it decomposes to benzoic acid, which remains in the flour after baking. The benzoic acid residue is not hazardous (see "sodium benzoate").

Lifetime feeding experiments have been conducted on rats and mice. No adverse effects were caused by concentrations of peroxide up to one thousand times as high as humans might encounter. In one experiment the testes of rats atrophied, but this, apparently, was because benzoyl peroxide destroys vitamin E. The rats whose diet consisted almost entirely of treated flour were simply suffering from vitamin deficiency. Short-term tests on dogs further supported the safety of benzoyl peroxide.

Ref.: FAO (35)-155; *Fd. Cos. Tox.* 2, 527 (1964); *Fd. Chem. Tox.* 20, 243 (1982); *21* CFR 137.105, 184.1157.

Beta-Carotene and Vitamin A   Safe

Beta-carotene is a yellow pigment that occurs in many fruits and vegetables, as well as in animal fat. Beta-carotene is important in a good diet because the body converts it to vitamin A. Food manufacturers add beta-carotene to margarine, nondairy coffee whiteners, shortening, butter, milk, cake mix, dessert toppings, and other products either as artificial coloring, as a nutritional supplement, or both. When foods are fortified with beta-carotene or vitamin A, the amount contained in the food is always listed in the nutrition labeling panel. We can also obtain vitamin A directly from liver or fish oil. While vitamin A overdoses may cause birth defects and poisoning, beta-carotene will at worst cause temporary skin yellowing. The average adult should consume at least 5,000 units of vitamin A or beta-carotene daily; pregnant women need 8,000 units. For additional information, refer to the discussion of vitamin A on page 91 in *Nutrition Scoreboard.*

Ref.: Fed. Reg. 47, 47435 (Oct. 26, 1982); *21* CFR 73.95, 182.5245, 182.5930–182.5936.

Brominated Vegetable Oil   ?

The soft drink industry seems to have nothing but headaches: exploding bottles, dentists at its throat, environmentalists angry about nonreturnable bottles and cans, and, of course, food additives. One such additive is brominated vegetable oil (BVO).

Chemically, BVO is vegetable oil (olive, sesame, corn, or cottonseed) whose density has been increased to that of water by being combined with bromine. Flavoring oils are dissolved in BVO, which is then added to carbonated or noncarbonated fruit-flavored drinks. The lighter-than-water oils are dispersed throughout the drink by BVO, without which they would float to the surface and form a ring at the neck of the bottle. BVO also makes the soft drink slightly cloudy, giving the illusion of thickness or "body." A few of the drinks that contain BVO are Mountain Dew, Shasta Orange, Orange Crush, and Mello Yello.

Beverage manufacturers used BVO for decades and, in the absence of any scientific studies, assumed that it was safe. In January 1969, Drs. Ian Munro, E. J. Middleton, and H. C. Grice, scientists at Canada's Food and Drug Directorate, published a study that indicated that this additive was not so safe after all. Rats that ate food containing 0.5 or 2.5 percent BVO for eighty days suffered heart, liver, thyroid, testicle, and kidney damage or changes.

Subsequent studies done in England showed that BVO (or fragments of BVO) accumulate in and become permanent residents of animal tissue. Organic bromine residues in human tissues are much higher in countries in which BVO is used than in other countries (e.g., West Germany).

A year after the Canadian study revealed that BVO was hazardous, FDA removed it from the list of food additives that are "generally recognized as safe" and gave it "interim" approval. This meant that manufacturers had to stop using BVO within six months, unless they submitted data supporting the substance's safety. When the deadline arrived, manufacturers were still using it in food, but had not filed the required safety data. A study that was supposed to be completed in 1973 was finally completed in 1975. A preliminary evaluation did not reveal any problems. However, the chronic effect of BVO residues in human tissues is not known. As of mid 1985, FDA still had not decided whether to give final approval to BVO.

High doses of BVO caused behavioral birth defects in an animal study done by Charles Voorhees at the Children's Hospital Research Foundation in Cincinnati. The dose that affected the central nervous system was lower than that which caused physical abnormalities, but it is unlikely that the low levels found in food would cause behavioral problems. Subtle or occasional problems in a sensitive fraction of the population, however, would never be detected.

Before the toxic effects of BVO were discovered, beverage manufacturers used it at levels of 300 parts per million. The legal limit in the United States and Canada is now 15 ppm. BVO was banned in Sweden in 1968 and in Great Britain in September 1970.

Brominated vegetable oil is used almost exclusively in snack-type products that are devoid of redeeming nutrients. The public would not suffer one whit if BVO were banned.

Ref.: Fd. Cos. Tox. 7, 25 (1969); *9,* 1 (1971); FAO (40)-13; *Food Chemical News,* November 9, 1970 (refers to 1970 FAO/WHO Committee meeting); *The Wall Street Journal,* January 25, 1970; New York *Times,* August 29, 1970; pers. comm. from FDA; *Food Product Development,* May 1971, page 90; *Fd. Chem. News* p. 15 (May 9, 1983); *21* CFR 180.30.

Butylated Hydroxyanisole (BHA)   Avoid

"Enter the ageless age," intones one advertisement for BHA, one of the chemical workhorses of the processed food industry. With preservatives like this, potato chips, presweetened cereals, bouillon cubes, and other vital components of our food supply will smell fresh for one, two, or even five years! Just think, in case you leave a bag of chips in your suitcase after summer vacation, they will be there, smelling fresh as can be, when you go on vacation the following year. The way in which BHA retards rancidity is discussed later (see entry for butylated hydroxytoluene—BHT).

Some companies recognize that BHA, BHT, and other synthetic antioxidants are not the sole route to quality products. Though chemicals like BHA can retard rancidity, they won't stop a food from going stale, losing its crispness, or losing some of its flavor. These other qualities usually deteriorate long before rancidity would set in, so companies try to sell the foods or take them off the grocery store shelves before an antioxidant would even be needed.

BHA has been used in foods in the U.S. since 1947. The average person now consumes several milligrams of this synthetic chemical daily. Except in a few foods, such as active dry yeast, BHA is limited to a level of 0.02 percent (together with other antioxidants). It is commony used in lard, chewing gum, vegetable oil, baked goods, pork sausage, dry mixes, as well as cosmetics, and other nonfood uses.

Most studies have indicated that BHA is safe. BHA is relatively nontoxic and does not appear to pose any problems during pregnancy. No serious doubts arose until early 1982 when Nobuyuki Ito, at the Nagoya City (Japan) University Medical School, threw a bombshell at the food industry. Ito found that BHA "induced benign and malignant forestomach neoplasms" in both male and female rats. Though humans do not have a forestomach, the causation of any kind of tumors in animals is cause for great concern. Oftentimes, a chemical that causes one kind of tumor in one species will cause another kind of tumor in a second species. Ito's finding was especially surprising, because previous, smaller tests did not indicate any problem, and in some studies BHA even had an anticancer effect.

The Japanese Government quickly proposed that BHA be outlawed, but American trade associations and the FDA persuaded Japan to wait until the unexpected result could be carefully analyzed and, they hoped, debunked. In 1983, a review committee of scientists from Japan, Canada, Britain, and the United States concluded that Ito's study was well-conducted. The committee also concluded, however, that BHA posed such a slight risk that it should not be banned until further studies were done. Only the Japanese representative disagreed with this conclusion. The majority believed that the cancers might be caused by some peculiar mechanism related to the high dosages used in the study. So the studies go on, and consumers continue to ingest BHA.

Cancer aside, studies have raised several small, additional questions. In studies on mice and rats, huge amounts of BHA (and also BHT)—0.25 to 0.5 percent of the diet—caused behavioral changes. The scientists reported that "BHA-treated offspring showed increased exploration, decreased sleeping, decreased self-grooming, slower learning, and a decreased orientation reflex." Occasional reports of allergic reactions pop up in medical journals. BHA, by itself, does not pose a great threat with regard to either behavioral or allergic reactions.

Chemicals like BHA provide a little extra insurance for food processors concerned about spoilage. However, other chemicals or methods could replace most or all uses of BHA. Vitamins C and E are perfectly safe antioxidants, though not quite as potent or cheap as BHA or BHT. Freezing, nitrogen gas to replace air, and dark glass instead of clear bottles could replace synthetic antioxidants in many foods. In sum, BHA appears to add a slight risk to the food supply and should be avoided.

Ref.: Report on health aspects of BHA (GRAS review), Fed. Am. Soc. Exper. Biol., Rockville, Md., (1978); *Neurobehav. Toxicol. Teratol. 3,* 321 (1981); *Toxicology 23,* 79 (1982); N. Ito *in Jap. J. Cancer Res.* (1982); *Food Chem. News,* p. 30, (July 5, 1982), p. 31 (Feb. 27, 1984); "Report of the Principal Participants of the Four Nations on the Evaluation of the Safety of BHA," (FDA, Feb. 28, 1983); *21* CFR 172.110, 181.24, 182.3169.

Butylated Hydroxytoluene (BHT)   Avoid

Almost as familiar to label readers as sugar and salt is the preservative BHT. "Freshness preserved with BHT," "BHT added to packaging," or just plain "BHT" is included on the labels of thousands of oil-containing foods. Companies naturally opt for the emotionally neutral initials, as opposed to the full—and to some, scary—chemical name: butylated hydroxytoluene.

BHT helps prevent rancidity, which results when the unsaturated portion of fats or oils reacts with oxygen. The oxidation process involves highly reactive chemical intermediates known as "free radicals." These free radicals promote chain reactions that convert fatty acids into chemicals called aldehydes and ketones. The characteristic odor of rancid foods is due chiefly to the aldehydes. BHT and other antioxidants, such as BHA and propyl gallate, react with the free radicals, thereby breaking the chain reaction. A mixture of antioxidants is often more effective than a single one. Thus, many products contain BHT plus BHA or propyl gallate.

BHT was approved for use in the United States in 1954. About a million pounds of BHT are added to processed foods each year. Treated foods include breakfast cereal packaging, (it migrates onto the cereal itself), chewing gum, convenience foods, vegetable oil, shortening, potato flakes, enriched rice, potato chips, candy, and a multitude of others. The total concentration of antioxidants (BHT plus BHA, propyl gallate, and others) ranges from as low as 0.0001 percent in gelatin desserts to 0.1 percent in chewing gum and dry yeast. The usual concentration is about 0.01 percent. If you are an average, processed food-eating American (and I hope you're not), you probably consume five or ten milligrams of BHT daily.

BHT is much cheaper than BHA (see previous entry), but its use is limited, because it is less stable at the high temperatures used to pasteurize food.

BHT is often used unnecessarily. For instance, some makers of vegetable oil and potato chips add BHT to their products, while some competitors do not. Perhaps manufacturers add them out of habit, because of outmoded manufacturing techniques, or to extend slightly the shelf lives of their products. In any case, the benefits BHT confers are clearly slight. If you wish, you can greatly reduce your intake of BHT and other preservatives by carefully reading food labels. Because of the public concern about chemicals, some companies appear to be relying less on BHT, preferring to advertise their products with the attractive phrases "no preservatives" or "natural."

More than a decade ago, two British biochemists discovered levels of BHT as high as 3 parts per million (ppm) in human fatty tissue. The average level of BHT was six times as high in the fat of Americans (1.3 ppm) as in the fat of Britons (0.2 ppm). The significance of this finding is unknown, but we should be suspicious of any synthetic chemical that accumulates in our body; we should be doubly suspicious when studies on the chemical have left a trail of warning signs.

The question of BHT's safety has had a stormy, complex history. Some studies indicate risks, while others have suggested benefits.

In 1959 Australian biologists reported that BHT caused rats' hair to fall out, increased cholesterol levels in the rats' blood, and caused rats to be born without eyes. These effects were seen when their diet contained 0.1 percent of BHT, a much higher level than humans consume.

The possibility that BHT caused birth defects alarmed—with good reason—a lot of people, and scientists dove back into their laboratories to learn more about the dubious compound. The outcome of this renewed interest was a barrage of reports published in 1965 that demonstrated that BHT caused neither birth defects nor balding. The reason for the discrepancy between the one 1959 report and later studies was never determined.

In other studies, toxicologists have found that high dosages of BHT caused the livers of lab animals to enlarge and develop high levels of enzymes. The changes reflect the liver's efforts to metabolize and dispose of the foreign chemical. Dr. Alvin Malkinson, assistant professor of biochemical pharmacology at the University of Colorado School of Pharmacy, has pointed out that the higher enzyme levels are a mixed blessing. He said that the enzymes:

> can detoxify dangerous drugs or metabolites, but at the same time can convert innocuous chemicals into potent carcinogens. These enzymes are highly sensitive to environmental changes and are induced to different extents by various agents.

Thus, the induction of some of these enzymes by BHT could upset a delicate balance and have unexpected side effects.

For this and other reasons, Malkinson concluded that the FDA should ban BHT. The FDA has acknowledged that the enzyme-inducing effect raises significant questions.

The most important question concerning BHT is whether it causes—or prevents—cancer. The studies are too numerous to explain individually, but the following discussion will give you a sense of the science. Neal Clapp and his colleagues at Oak Ridge National Laboratory have studied BHT in combination with various other agents. In one study, BHT reduced the incidence of tumors induced in female—but not in male—mice by a potent carcinogen (diethylnitrosamine) fed to the animals. In another study, Clapp found that BHT alone, or in combination with diethylnitrosamine, more than doubled the incidence of lung tumors in mice. Clapp also found that when mice were exposed to a stiff dose of X rays, BHT increased the death rate in one strain of mouse, but decreased the death rate in another. In a study on rats that were exposed to two carcinogenic chemicals, B. M. Ulland, J. H. Weisburger, and their colleagues discovered that BHT reduced the number of liver and mammary tumors.

One of the larger cancer studies on BHT was conducted by the National Cancer Institute in the late 1970s. The researchers concluded that "under the conditions of this bioassay, BHT was not carcinogenic" for the strain of mouse and rat used. However, the original data suggest a less cheerful conclusion. Four male mice and two female mice that had been fed BHT developed tumors of their tear glands. None of the mice not consuming BHT developed such tumors. More significantly, female, BHT-eating mice had five times the rate of lung tumors as their luckier sisters whose diet lacked BHT. A subsequent and equally large study done in Japan on the same strain of mouse did not detect an increased risk of lung tumors.

Finally, Dr. Preben Olsen, of Denmark's National Food Institute, reported in October 1983 that BHT caused cancer of the liver in both male and female rats. This new study did not elicit any visible reaction from the Food and Drug Administration.

The laboratory evidence on whether BHT causes, prevents, or has no effect on cancer in mice and rats is mixed, but because of the possibility that this unnecessary chemical additive might be increasing slightly the risk of cancer, it should be phased out of our food supply.

Researchers and physicians have raised other, smaller questions about BHT, including behavioral and allergic reactions. Enormous doses (0.23–0.5 percent in food) of BHT affect the behavior of mice. The mice "showed decreased sleeping, increased social and isolation-induced aggression, and a severe deficit in learning." One study correlated the behavioral changes with changes in brain chemistry. Other studies showed slight behavioral effects on rats at a lower dosage (0.1–0.25 percent BHT). Such studies led the Joint FAO/WHO Expert Committee on Food Additives in 1980 to call for additional behavior-oriented tests. Whether the small amount of BHT in food might affect sensitive people in subtle ways is an open question.

BHT provides a good example of how slowly the FDA moves to control possibly hazardous additives. In July 1973 the Select Committee on GRAS Substances (SCOGS) sent FDA its final evaluation of BHT. SCOGS recommended further testing. Four years later, on May 31, 1977, the FDA finally took a toothless action: it proposed that BHT be removed from the GRAS list of additives and considered a regulated food additive. Eight years later, the "proposed" action had never been finalized, and BHT continues to be regulated and used exactly as if no review or studies had ever been conducted.

The questions raised about this preservative have led some companies to stop using it. Until any new studies conclusively exonerate or indict BHT, FDA is unlikely to take action. That leaves it to each of us to weigh the merits of the case. I find BHT easy to avoid, because it is used primarily in foods that are high in fat or sugar and that I would not want to eat for a variety of other reasons.

Ref.: Aust. J. Exp. Biol. 37, 533 (1959); *Fd. Cosmet. Tox. 8,* 409 (1970); *12,* 367 (1974); *Ann. Allergy 31,* 126 (1973); *Development. Psychobiol. 7,* 343 (1974); *Fed. Reg. 42,* 27603 (May 31, 1977); *Colo. J. Pharm. 21,* 43 (1978); *J. Nat. Cancer Inst. 61,* 177 (1978); *NCI Tech. Rep. Series No. 150* (1979); *Fd. Cosmet. Toxicol. 19,* 153 (1981); *Environ. Res. 29,* 1 (1982); *Fd. Chem. Toxicol. 20,* 861 (1982); *Food Chem. News* p. 3 (Oct. 31, 1983), p. 42 (Nov. 28, 1983); *Acta Pharmacol. et Toxicol. 53,* 433 (1983); *21* CFR 137.350, 16.110, 172.115, 180.20, 181.24, 182.3173.

Caffeine

Children, Pregnant women: **Avoid**
Others: **?**

Caffeine, a stimulant of the central nervous system, occurs naturally in tea leaves and in coffee, cocoa, and kola beans. The discovery that coffee beans contain a substance that wards off sleep has been credited to residents of an Arabian monastery. Shepherds noted that goats that ate coffee beans pranced about all night long. The abbot, learning of this, made from the beans a drink that kept him awake during long, prayerful nights.

In all probability, you've been consuming caffeine since childhood. Your first Coke or Pepsi was laced with it. So was the tea you sipped when you had a cold. As you got older, you learned to love a cup of coffee. If you ever ate a chocolate bar, you ate caffeine. In school, you may have stayed up late studying for exams with the help of over-the-counter caffeine pills. And unless you were one of those who suffered from jumpy nerves or insomnia, or belonged to one of the religious groups that forbids its use, you probably consumed caffeine without a second thought. And why not? Caffeine was always thought to be harmless.

In recent years, caffeine has joined the ranks of common chemicals we worry about. It gets a high priority, too, because caffeine is one of the few drugs that shows up regularly in our food supply (alcohol and quinine are two others).

Even before we started to get uneasy about caffeine, we knew it affected the central nervous system in ways that fought fatigue. We knew it increased the secretion of gastric acids and probably increased the number and misery of persons suffering from peptic ulcers. We knew it raised blood pressure, had a diuretic effect, and dilated some blood vessels while constricting others.

We knew, but we didn't worry. Tens of millions of Americans drank, and still drink, substantial quantities of coffee and tea. The average coffee drinker consumes about 675 cups a year. High as that may seem, per person coffee consumption has actually decreased by 52 percent since 1946, because of rising prices, declining quality, and the enormous increase in the consumption of soft drinks.

Soft drinks are the major source of caffeine for most children and some adults. The Food and Drug Administration has actually required that caffeine be added to cola and "pepper" drinks. In recent years, caffeine has found its way into orange, apple, and other flavored drinks. A 12-ounce can of soda contains only about a third as much caffeine as a cup of coffee (see table following), but because a child weighs much less than an adult, a can of soda drunk by a child is roughly equivalent to a cup of coffee drunk by an adult. In 1983, the average American drank more than 14 ounces of soft drinks per day, double the amount consumed in 1966. About half of all soda pop contains caffeine. Caffeine is not added to any food besides soda pop.

The reason companies add caffeine to soda pop is a matter of debate. Manufacturers say that caffeine's bitter flavor is a vital component of the product's overall taste. Observers outside the industry suggest other rationales. Most obviously, caffeine is a stimulant and adds some of the much advertised "life" to cola and other beverages. More insidiously, some point out that caffeine is mildly addictive—many people are familiar with the headaches that are the most common withdrawal symptom—and that companies hope that some consumers will get hooked. (In 1980 a report commissioned by the Federal Trade Commission contemplated the possibility that unscrupulous manufacturers might someday add caffeine or other mildly addictive chemicals to a variety of foods to promote brand loyalty.)

In 1978, an official review committee reported to the FDA that caffeine in soft drinks had not been proved hazardous, but pointed out:

> It is inappropriate to include caffeine among the substances generally recognized as safe. At current levels of consumption of cola-type beverages, the dose of

Caffeine Content of Soft Drinks*

Brand	Milligrams Caffeine (12 oz. serving)
Sugar-Free Mr. Pibb	58.8
Mountain Dew	54.0
Mello Yello	52.8
Tab	46.8
Coca-Cola	45.6
Diet Coke	45.6
Shasta Cola	44.4
Shasta Cherry Cola	44.4
Shasta Diet Cola	44.4
Mr. Pibb	40.8
Dr. Pepper	39.6
Sugar-Free Dr. Pepper	39.6
Big Red	38.4
Sugar-Free Big Red	38.4
Pepsi-Cola	38.4
Aspen	36.0
Diet Pepsi	36.0
Pepsi-Light	36.0
RC Cola	36.0
Diet Rite	36.0
Kick	31.2
Canada Dry Jamaica Cola	30.0
Canada Dry Diet Cola	1.2

* *Ref.:* "FDA Consumer," March 1984

caffeine can approximate that known to induce such pharmacological effects as central nervous system stimulation.

The FDA then proposed that caffeine no longer be required in cola and "pepper" drinks. Some companies soon began marketing highly advertised caffeine-free beverages. In 1981 the 7-Up Company riled competitors by bragging that 7-Up never had caffeine and never would. 7-Up followed up in 1982 by introducing caffeine-free Like cola. Other companies, including Coca-Cola and PepsiCo, quickly developed their own caffeine-free colas. The loophole in the law that enables companies to ignore the caffeine requirement is that the law does not say how much caffeine must be present—one molecule would suffice (the upper limit is 0.02 percent).

Large amounts of caffeine can cause a syndrome dubbed "caffeinism." The symptoms, according to Dr. John F. Greden, a psychiatrist at the University of Michigan, read like a classic description of an anxiety attack: nervousness, anxiety, irritability, muscle twitching, jitteriness, and insomnia. Office workers and waitresses who have free access to a continuous supply of freshly brewed coffee are prime candidates for caffeinism. The problem can get so severe that

Caffeine Content of Beverages and Foods†

Item	Milligrams Caffeine Average	Range
Coffee (5-oz. cup)		
Brewed, drip method	115	60–180
Brewed, percolator	80	40–170
Instant	65	30–120
Decaffeinated, brewed	3	2–5
Decaffeinated, instant	2	1–5
Tea (5 oz. cup)		
Brewed, major U.S. brands	40	20–90
Brewed, imported brands	60	25–110
Instant	30	25–50
Iced (12 oz. glass)	70	67–76
Cocoa beverage (5-oz.cup)	4	2–20
Chocolate milk beverage (8 oz.)	5	2–7
Milk chocolate (1 oz.)	6	1–15
Dark chocolate, semisweet (1 oz.)	20	5–35
Baker's chocolate (1 oz.)	26	26
Chocolate-flavored syrup (1 oz.)	4	4

† Ref.: "FDA Consumer," March 1984

some sufferers, fearing an underlying mental disorder, have gone to psychiatrists. In several cases reported in medical journals, astute psychiatrists, having discovered that their patients were drinking ten to twenty cups of coffee daily, advised them to quit. Recovery was almost immediate.

Interestingly, many heavy coffee consumers (five or more cups per day) seem to develop a partial tolerance for caffeine's sleep-disturbing effects. But children, says one prominent researcher, J. Murdoch Ritchie, a pharmacologist at Yale University, "are more susceptible to excitation [by caffeine] than adults."

Because caffeine is a psychoactive chemical, its effects on the body are being carefully examined. Some studies demonstrate scientifically that as little as one cup of coffee can cause sleeplessness. Other studies show that small amounts can disrupt normal sleep patterns. Others demonstrate that caffeine increases alertness.

Robert Elkins, Judith Rapoport, and their colleagues at the National Institute of Mental Health recently fed caffeine (equivalent to either two or seven cans of soda pop) to a group of 8- to 13-year-old boys who normally consumed little caffeine. The result? The boys experienced restlessness, nervousness, nausea, and insomnia. Their learning ability was mildly affected as well. Because millions of children consume large quantities of soda pop, FDA should simply prohibit caffeine as an additive in soft drinks.

Caffeine belongs to the class of chemicals called purines, some of which are important constituents of chromosomes and genes. Geneticists knew that some purines caused mutations and feared that caffeine might also do so. The earliest studies, done around 1950, showed that caffeine was weakly mutagenic in bacteria. This finding encouraged scientists to do experiments on mammals and insects. In 1968 a German researcher claimed to have shown that caffeine caused mutations in mice. However, other scientists found flaws in both his data and his conclusions. Subsequent studies all gave negative results, so caffeine does not appear to pose any real threat as a mutagen in humans. Other studies indicate that caffeine does not cause cancer.

The most controversial question about caffeine concerns its possible effects on reproduction. Since 1964, a dozen animal studies have demonstrated that caffeine can cause reduced fertility and a wide variety of birth defects in rats, mice, and rabbits, including cleft palate, ectrodactyly (missing fingers and toes), and skull malformations. In one coffee industry-sponsored study, as little as the equivalent of five cups of coffee a day caused birth defects, though in most studies defects did not appear until the animals consumed about five or ten times as much. In 1976 the Center for Science in the Public Interest (CSPI) petitioned the FDA to conduct further research, advise pregnant women to avoid caffeine, and require a warning label on coffee labels.

The growing controversy over caffeine led FDA to conduct the most sensitive animal study yet performed. Thomas F. X. Collins, FDA's animal teratology expert, found that the equivalent of about twenty-four cups of coffee a day or more given as one dose caused ectrodactyly, while as little as three cups of coffee delayed bone formation. With this study in hand, FDA Commissioner Jere Goyan, in September 1980, said,

> I believe that prudence dictates that pregnant women avoid caffeine-containing products or use them sparingly.

The FDA then commenced an educational campaign.

Another indication that caffeine promotes birth defects comes from a recent animal study done at Children's Hospital in Cincinnati. This time, caffeine itself caused few birth defects, but greatly increased the rate of birth defects caused by several other chemicals. For instance, caffeine alone caused malformations in 2.5 percent of the offspring, while the drug cycloheximide alone caused malformations in 17.2 percent of the offspring. When the two chemicals were administered together, birth defects occurred in 96.6 percent of the offspring.

Determining whether a chemical has caused human birth defects is difficult, unless, as in the case of thalidomide, some women consume huge amounts of a drug or the chemical causes highly unusual birth defects. Because a common defect, such as cleft palate, might be caused by dozens of different chemicals, and because a chemical might cause defects in only a small percentage of babies, human studies are expensive and insensitive. Despite their limitations, several studies concerning coffee and human birth defects have been done.

Shortly before FDA's warning to pregnant women, CSPI opened a Caffeine/Birth Defects Clearinghouse and heard from numerous parents of babies with birth defects. In most cases, mothers had smoked, drank alcohol, and used various prescription drugs, in addition to drinking coffee, so the likely cause of birth defects could not be determined. However, in three cases, coffee appeared to be the culprit. Jonquil Prevette was born with multiple defects, including cleft palate and missing fingers and toes, both seen in animal studies on caffeine. Jonquil's mother was a ten-to-twelve-cup-a-day coffee drinker, but otherwise she scrupulously avoided drugs, cigarettes, and alcohol. She was not exposed to any workplace pollutants. The other two cases were quite similar. Mrs. Prevette explained:

> I know that my experience does not absolutely prove that coffee was the cause of my baby's birth defects. But it seems to offer the only reasonable explanation. I think common sense says that pregnant women should consume as little caffeine as possible.

In 1982 two human studies were published. One, supervised by Dr. Shai Linn at Brigham and Women's Hospital in Boston, involved 12,205 babies. The researchers compared five-cup-a-day coffee drinkers to abstainers and looked primarily at the effects in late pregnancy. They saw no effect on birth weight, length of gestation, and birth defects (which are typically caused in the first trimester of pregnancy). One of the interesting findings in this study was that very few women drank more than three cups of coffee a day. This probably reflected the overall decline in coffee drinking and the aversion to coffee that many women develop during pregnancy. The body seems to have a built-in warning mechanism.

The second study was overseen by Dr. Lynn Rosenberg of Boston University School of Medicine. In this study, doctors examined the coffee-drinking habits of mothers of 2,030 babies born with specific types of birth defects. Like the Linn study, few mothers consumed four or more cups of coffee a day and no link was seen between the coffee and the birth defects. The authors acknowledged that they could not have detected an effect of coffee that caused less than a doubling or tripling in birth defects. Only twenty-two of the babies had missing fingers and toes, a group too small to allow any meaningful statistical analyses.

One can conclude from the various studies that coffee does not cause a large number of birth defects, but may well be causing occasional ones. I don't think that definitive human studies will ever be done—there are just too many confounding factors in a woman's life, such as drugs, pollution, anxiety, alcohol, genetic susceptibilities, and cigarette smoking. I think that a prudent woman would follow FDA Commissioner Goyan's advice: avoid caffeine or use it sparingly. One or two cups of coffee is highly unlikely to cause any problem, but, just to be on the safe side, isn't it worth consuming as little caffeine as possible for the sake of the developing baby?

Many women who are not pregnant should also be careful about caffeine. Research by Dr. John Minton, a surgeon at Ohio State University, has indicated that caffeine is one cause of fibrocystic breast disease (benign breast lumps). Breast lumps are not only often extremely painful but, because they may camouflage—or increase the risk of—malignancies, they often necessitate biopsies.

When Dr. Minton studied eighty-eight women with breast lumps, he found that out of forty-five patients who abstained completely from caffeine (and similar chemicals), thirty-seven experienced total disappearance of breast lumps, and seven of the remainder reported improvement. Among twenty-eight women who reduced their consumption of caffeine, seven reported that their cysts disappeared and fourteen reported improvement. Of the fifteen women who went on consuming their usual amount of caffeine, only two found that their breast lumps disappeared spontaneously.

Doctors at the University of Southern California School of Medicine did an even better study and came up with identical results. They used the technique of telethermometry to objectively measure the presence of cysts. Philip Brooks and his colleagues concluded, "This study dramatically shows the improvement in fibrocystic breast disease with restriction of caffeine ingestion."

Although the ideal double-blind controlled study of caffeine and breast lumps is yet to be done, and one study did not confirm Minton and Brooks's work, many doctors are urging patients with fibrocystic breast disease to try giving up caffeine. Many additional women are swearing off on their own.

According to Minton, complete relief may take up to six to eight months in young women and two years in older women. Minton stresses that women with breast lumps should discuss their condition with their doctors rather than simply self-treat, because lumps may be malignant.

The large and still growing pile of scientific investigations clearly indicates that small amounts of caffeine present little risk to the general population, but that certain people should make a special effort to minimize their caffeine intake: children, because of the chemical's influence on sleep and behavior; women who are or may become pregnant; women with fibrocystic breast disease; anyone who is tense, jittery, or has trouble falling asleep; and those with heart disease.

Exactly what constitutes a reasonable or unreasonable amount of caffeine for the rest of us varies from person to person. But youngsters who drink more than one or two caffeine-containing sodas per day, and adults who regularly drink more than a cup or two of coffee or several cups of tea per day should certainly consider modifying a habit that may not be as harmless as once thought.

Ref.: *Arzneimittel-Forschung 14*, 415 (1964); *New Eng. J. Med. 304*, 630 (1981), *306*, 141 (1982); *Lancet i*, 1415 (1981); *Consumer Reports*, October 1981; *Surgery, 90* 299 (1981), *91*, 263 (1982); *J. Reprod. Med. 26*, 279 (1981); *Reg. Toxicol. Pharmacol. 1*, 355 (1981); *J. Am. Med. Asso. 244*, 1078 (1980), *247*, 1429 (1982); *Teratology 25*, 95 (1982); *J. Psychiat. Res. 17*, 187 (1982–83); *Tox. Appl. Pharmac. 74*, 364 (1984); *21* CFR 182. 1180.

Calcium compounds   Safe

Calcium compounds are used in many different foods for many different purposes. The calcium part of the chemicals is safe and, indeed, acts as a nutrient, providing the body with extra calcium. The "last name" of the compound determines the function of the calcium, as indicated in the following listing. These substances are all safe:

calcium acetate	sequestrant
calcium carbonate	alkali, white coloring excipient, yeast food
calcium chloride	firming agent in canned fruits and vegetables
calcium gluconate	buffer, sequestrant
calcium hexametaphosphate	sequestrant
calcium hydroxide	alkali
calcium lactate	firming agent, flavoring, nutrient
calcium phosphate (mono-, di-, tribasic)	sequestrant, acid in baking powder (mono), anticaking agent (tribasic)
calcium phytate	sequestrant
calcium pyrophosphate	sequestrant
calcium stearate	anticaking agent
calcium sulfate	alkali, yeast food, dough conditioner

Ref.: 21 CFR 182. 1191–182.1217, 182.5191–182.5223, 184.1185–184.1230.

Calcium and Sodium Propionate   Safe

Almost everyone has heard of the food additive calcium propionate. It is the chemical most often used to prevent the growth of mold and certain bacteria in bread and rolls. While preserving the baked goods, it also provides a calcium supplement to the diet. Sodium propionate, the sodium salt of propionic acid, is preferred in pies and cakes, because calcium alters the action of chemical leavening agents.

Propionic acid occurs naturally in many foods and acts as a natural preservative in Swiss cheese, in which it may occur at a 1 percent level. Propionate is also formed and used as a source of energy when the body metabolizes certain fats and amino acids.

Because most germs are killed when cakes and breads are baked, one might wonder why preservatives are needed at all in these foods. The most obvious reason is that molds may contaminate a food after it is removed from the oven. Secondly, during baking the interior of a loaf of bread may never rise above 100° C (212° F), which is not hot enough to kill all bacterial spores. Were it not for a preservative these bacteria would multiply and soften and discolor the bread and cause off-odors.

Propionates inhibit the growth of, but do not kill, microorganisms. Although microorganisms tolerate small amounts of propionate, the moderate levels (0.1 to 0.2 percent) used in food appear enormous from the humble perspective of a microbe. When molds and bacteria are confronted with the onslaught of propionate, they are excessively occupied with one metabolic function and cannot perform other vital functions. Consequently, the microbes grow slowly or not at all. The yeast used to make bread rise is added at levels high enough to resist the effects of the preservative; the yeast is killed during baking.

Propionate is one of the most innocuous food additives. Fed to rats as 3.75 percent of their diet for a year, sodium propionate had no ill effects.

Ref.: FAO (31)-84; CRC-249; *Chem. Abst. 69,* 33733; *Fed. Reg. 49,* 13139 (April 3, 1984); *21* CFR. 184.1081, 184.1221.

Calcium and Sodium Stearoyl Lactylates and Sodium Stearoyl Fumarate — Safe

Stearoyl lactylates and stearoyl fumarate are closely related chemicals that were first used commercially in the early 1960s. These substances strengthen bread dough so that it can withstand the mechanical punishment it receives in modern bread-making machinery; moreover, bakers do not have to control mixing times as precisely. Bread and cake made with these additives (plus mono- and diglycerides) stay soft longer and have a more uniform grain and greater volume than untreated products.

Manufacturers use stearoyl lactylates and fumarate in bread dough, cake fillings, and other starch-containing foods at levels up to 0.5 percent. These chemicals also serve as whipping agents in dried, liquid, and frozen egg whites and in artificial whipped cream. Companies use about one million pounds of this additive annually.

Digestive enzymes in animals break these additives down to stearic alcohol and either lactic or fumaric acid, all of which are harmless, easily metabolized substances.

Ref.: FAO(40)-15; FAO(46A)-109; CUFP-26; *21* CFR 172.826, 172.844–172.848.

Caramel   Safe

Caramel, one of the most familiar food additives, is a complex mixture of compounds that form when sugar or starch is heated. Not only is caramel produced commercially for use as a coloring and flavoring in a wide variety of foods, but it can be made right on the kitchen stove. Sugars are sometimes added to baked goods so that they caramelize and turn brown when they are heated.

Three fourths of all caramel used in the United States serves as artificial brown coloring in soda pop, especially colas and root beer. Smaller amounts are used in candy, baked goods, soy sauces, syrups, dark beers and certain whiskies, and a range of other foods. Approximately 37 million pounds are produced a year.

Manufacturers have developed a variety of caramels to meet the needs of specific food industries. Most caramel is produced by heating sugar or corn syrup in the presence of ammonia and/or sulfite, which assist caramelization and confer particular properties. Caramel intended for soda pop, an acidic food, is prepared with both the ammonia and sulfite. Caramel intended for use in baked goods, beer, sauces, and meat products is produced with the ammonia, but without the sulfite. A small amount of plain caramel (no catalysts at all) is also made.

While long thought to be safe, the caramel made with ammonia came under suspicion in the early 1970s. Tests indicated that a contaminant, 4-methylimidazole, might be toxic. The ammonia-caramel caused reduced body weight, reduced organ weights, and reduced numbers of white blood cells in laboratory rats. Subsequent studies gave indications of pituitary gland and breast tumors, but the effects were not strong enough to be considered definitive. FDA has limited the contaminant to 0.02 percent or less, a level that is presumably safe, and has asked the industry to undertake additional tests.

Ref.: Fd. Cosmet. Toxicol. 15, 509, 523 (1977); *Fd. Chem. Toxicol. 21,* 237, 701 (1983); International Technical Caramel Association (Washington, D.C.).; *21* CFR 73.85, 182.1235.

Carbon Dioxide (Carbonated Water) Safe

Carbon dioxide, a harmless gas, is responsible for the bubbles in beer, soda pop, mineral water, and the like.

Ref.: 21 CFR 182.1240.

Carboxymethylcellulose (CMC, Cellulose Gum), Safe
Cellulose, and related compounds

Cellulose is a safe and inexpensive carbohydrate that comprises the woody parts and cell walls of plants. Chemists have learned how to modify cellulose to generate derivatives with a variety of properties. The nature and degree of modification affect the thickness of solutions, solubility, or concentration or temperature at which a solution gels.

One well-known product that contains powdered cellulose itself is Fresh Horizons bread. This is a cousin of Wonder Bread in which cellulose—or, more recognizably, powdered sawdust—is used to increase the fiber content and reduce the calorie content. The baker has advertised that Fresh Horizons has several times the fiber content of whole wheat bread, which, if true, would be significant. However, cellulose is the least useful form of fiber, because intestinal bacteria can digest a sizable fraction of it.

Carboxymethylcellulose (CMC), the most widely used cellulose derivative, is made by reacting cellulose (wood pulp, cotton lint) with a derivative of acetic acid (the acid in vinegar). It is also called cellulose gum. Manufacturers first used CMC as a food additive in 1924, but it was not used widely until the early 1940s, when natural vegetable products were in short supply due to the war. Some of the functions CMC serves in food include:

- in ice cream: adds body and improves the texture, controls the formation of ice crystals; because CMC causes whey to separate out, it is often used in combination with carrageenan or gelatin (up to 0.3 percent);
- in beer: to stabilize the foam;
- in pie fillings and jellies: prevents fruit from settling or floating (up to 0.5 percent);
- in cake icings: prevents sugar from crystallizing and water from evaporating; helps maintain a smooth, glossy appearance;
- in diet foods: the water-binding capacity of CMC gives the dieter a feeling of fullness and satiety without adding any calories; adds body to artificially sweetened beverages (up to 3 percent);

- in bread doughs: helps hold in moisture, increases volume;
- in candy; prevents the sugar from crystallizing.

Animals cannot absorb or digest carboxymethylcellulose; when ingested it is totally excreted in the stools. Massive amounts (more than 5 percent) of CMC in food diminish an animal's rate of growth but have no apparent effect on internal organs, cancer incidence, or reproduction.

Tumors have never been induced in experimental animals by food containing as much as 20 percent CMC, but when researchers injected the additive under the skin of rats, tumors formed at the site of injection. The FAO/WHO Expert Committee on Food Additives and most scientists, however, agree that CMC is not carcinogenic, because it passes right through the gastrointestinal tract and never enters the blood or internal organs. Injection-site tumors are probably caused by physical irritation.

CMC has been used as a laxative and antacid. No undesirable side effects were caused by doses ranging as high as ten grams a day for six to eight months.

The food industry also uses the ethyl, methyl, methyl ethyl, hydroxypropyl, and hydroxypropyl methyl† derivatives for many of the same purposes as carboxymethylcellulose. These compounds are used to improve the clarity of berry pie fillings, retard melting of ice cream, reduce absorption of water by pie crust, substitute for a portion of the egg ingredient in cake batter, and artificially thicken many foods. An unusual feature of solutions containing methyl cellulose is that they become thicker rather than thinner upon heating; above a certain temperature they may gel. The body does not absorb or digest any of these substances.

Unmodified cellulose is sometimes used as an inert filler in solid and liquid diet foods, but ordinarily it gives foods an unacceptably grainy texture. Food technologists have overcome this problem by treating cellulose with carefully controlled amounts of acid. They call the product microcrystalline cellulose (MC) and use it as a food additive.

Microcrystalline cellulose's properties are interesting enough to suggest that it may become an increasingly familiar name on food labels. Particles of MC, which are extremely porous, can absorb such liquid foods as syrup, melted cheese, and liquified peanut butter and convert them to dry granular forms. Solutions of microcrystalline cellulose in water have a creamy consistency at low concentrations and form smooth spreading gels at high concentrations. According to the manufacturer of MC, unpublished animal feeding studies show that MC does not impair the availability of nutrients in the diet. The World Health Organization has concluded that MC does not pose a hazard to health.

† The full names of these chemicals are ethyl cellulose, hydroxypropyl cellulose, etc.

Ref.: WHO (8)-47; FAO (40A)-75, 79, 82; FAO (46A)-131; CRC-Ch. 8; *Food Engineering 33*, 44 (August 1961); *Fd. Cos. Tox. 2*, 539 (1964), *6*, 449 (1968); *Washington Post* (food section) Oct. 28, 1976; *21* CFR 172.868–172.874, 182.1480, 182.1745.

Carnauba Wax   ?

Wait a minute, isn't carnauba wax the stuff used on cars, not food? In fact, it is used on both. Over the years, I have seen some people raise suspicions about certain food additives, because they were used in explosives as well as foods, as if that double use constituted proof of great harmfulness. Chemicals can have many uses, and only toxicological tests, not false logic, can determine if they are really safe or dangerous.

In the case of carnauba wax, which is derived from the leaves and buds of the Brazilian wax palm, the meager testing that has been done suggests safety. The wax is a highly insoluble mixture of long-chain fatty acids, which, in theory, should be either digested or passed right through the body. Better studies ought to be done to test for long-term effects and the presence of contaminants. Carnauba wax is used on fresh fruits and in baked goods, candies, and other processed foods.

Ref.: Fed. Reg. 47, 34164 (1982); *21* CFR 182.1978.

Carrageenan   Premature Infants: **Avoid**
                                                              Others: **Safe**

For centuries, housewives living near the coasts of Ireland and France have used a substance obtained from the sun-bleached fronds of a local seaweed, Irish moss, as an ingredient in blancmange pudding. Europeans have also used the same seaweed to treat peptic and intestinal ulcers. The active chemical in Irish moss is the carbohydrate carrageenan, named after Carragheen, Ireland.

Irish moss grows along the shores of Maine, the Maritime provinces of Canada, the British Isles, Scandinavia, and France. Fishermen scrape the red, bushy seaweed from coastal rocks with special long-handled rakes, or simply collect it on the beach. Carrageenan is extracted from the plant with hot water. The United States imported over 2 million pounds of carrageenan in 1982.

Food manufacturers use carrageenan because of the unique way it reacts with milk protein. A weak gel that forms in the milk prevents cocoa particles from settling in chocolate milk and prevents butterfat from separating out of evaporated milk. The seaweed derivative has similar stabilizing effects in canned milk drinks, "instant breakfast," and infant formula. Manufacturers use carrageenan to add "body" to soft drinks, to thicken ice cream, jelly, sour cream, and syrup, to stabilize the foam in beer, and to prevent the oil from separating out of frozen whipped topping.

Carrageenan is sometimes used as the gelling component of gelatin-type desserts and milk puddings. A carrageenan gel forms more readily and melts less readily than a gel made of gelatin, and it does not develop a thick skin on standing. The gels have a natural brittleness which may be tempered by adding a small amount of locust bean gum. Carrageenan-based products are used by vegetarians, because gelatin is made from animals.

Scientists have fed carrageenan to animals and observed that it is poorly absorbed by the body and is apparently harmless at levels as high as 15 percent of the diet for short periods of time. When guinea pigs and rabbits consume carrageenan for several months, however, they often develop ulcers of the colon. When carrageenan is treated with acid, which decreases the size of the molecules, and fed to rabbits and guinea pigs, levels as low as 0.1 percent of the diet cause intestinal ulcers.

Companies that manufacture canned infant formula use carrageenan to keep the fat and protein in solution. Though the animal studies suggest a hazard, one factor that reduces the risk to babies is that they always consume carrageenan with milk, which reduces its acidity; in the animal studies carrageenan was added to the drinking water. That the sensitive laboratory animals were herbivorous may also be significant.

Dr. Paul M. Fleiss, a professor of pediatrics at the University of Southern California, believes that carrageenan poses a special risk to premature infants. The carrageenan in formula may disrupt the development of the gastrointestinal tract of these babies and cause necrotizing enterocolitis. Fleiss says, "We therefore believe carrageenan should not be fed to developing premature infants . . . until data prove it does not cause the mucosal changes it causes in laboratory animals."

Carrageenan has been tested for its ability to cause cancer or to enhance the carcinogenicity of other chemicals. Some of the tests, including ones done at the highly regarded American Health Foundation, indicate that large amounts of carrageenan increase the potency of chemicals that cause colon cancer. One must be cautious in interpreting these studies, because the large doses of carrageenan can cause ulcerative colitis, which may be the true cause of the cancer risk. The World Health Organization's International Agency for Research on Cancer concluded in 1983 that carrageenan, by itself, is not carcinogenic.

Ref.: *J. Pharm. Pharmacol. 21,* 187S (1969); *Cancer Res. 38,* 4427 (1978); *Gastroenterology 74,* 161–2 (1978); *Fed. Reg. 44,* 40343-5 (July 10, 1979); *Lancet i,* 338 (1981); *West. J. Med. 132,* 365–6 (1980); *Fd. Cosmet. Toxicol. 19,* 779–781 (1981); *IARC Monographs on the Evaluation of the Carcinogenic Risk of Chemicals to Humans 31,* 79 (1983); *21* CFR 172.620–172.626.

Casein   Safe

A science experiment that millions of children have conducted at their breakfast tables is to add grapefruit juice or lemon juice to milk. Like in a magic trick, mixing the two liquids together causes the milk to curdle. The curd is primarily casein, the principal protein in milk.

Casein is a nutritious protein, because it contains significant amounts of all the essential amino acids. Food manufacturers add casein to ice cream, ice milk, frozen custard, and sherbet to improve their texture. In nondairy coffee creamers, casein adds body and acts as an emulsifier and whitener. One of the most "important" uses is as a binder in imitation cheeses. Casein is a safe and nutritious food additive.

Ref.: 21 CFR 182.1748.

Cellulose Gum: *see* carboxymethylcellulose

Chewing Gum Base   ?

Chewing gum base is the tasteless wad that is left in your mouth when all the flavor is gone from a stick of gum. Gum base is composed of natural (chicle, natural rubber, etc.) or synthetic (butyl rubber, paraffin, polyethylene, etc.) masticatory substances, synthetic softeners (glycerated gum resin, stearic acid, etc.), resins, antioxidants, and other goodies. Chewing gum bases have no nutritive value, and they have not been adequately tested.

Turn to the discussions of mannitol, sorbitol, and xylitol for a word about noncariogenic ("sugarless") chewing gum.

Ref.: 21 CFR 172.615 lists some of the dozens of substances that gum manufacturers use.

Chlorine (Cl_2)   Safe

Before bakers can use flour, they must "age" it, either by storing it for several months or by treating it with a chemical. The best agent for aging cake flour is chlorine gas, which, at a level of 400 parts per million, instantly ages the flour and bleaches it white. The chlorination process prevents cakes from collapsing when they're removed from the oven and prevents fruit from sinking in fruit cakes.

Chlorine affects the flour by causing changes in both the protein and starch. In addition, chlorine reacts to a limited extent with the small amount of unsaturated oil that is present in white flour. Toxicologists were suspicious of the chlorinated flour oil (CFO) that forms and therefore conducted tests on rodents to determine its possible effects.

In one series of experiments, British scientists treated flour with chlorine and then extracted the CFO. They fed the modified oil at high concentrations (up to a thousand times the amount to which a person might be exposed) to four generations of rats and mice. CFO did not accumulate in body fat and had an adverse effect (on lactation) only at the highest concentration. While CFO appeared to be innocuous, it should be noted that very few animals (2 to 6 mother rodents per dosage level per generation) were used in the experiment.

A good study on rats and not quite as good a study on mice indicated that chlorinated flour does not cause cancer or other problems.

Ref.: FAO (40A)-109; *Proc. Nutr. Soc. 25,* 51 (1966); *Fd. Chem. Tox. 21,* 427, 435 (1983); *21* CFR 137.105.

Chlorine Dioxide (ClO$_2$)   Safe

In 1946 the baking industry in the United States and abroad was rudely shocked. Sir Edward Mellanby, an English biochemist, demonstrated that ordinary flour or bread that had been treated with agene (nitrogen trichloride) made dogs stark raving mad and was sometimes even fatal. At the time, agene was used to bleach and age 80 to 90 percent of the bread flour in the United States and England. Cereal chemists anxiously sought an economical, effective, and safe substitute and found that one of the lesser used flour treatment agents, chlorine dioxide, filled the bill. After agene was banned in 1949, chlorine dioxide gas became the most widely used bleaching and maturing agent. However, in 1983, the American Institute of Baking reported that it is "probably not used" anymore.

Since 1975, chlorine dioxide has been used in the processing of fresh fruits and vegetables. According to the Food and Drug Administration, no residue remains on the produce after washing by the processor, and "the annual poundage of the substances consumed via food appears to be negligibly small."

Chlorine dioxide has been rather well tested, because no one wanted a repeat of the agene scare. In one of the more complete experiments, four generations of rats were fed diets consisting mainly of heavily treated (300 ppm) flour or bread. No adverse effects on growth, survival, internal organs, or reproduction were observed. Short-term tests have been done on rats, rabbits, dogs, and monkeys with no indication of any problems.

Ref.: FAO (35)-159; *J. Sci. Fd. Agr. 7,* 464 (1956), *15,* 725 (1964), *18,* 203 (1967); pers. comm. from FDA and American Institute of Baking; *21* CFR 137.105.

Cinnamaldehyde   Avoid

The taste and fragrance of cinnamon in chewing gum or candy may come from the chemical cinnamaldehyde rather than real cinnamon. Americans ingest about 500,000 pounds of this flavoring annually. But don't bother looking for cinnamaldehyde in the list of ingredients on the label—it would only be listed as "artificial flavoring."

Cinnamaldehyde is closely related to cinnamic acid and cinnamyl anthranilate, two other artificial flavorings that are rarely used (no more than a few hundred pounds a year). In 1980 the National Cancer Institute announced that cinnamyl anthranilate, which is used in grape- and cherry-flavored ice cream, beverages, chewing gums, and other processed foods, caused liver cancers in male and female mice. It also caused kidney and pancreatic cancers in male rats. A year and a half later, in May 1982, the Food and Drug Administration proposed banning this flavoring. While the ban has not been finalized, companies have stopped making and using the additive. However, the flavoring industry's trade association, the Flavor Extract Manufacturers' Association, is trying to persuade the FDA that any possible risk from cinnamyl anthranilate is so small that the additive should be allowed.

As soon as cinnamyl anthranilate was found to be carcinogenic, the FDA said that "it now becomes imperative that cinnamaldehyde be examined for its carcinogenic potential as soon as possible." FDA was especially concerned, because previous tests showed that methyl anthranilate and anthranilic acid did not promote cancer. These negative tests threw suspicion on the cinnamyl portion of cinnamyl anthranilate . . . and on cinnamaldehyde. Four years later the urgency had evaporated. Cinnamaldehyde still had not been tested. FDA's own tests were never done for lack of funding, and FDA never demanded that industry conduct the tests. In 1984 the World Health Organization added its voice to others calling for new cancer tests.

If cinnamaldehyde is ever tested and found to promote cancer, the public will be faced with another dilemma. It would be easy to ban the artificial flavoring, but what about *natural* cinnamon, whose chief flavor component is the very same chemical? We consume about 600 tons of cinnamon annually. The Delaney Clause bans cancer-causing additives only, not foods, but the *spirit* of the law would cover cinnamon. A similar situation arose in 1960 when safrole, a carcinogenic flavoring present in root beer, was outlawed. This may be one of the few situations in which it might be appropriate to put a warning label on a natural food, thereby encouraging consumers to switch from cinnamon to other seasonings. So much for hot apple cider with cinnamon sticks!

Ref.: The Book of Spices, Rosengarten, F., rev. ed., Pyramid Books, New York (1973); NIH Publication No. 80-1752 (August 1980); *Fed. Reg. 47*, 22545 (May 25, 1982); *Food Chem. News* p. 31 (Jan. 7, 1985); FDA files; *21* CFR 172.515.

Citric Acid — Safe
Isopropyl citrate
Sodium citrate
Stearyl citrate
Triethyl citrate

Citric acid is one of the most versatile, commonly used, and unquestionably safe food additives. It is an important metabolite in virtually all living organisms and occurs in high concentrations in citrus fruits and berries. It comprises as much as 8 percent of the juice of unripe lemons and a somewhat smaller proportion of the juices of many ripe fruits.

Chemical companies have been producing citric acid since 1860. They normally make it by the fermentative action of fungus *(Aspergillus niger)* on beet molasses. The growing conditions are carefully controlled so that the fungus produces but does not metabolize the acid.‡ A small amount is also isolated from pineapple by-products and from low-quality lemons. American food companies use one hundred million pounds of citric acid and its salts annually.

Citric acid is an important food additive because it is a strong acid, is inexpensive, has a tart flavor, and serves as an antioxidant. Food processors use it in ice cream, sherbet, fruit juice drinks, carbonated beverages, jellies, preserves, canned fruits and vegetables, cheeses, candies, and chewing gum. In soft-centered candy citric acid has the added function of solubilizing the sugar (see "invert sugar").

Manufacturers use citric acid as an antioxidant in instant potatoes, wheat chips, and potato sticks. Citric acid prevents spoilage by trapping metal ions which might otherwise promote reactions that spoil or discolor the food. It is often used together with "primary" antioxidants (BHA, BHT, propyl gallate), which inhibit oxidation by a totally different mechanism. The combined effect of the different kinds of antioxidants is synergistic. Wine producers make good use of citric acid's ability to trap metal ions; the acid combines with iron, which might otherwise form iron-tannin complexes that make wine cloudy.

‡ Before trying to make citric acid in your bathtub, you should know the following tricks of the trade. Copper is added to inhibit aconitase, the enzyme that metabolizes citrate; metal atoms that are components of enzymes that promote the degradation of citrate are preferentially removed; the acidity of the growth medium is kept below pH 3.5.

The sodium salt of citric acid is used as a buffering agent to control the acidity of gelatin desserts, jams, jellies, candies, ice cream, and other products.

Several other forms of citric acid that are occasionally used by food manufacturers include isopropyl citrate, stearyl citrate, and triethyl citrate. They are generally used in oily foods to retard spoilage. They are safe.

Ref.: ECT 5, 524; CRC-Ch. 7; *Fed. Reg.* 48, 834 (Jan. 7, 1983); 21 CFR 182.1033, 182.1751, 182.6033, 182.6195, 182.6386–182.6751.

Corn Syrup, High Fructose Corn Syrup

Moderate amounts: **Safe**
Large amounts: **Avoid**

Corn syrup is a sweet, thick solution made by "digesting" cornstarch with acids or enzymes. It contains dextrose, maltose, and dextrin. Food manufacturers use corn syrup to sweeten and thicken foods and beverages. It also retards the crystallization of sugar in candy, icings, and fillings and prevents the loss of moisture from cakes, cookies, and whipped foods.

Corn syrup may be dried and used in powdered products, such as nondairy coffee whiteners, in which case it is called corn syrup solids.

Because corn syrup is a cheaper source of sweetness than cane or beet sugar, its use is soaring. On a per capita basis, corn syrup consumption shot up from 10.1 pounds in 1960 to 66 pounds in 1983.

One drawback of regular corn syrup is that it is not quite as sweet as sugar. Chemists have overcome this problem by treating corn syrup with an enzyme that converts some of the dextrose to fructose, which is relatively sweet. The final product, called "high fructose corn syrup," has enabled the corn sugar industry to capture an ever increasing share of the sweetener market. Over 8 billion pounds—43 pounds per person—of high fructose corn syrup were produced in 1983. It is used in soda pop, baked goods, and other processed foods.

The cane and beet sugar industries in the United States survive in the face of the availability of much cheaper foreign sugar only because of subsidies or import restrictions. It has been amusing to see the corn sugar industry gleefully support higher sugar prices (which add billions to consumers' food bills). The higher prices persuade food processors to switch from sugar to corn sweeteners.

All forms of corn syrup represent "empty calories" and promote both obesity and tooth decay.

Ref.: ECT 9, 926; *Fed. Reg.* 48, 5716 (1983); 21 CFR 182.1866.

Cysteine   Safe

Cysteine is an amino acid and a natural constituent of protein-containing foods. Manufacturers occasionally add small amounts of cysteine to foods to prevent oxygen from destroying vitamin C. Bakers use cysteine to reduce the mixing time for dough.

Ref.: Baker's Digest 41 (3), 34 (1967); *21* CFR 184.1271–184.1272.

Dextrin   Safe

The mixture of fragments that results from treating starch with acid, alkali, or enzymes is called dextrin. Dextrin is as safe as starch itself. See the entry for starch.

Food manufacturers use dextrin to prevent sugar from crystallizing in candy, to encapsulate flavor oils used in powdered mixes, and as a thickening agent.

Ref.: Fed. Reg. 44, 18246 (March 27, 1979), *47,* 3647 (August 20, 1982); *21* CFR 184.1277.

Dextrose (glucose, corn sugar)   ?

Dextrose is one of the most important and ubiquitous chemicals in living organisms. This chemical is present in every living cell. Plants produce dextrose by photosynthesis, while animals make dextrose from a variety of different chemicals or obtain it from food. Dextrose has a key position in the metabolic pathways of both plants and animals; when an organism converts chemical "A" to chemical "Z," it often converts "A" to dextrose, and then dextrose to "Z." Dextrose is a sugar and a source of sweetness in fruits and honey.

In 1811 a Russian chemist named Kirchoff discovered that he could produce dextrose simply by heating starch in the presence of acid. For this valuable discovery the Russian czar awarded Kirchoff with a lifetime pension of five hundred rubles a year and the Order of St. Anne. Subsequently, organic chemists found that starch, cellulose, and glycogen (animal starch) consist of great numbers of dextrose molecules linked end to end. When we eat plant or animal starch our digestive enzymes break it down to dextrose. Our body uses the dextrose for energy or converts it to glycogen, which is stored in our liver and muscles. When we need energy our body converts glycogen back to dextrose. Man and most other animals cannot digest cellulose, because we lack certain enzymes.

Food manufacturers use dextrose primarily as a sweetener, but it serves additional functions in certain foods. Dextrose (and other sugars) turns brown when heated and contributes to the color of bread crust and toast. The same browning reaction accounts for the brown color of caramel. In soft drinks, dextrose contributes "body" and "mouth feel." Dextrose is only three fourths as sweet as table sugar (sucrose) and may be used in place of table sugar when oversweetness is a problem.

Like other refined sweeteners, dextrose can promote tooth decay, especially when used in sticky foods. See further discussions under "sucrose" and the sugar section of *Nutrition Scoreboard* (pages 41–53).

Dimethylpolysiloxane (methyl silicone, methyl polysilicone) — Safe

Silicon, which is present in sand and rock, is the second most abundant element in the earth's crust. Compounds containing silicon, despite their ready availability, are not utilized by living organisms and are not necessary for their growth (except for diatoms, which make their delicate shells from silica, the dioxide of silicon).

Silicon is chemically closely related to carbon and, like carbon, can form the backbone of an infinite number of compounds. In the last thirty years chemists have synthesized—and engineers have developed uses for—an incredible variety of silicon compounds, many with highly unusual properties. The silicones, which are long polymers containing silicon, oxygen, and organic groups, are the most important of the synthetic silicon compounds.

The assortment of jobs to which silicones have been applied boggles the mind. Silicones are used in bouncing putty, ironing spray, water-repellent coatings, and electrical insulation; silicone fluids are used to supplement soft tissues of the body and to lubricate arthritic joints; silicone rubber tubing is used to replace damaged tissues in the body, such as the urethra. Most of these applications depend upon silicone's properties of being insoluble in water and chemically inert.

The use of silicone by food manufacturers is trivial compared to its other uses. Dimethylpolysiloxane, the basic silicone, prevents the formation of troublesome foam during the manufacture of wine, refined sugar, yeast, gelatin, and chewing gum. Vegetable oil makers add it to their products, under the name methyl silicone or methyl polysilicone, to prevent foaming and spattering when the oils are cooked. This synthetic compound is used at levels between 0.9 and 10 parts per million.

The safety of silicones, which would be expected on the basis of their inertness, has been supported by feeding tests in animals (up to 0.1 percent of the diet) and by clinical usage in man. In a chronic feeding study done on rats,

0.1 percent silicone had no visible effect on growth, blood composition, tissues, and reproduction.

The one caution is that formaldehyde is used as a preservative in dimethyl polysiloxane. In fact, this is the only approved use of formaldehyde in our entire food supply. The risk is trivial, because of the small amounts involved.

Ref.: FAO (46A)-151; *AMA Arch. Ind. Health 21,* 514 (1960); *Chemistry and Technology of Silicones,* Noll, W., Academic Press, New York (1968); CUFP-21; *21* CFR 121.1099; *21* CFR 173.340.

Dioctyl Sodium Sulfosuccinate (DSS)   ?

A recurring problem that manufacturers have in the factory and cooks have in the kitchen is getting certain powdered foods to dissolve in water. Starch, cocoa, and other items sometimes just refuse to get wet! The difficulty has to do with the surface tension of water, and the solution is to coat the powder with a very small amount of a detergent-like chemical, such as dioctyl sodium sulfosuccinate (DSS).

The most likely place in the pantry to encounter DSS is in powdered soft drink mixes, in which it helps fumaric acid dissolve in water. Manufacturers also use it in some canned milk beverages containing cocoa fat and in foods that contain hard-to-dissolve thickening agents. DSS has a wide variety of industrial applications, such as in sugar refining, cleaning fruits and vegetables, and washing bottles.

DSS has been poorly tested. Only one long-term cancer test has been done in animals. That was conducted in the 1940s and is totally inadequate by current standards. For what it's worth, that study on rats did not indicate any problem. In 1976, new reproduction studies were completed. The tests indicated that near-toxic levels of DSS caused birth defects but it is unlikely that the tiny amounts of DSS in food would cause a problem. In 1984, an FDA review panel concluded that the additive should not be considered a potential human teratogen, but recommended that additional studies be conducted.

Ref.: J. Am. Pharm. Asso., 37, 29 (1948); *Food Prod. Development,* May 1972, p. 54; CRC-256, 498, 622; pers. comm. from American Cyanamid Co. and Hoechst-Roussel Pharmaceuticals, Inc. regarding testing data; *Food Chem. News,* p. 50 (March 31, 1980), p. 2 (Dec. 20, 1982); *Report,* DSS Scientific Review Panel; FDA Docket No. 84N-0184 (June 1984); *21* CFR 172.520, 172.810.

Disodium Guanylate (GMP)   Sufferers of Gout: **Avoid**
Disodium Inosinate (IMP)   Others: **Safe**

Disodium guanylate and disodium inosinate belong to the same family of food additives as monosodium glutamate: flavor enhancers. They get the abbreviations, GMP and IMP, from their chemical synonyms, guanosine monophosphate and inosine monophosphate. Flavor enhancers have little or no taste of their own, but accentuate the natural flavor of foods. They are often used by manufacturers in place of more expensive natural ingredients. "Save substantial sums of money" was the catchphrase in an ad that Takeda, Inc. once ran.

The taste-enhancing effect of GMP and IMP was discovered in 1913 by Dr. Shintaro Kodama, a scientist at Tokyo University. Dr. Kodama isolated a close relative of IMP (histidine salt of inosinate) from dried bonito tuna, a traditional condiment in Japan. Since then, IMP has been found in a wide variety of fish and animal meats at levels up to 0.3 percent, and GMP has been found at high concentrations in some kinds of mushrooms and several species of fish. They contribute greatly to the natural flavor of these foods. The IMP in meat forms when ATP, the "energy" molecule in living organisms, breaks down after an animal dies. In properly aged meat most of the ATP has changed to IMP; if aging is too prolonged, the IMP decays to inosine and hypoxanthine and the flavor is lost.

GMP and IMP have been sold commercially as food additives since 1960. The FDA estimates that about 30,000 pounds of each are used each year. You will find them in powdered soup mixes, ham and chicken salad spread, sauces and canned vegetables. Levels of usage vary from 0.003 to 0.05 percent. Manufacturers often use them together with monosodium glutamate, because of a synergistic action that exists between the three chemicals. GMP and IMP cannot be used in many moist foods, because enzymes in the food slowly digest the flavor enhancers.

These two additives are not quite interchangeable with MSG. IMP and GMP are about ten to twenty times as potent and forty times as expensive and have a subtly different taste effect. But like MSG, these flavor enhancers impart the impression that the food containing them has extra thickness and "meatiness." These qualities enable manufacturers to reduce the amount of expensive meat extract in their products.

Chemically, both GMP and IMP are related to the nucleic acids (DNA, RNA) of which our genes are composed, whereas MSG is an amino acid and a constituent of proteins. IMP and GMP are made from a natural product, yeast ribonucleic acid (RNA).

The way the body handles GMP and IMP is well understood. The IMP is degraded in the small intestine to hypoxanthine, while GMP is degraded to guanine. Both compounds are then absorbed by the body, converted to uric acid, and excreted. Persons who must avoid purines and uric acid, such as sufferers of gout and certain other genetic diseases, should not eat foods containing these additives. In gout, painfully large deposits of uric acid accumulate in joints.

Under normal circumstances, IMP and GMP are safe. However, they are closely related to adenosine, a chemical that acts as a neurotransmitter in the brain. These food additives should be tested to insure that they do not have subtle effects on behavior.

Ref.: Food Tech. 18, 287, 298 (1964); *Toxicology 2,* 185 (1974), *3,* 333, 341 (1975); *21* CFR 172.530, 172.535.

EDTA (Ethylene diamine tetraacetic acid);   Safe
Calcium disodium EDTA; Disodium EDTA

Modern food manufacturing technology, which involves metal rollers, scrapers, blenders, and containers, guarantees that tiny amounts of metal contamination will be present in food. These contaminants are undesirable, not only because they may be dangerous, but because they may impair the taste, odor, or appearance of food. Minute amounts of metal cause beverages to become cloudy, fruits and vegetables to discolor, and fats to spoil.

EDTA is extremely efficient at trapping the inevitable metal impurities. The structure of this molecule is such that positively charged metal ions—aluminum, copper, iron, manganese, nickel, zinc—are attracted to and trapped within a cage of negative charges. Manufacturers frequently use EDTA in combination with other antioxidants, such as BHT and propyl gallate, for a highly effective two-pronged attack on oxidation.

EDTA functions well in water and in oil-water mixtures. It does not dissolve in pure fats and oils so is not used in them.

You will find EDTA in many commerical salad dressings, margarine, mayonnaise, and sandwich spreads, in which it prevents the vegetable oil ingredient from going rancid. EDTA inhibits the metal-catalyzed browning of processed fruits and vegetables (potatoes, peas, corn, mushrooms, etc.) and prevents oxygen from destroying vitamin C in fruit juices. Canned shellfish—crabs, clams, and lobsters—usually contain large amounts of metal, often as high as 500 ppm, which promote discoloration and unpleasant odors and tastes; again, it's EDTA to the rescue. In beer, EDTA traps trace amounts of iron, which might otherwise cause a geyser of foam when the container was first opened, and copper, which causes clouding. Finally, soft drink companies use this versatile chemical to prevent artificial colors from fading.

Manufacturers are expected to add to a food only that amount of EDTA needed to trap metal impurities. Large excesses would combine with calcium, iron, and other nutrients and prevent them from being utilized by the body. EDTA is most often used at a concentration of 0.01 percent, but some products require as little as 0.0025 percent, others as much as 0.05 percent, depending on the amount of trace metal present.

Doctors used EDTA for medical purposes long before food chemists recognized its usefulness as an additive. Physicians treat acute metal poisoning by giving patients large intravenous injections of EDTA. The EDTA captures the noxious metal ions in the blood, and the EDTA-metal complex is then excreted in the urine. This treatment is not 100 percent effective, but hundreds of lives have been saved by it.

A second clinical application is to prevent the clotting of blood that is drawn for transfusions. The EDTA works by binding calcium, which is an essential component of the clotting reactions.

Occasional patients have suffered kidney damage from the injection of large doses of EDTA, but two lifetime feeding studies on rats and one on mice indicated that EDTA does not affect bones or teeth (which need calcium), growth, organs, tumor incidence, or reproduction. Metabolic experiments have shown that the body absorbs only about 5 percent of an oral dose and that this small amount is subsequently excreted in the urine.

Large doses of EDTA damage chromosomes in plant and cultured animal cells, but this damage appears to be due to a general disruption of cellular metabolism rather than any intrinsic mutagenicity of EDTA. Huge amounts did not cause birth defects in rats.

Ref.: FAO (40A)-39; *J. Am. Med. Asso. 174,* 263 (1960); *Tox. Appl. Pharm. 5,* 142 (1963), *40,* 299 (1977), *61,* 423 (1981); *Fd. Cos. Tox. 10,* 697 (1972); DHEW Pub. No. (NIH)77-811; *21* CFR 172.120, 172.135.

Ergosterol   Safe

Ergosterol is a natural steroid in yeast and mold that is converted by ultraviolet radiation to vitamin D. Irradiated ergosterol or other forms of vitamin D are added to most milk to insure that people get an adequate amount of the vitamin. Too little vitamin D can cause rickets, a serious bone disease.

Too much vitamin D can also be harmful, causing kidney and other damage. The American Academy of Pediatrics has urged that foods other than milk not be fortified with this vitamin, but the breakfast cereal producers have ignored this advice. You should avoid taking vitamin supplements that contain more than the recommended daily allowance of 400 I.U.

Ref.: Dairy Council Digest, 47 (3) (1976); *Recommended Dietary Allowances,* Nat. Acad. Sci., Washington, 1980; *21* CFR 182.8950–182.8953.

Ferric and Ferrous compounds—see Iron Compounds

Ferrous Gluconate   Safe

Ferrous gluconate is the iron salt of gluconic acid, a chemical that is present naturally in the body. Ferrous gluconate is used by the pharmaceutical industry as a source of iron for nutrient supplements and, since about 1960, by olive growers as an artificial coloring.

The black olive, surprisingly, is a highly processed fruit. Olives destined to be black olives are immature at the time of harvest, and are straw yellow to light green in color and extremely bitter. Treating them with 1–2 percent lye (sodium or potassium hydroxide) destroys the bitter chemical constituent, and exposing them to air turns the skin brown. Variations in color from one olive to another are remedied by ferrous gluconate, which darkens the fruit to a uniform, jet-black color.

Treating olives with ferrous gluconate is perfectly safe from a health standpoint, but too much can detract from the flavor. According to the Department of Agriculture, several processors have stopped using this additive, because they found that it sometimes makes olives unacceptably soft.

Ref.: 21 CFR 73.160.

Food Starch, modified—see Starch, Modified

Fructose   Safe

One of the recent gimmicks that health food companies are using to enhance the image of their products is to tout the sweetener fructose. An ad for General Nutrition Corporation said, "We have fructose! The miracle sweetener. No fat, no sodium, no empty calories." Sounds great, doesn't it? But miracles ain't what they used to be.

Fructose is a sugar that occurs primarily in fruits, though fruits also contain sucrose, glucose, and other sugars. Fructose constitutes one half of a molecule of sucrose (cane or beet sugar); glucose (corn sugar) makes up the other half.

Fructose has gained favor in recent years, because it has certain advantages over sucrose, glucose, or corn syrup. First, in certain cold, acidic beverages, but not other foods, it tastes almost twice as sweet as sucrose. This means that less can be used. Second, it is metabolized by the body somewhat differently from sucrose or glucose. Fructose has relatively little effect on blood sugar levels, whereas sucrose or glucose makes the blood sugar levels of most people rise significantly, then drop back down. The health significance of those swings in blood sugar levels is unclear, but a stable level is probably a benefit for diabetics and hypoglycemics.

Pure fructose is relatively expensive, as a trip to the health food store would reveal. It is made by chemically splitting sucrose into its two component sugars and then separating out and purifying the fructose. Food manufacturers usually resort to "high fructose corn syrup" (HFCS) for a sweetener. This product, which is cheaper than ordinary sugar, is made by treating corn syrup with enzymes to convert some of its glucose to fructose. It generally contains anywhere from 42 to 90 percent fructose, the rest being glucose and other compounds. (Recall that table sugar, when absorbed by the body, contains half fructose, half glucose.) Though fructose is advertised as being "natural" and often associated with a picture of a piece of fruit, it is at least as highly processed as other sugars.

Fructose does not pose any serious safety problems, other than contributing to one's general intake of sugar. It is no less of a threat to teeth than ordinary table sugar, and it is unencumbered with any vitamins or minerals.

Ref.: *Sugars in Nutrition,* Sipple, H. L. & K. W. McNutt, Academic Press, New York (1974); "Dietary Sugars in Health and Disease. I. Fructose", Fed. Am. Soc. Exp. Biol., Bethesda, Md. (1976); *J. Am. Diet. Asso.* *74,* 41 (1979); *Nutrition Action,* p. 7 (Feb., 1980); *21* CFR 182.1855.

Fumaric Acid   Safe
(calcium fumarate, magnesium fumarate, potassium fumarate, sodium fumarate)

Fumaric acid is a solid at room temperature, inexpensive, highly acidic (more acidic than citric acid, for instance), and does not absorb moisture readily. This set of qualities makes fumaric acid the ideal source of tartness and acidity in such dry products as gelatin desserts, pudding, pie fillings, candy, instant soft drinks, and leavening agents. Americans consume several million pounds of this additive annually.

One drawback of fumaric acid is that it dissolves very slowly in cold water. For a time this property prevented food manufacturers from using it in powdered, cold beverage mixes. However, Monsanto chemists discovered that the acid would dissolve readily in cold water if it were mixed with 0.3 percent dioctyl sodium sulfosuccinate (DSS), a "wetting agent."

Fumaric acid is an important metabolite and is present in every cell of the body. Biologists first examined the toxicity of the acid during World War II, when food manufacturers began to use fumaric acid in place of tartaric acid, which had become difficult to obtain from its manufacturers in the wine-producing countries of Europe. Experiments on a variety of mammals, including man, indicate that fumaric acid is harmless.

Ref.: 21 CFR 172.350.

Furcelleran ?

Furcelleran is a vegetable gum whose composition and properties are similar to carrageenan's. Like carrageenan, this food additive is obtained from seaweed. It is occasionally used by food manufacturers as a gelling agent in milk pudding and as a thickening agent in other foods. It has never been carefully tested.

Ref.: FAO (46A)-93; *21* CFR 172.655–172.660.

Gelatin Safe

The first lesson in modern "cooking" that many children have is preparing gelatin dessert. Kids are often amazed when they add a brightly colored powder to water and see the solution turn into a firm gel. The magic ingredient is, of course, the protein called gelatin.

Gelatin is obtained from collagen, the most abundant protein in animals and the major constituent of tendons and ligaments (gristle in cooked meat). The structure of collagen may be likened to a many-stranded rope. When it is heated the collagen (rope) breaks up into gelatin molecules (the strands). When the gelatin is dissolved in hot water, which is then allowed to cool, the molecules react weakly with one another to form a gel. If you could see a gel under a powerful microscope, it would look like a vast, tangled three-dimensional network of long, skinny molecules.

In addition to gelatin, powdered dessert mixes also contain sugar or dextrose for sweetness, an acid for tartness, sodium citrate to control the acidity, artificial coloring, artificial or natural flavoring (depending on the brand), and in some brands and flavors a pinch of the preservative BHA to protect the flavoring. Commercial gelatin desserts clearly belong in the junk food category, because of the sugar and food dyes and lack of vitamins and minerals. Homemade gelatin dessert, prepared with fruit juice and real fruit, would be a far better choice.

Gelatin is not the only natural substance that can form a gel—agar, carrageenan, and other carbohydrates extracted from seaweed also can—but it is perfect for foods because its gel melts at body temperature. On the other hand, in hot climates gelatin desserts may melt prematurely unless they are refrigerated.

Food manufacturers sometimes use gelatin at low concentrations to thicken yogurt, ice cream, cheese spreads, and beverages. Gelatin is pure protein but has little nutritive value, because it contains little or none of the essential amino acids.

Gluconic Acid, Glucono Delta-Lactone, Magnesium Gluconate, Sodium Gluconate, Zinc Gluconate Safe

Gluconic acid is a metabolite of glucose (blood sugar) and far larger amounts occur naturally than are ingested in the form of additives. Gluconic acid itself is occasionally used as a component of bottle rinsing solutions, but the various gluconate salts are more widely used. Sodium gluconate is used in nonalcoholic beverages and in processed fruit and fruit juices to bind metal ions that might otherwise promote spoilage. Magnesium and zinc gluconates are used in mineral supplements, because they are highly soluble and readily absorbable.

The most widely used of this family of compounds is glucono delta-lactone, which is produced by oxidizing glucose (corn sugar, dextrose). When the lactone is dissolved in water, gluconic acid forms. Glucono delta-lactone is used to adjust the acidity or as a leavening agent in baked goods, cheeses, processed fruits and juices, and real and imitation dairy products. It is used in some cured meats to speed the formation of the pink color.

All of these substances are quite safe. See also ferrous gluconate.

Ref.: Fed. Reg. 47, 35778 (August 17, 1982), 49028 (October 29, 1982); *21* CFR 182.6757.

Glycerin (glycerol) Safe

Glycerin—also called glycerol—is a clear, thick liquid that manufacturers add to foods to maintain a certain moisture content and prevent foods from drying out and becoming hard. You will find it in marshmallows, candy, fudge, and baked goods in amounts ranging from 0.5 to 10 percent. Manufacturers also use glycerol as a solvent for oily chemicals, especially flavorings, that are not very soluble in water.

Glycerin is safe. It forms the backbone of fat and oil molecules and is a familiar chemical to the body. The body uses glycerin either as a source of energy or as a starting material in making more complex molecules. Combining glycerin with three molecules of nitric acid results in nitroglycerin; fortunately, this reaction does not occur in living organisms.

Ref.: 21 CFR 182.1320.

Glycine (aminoacetic acid) Safe

Glycine is an amino acid that is present in all proteins. It is especially abundant in collagen (20–35 percent), the protein that makes up much of the body's connective tissue. Bottlers sometimes add glycine (0.2 percent) to artificially sweetened soft drinks to mask the bitter aftertaste of saccharin.

Ref.: Fed. Reg. 39, 25484 (July 11, 1974); *21* CFR 172.812.

Guar Gum Safe

Guar gum is one of the most widely used, cheapest, and most effective of the vegetable gum stabilizers. A given weight of guar will form a thicker solution than any other stabilizer. Guar is also unusual among gums, because it dissolves in cold water. As an added bonus, if this feature fits into your culinary preferences, a guar gum solution will turn into a rubbery gel if borate is added as a cross-linking agent.

The guar plant, which resembles the soybean plant, is grown mainly for use as cattle feed in the United States (Texas and Oklahoma), Pakistan, Iran, and India. The endosperm of the seed of this plant is virtually pure guar. The remainder of the seed is a valuable source of protein for livestock. The United States imported 135 million pounds in 1982 (not all of it is used in food).

Guar gum serves as a thickening agent in beverages, ice cream, frozen pudding, and salad dressing. Manufacturers also use it to increase the resiliency of doughs and batters and in the production of artificial whipped cream.

Biochemists have shown that guar gum is largely digestible. Long-term feeding studies on mice and rats indicate that guar gum is safe.

Ref.: FAO (46A)-100; *Tox. Appl. Pharm. 5,* 478 (1963); WHO(8)-38; *Fd. Chem. Toxicol. 21,* 305 (1983); *21* CFR 184.1339.

Gum Arabic (acacia gum, gum senegal) Safe

Gum arabic is obtained from a short, Middle Eastern tree, the acacia, in which it serves as a wound sealant. The gum oozes out and is collected from trees whose bark has split open because of drought, microbial infection, or intentional cuts. American firms obtain virtually all their gum arabic from Sudan. The United States imported 14.7 million pounds of this gum in 1982.

Archeologists have discovered that the Egyptians used gum arabic four thousand years ago in paint. These days, food processors use it to prevent sugar crystals from forming in candy, to help citrus oils dissolve in drinks, to encapsulate flavor oils in powdered drink mixes, to stabilize the foam in beer, and to improve the texture of commercial ice cream.

Gum arabic is unusual among vegetable gums because it is very soluble in water; solutions become viscous only when they contain 10–20 percent gum. Another unusual property of gum arabic is that it is completely digested by rodents (rat, guinea pig) and, presumably, man. Gum arabic does not cause cancer in rats or mice, but has not been tested for effects on reproduction. Gum arabic is known to cause occasional allergic reactions.

Ref.: Fd. Chem. Toxicol. 21, 305 (1983); *21* CFR 184.1330.

Gum Ghatti   ?

Gum ghatti is a vegetable gum produced by a tree indigenous to India. Like karaya gum and gum arabic, it serves as a wound sealant in the tree. Food manufacturers use gum ghatti to keep the oil and water ingredients from separating out into two layers in such products as salad dressing and butter-in-syrup. Only a few thousand pounds are used each year.

So few tests have been conducted on gum ghatti that a European Economic Community scientific committee recommended that the gum be phased out of use unless a whole series of studies is conducted.

Ref.: Food Chem. News, p. 6 (Aug. 6, 1979); Tragacanth Importing Corporation (N.Y.); *21* CFR 184.1333.

Gum Guaiac   Avoid

Gum guaiac is a greenish brown resin obtained from the tropical guaiacum tree. Though it has been used to prevent oil-containing food from spoiling, it is not clear if any company is still using it. This antioxidant has not been adequately tested and should not be permitted in foods.

Ref.: Fed. Am. Soc. Exp. Biol., "Evaluation of the Health Aspects of Guar Guaiac as a Food Ingredient," Washington (1975); pers. comm. from FDA (June 6, 1983); *21* CFR 172.510, 181.24.

Helium Safe

Helium is an inert, safe gas that is used to float balloons or sometimes to force foods out of pressurized containers.

Ref.: 21 CFR 182.1355.

Hesperidin Safe

Hesperidin is a bioflavonoid that occurs in the pulp of citrus fruits. Aside from a minor use as a flavoring, hesperidin may be used therapeutically to strengthen blood capillaries. It is sometimes called "vitamin P," but is not a true vitamin.

Ref.: Ann. N.Y. Acad. Sci. 61 (3) (1955); pers. comm. from Sunkist Growers, Ontario, Calif.

High Fructose Corn Syrup *see* Corn Syrup, Fructose

Hydrolyzed Vegetable Protein (HVP) ?

Food makers use hydrolyzed vegetable protein (HVP) to bring out the natural flavor of food. HVP consists of vegetable (usually soybean) protein that has been degraded by chemicals or enzymes to the amino acids of which it is composed. Some of the products in which you will find it are instant soups, beef stew, frankfurters, gravy and sauce mixes, and canned chili.

HVP is safe for adults, but might pose the same sort of risk for infants that MSG (monosodium glutamate) poses. HVP is largely a mixture of amino acids, one being glutamate. Judging from studies on infant animals, imbalances of amino acids can cause brain damage. Due to vigorous public controversy a decade ago, baby food producers stopped adding flavor enhancers to their products. However, scientists at Washington University who have studied this problem have suggested banning the use of amino acids as additives in *any* food to protect infants that might eat homemade foods containing the chemicals.

Hydroxylated Lecithin   Avoid

Hydroxylated lecithin is manufactured by treating soybean lecithin with peroxide. The food industry uses it as an emulsifier and antioxidant in baked goods, ice cream, and margarine.

Scientists at Central Soya Company have fed this additive to small groups of laboratory animals for brief periods of time and did not detect any adverse effects, but much more thorough studies are needed to prove that hydroxylated lecithin does not cause cancer, mutations, birth defects, or other problems. The FAO/WHO Expert Committee on Food Additives has reported that "hydroxylated lecithin has not been adequately studied from the toxicological point of view and there are not satisfactory data available on which an evaluation could be based." Until "satisfactory data" are available, the American public should not be eating this synthetic chemical, safe though it may be.

Ref.: FAO (53)-229; pers. comm. from FDA, Central Soya, Ft. Wayne, Ind.; *21* CFR 172.814.

Invert Sugar

Invert sugar is a 50-50 mixture of two sugars, glucose and fructose, that is used by candy and other manufacturers because it is sweeter, more soluble, and crystallizes less readily than sucrose (ordinary table sugar). Invert sugar forms when sucrose is split in two by an enzyme (invertase) or an acid. It is called "invert" because chemists discovered that a solution containing the 50-50 mixture and a solution containing sucrose affect light in opposite ways. Like other sugars, invert sugar promotes tooth decay. It has no nutritional merit other than providing "empty" calories.

Iodine—*see* Potassium Iodide

Iron Compounds   Safe
(ferric ammonium citrate, ferric phosphate, ferric pyrophosphate, ferric sodium pyrophosphate, ferrous citrate, ferrous lactate, ferrous sulfate, reduced iron)

Everybody needs iron. This vital element holds oxygen in red blood cells and muscle cells. Severe deficiencies of iron can prevent the formation of adequate levels of hemoglobin (the protein molecule of which iron is a key part, and which carries oxygen in red blood cells). This would result in anemia, which causes fatigue, listlessness, heart palpitations, and decreased resistance to infections. Though anemia is thought to be rather widespread, no one really knows how many people suffer from mild anemia, because the dividing line between "healthy" and "anemic" is fuzzy. However, several decades ago, cautious public health experts advised that "harmless and assimilable" iron be added to white flour to replace that lost in the refining process. Now, not only is iron added to enriched flour, but to breakfast cereals and other heavily fortified foods.

Different forms of iron may be added to foods. The Latin word for iron is *ferrum,* and all chemicals beginning with "ferric" or "ferrous" are iron compounds. Powdered iron, sometimes called reduced iron, is used in some foods. While all forms of iron are supposed to be "harmless and assimilable," some are more stable than others, and some are more metabolically available to the eater.

Ferrous sulfate is the most biologically available form of iron. Half the amount added to food can be assimilated. It would undoubtedly be used frequently to enrich flour were it not that it has a reputation for causing rancidity (oxidation of fats), off-flavors, and discoloration if the products are stored at high temperatures. On the other hand, ferric sodium pyrophosphate and ferric phosphate are poorly absorbed, sometimes less than 5 percent of the amount added.

With such a wide range of bioavailability, the amount of iron added to a food may be less significant than the form in which it is added. I would like to provide a simple chart of bioavailability, but it turns out that many factors affect this important property. Particle size is one key factor. For instance, the bioavailability of iron filings jumps by one third when their size is reduced from 44 to 14 microns (one micron is one thousandth of a millimeter). Ferric phosphate, normally poorly absorbed, becomes much more available if it is more finely powdered. The presence of vitamin C or meat in the same food or meal can also enhance bioavailability. Thus, there is no way of knowing how useful most iron additives are just by reading the label, other than to say that ferrous sulfate is an excellent form.

Dr. Myron Winick, professor of nutrition at Columbia University, has said that "iron deficiency is the most prevalent nutritional deficiency in the United States today." Some people have urged that the deficiency be prevented by fortifying more foods and using higher levels of iron. In 1973 the FDA proposed just this, but the plan was scuttled when Dr. William Crosby, chief of hematology at the Scripps Clinic in California, and other blood experts argued that the higher levels of iron might cause hemochromatosis, particularly in men. This rare disease is associated with cirrhosis of the liver, heart failure, and sterility.

Though FDA did not act, many food companies are adding rather high levels of iron to more and more foods. Total breakfast cereal, a General Mills product, contains 100 percent of the recommended daily allowance of iron. The iron is added to such products more as a marketing gimmick than as a public health measure. The soundest way to get iron is from a variety of natural foods. That way you don't have to worry that the iron would be, on one hand, virtually unavailable—"shooting nutritional blanks," says Crosby—or, on the other hand, so available that it might cause iron overload. (See also discussion on page 98.)

Ref.: 21 CFR 182.5301–182.5315, 182.5375.

Karaya Gum ?

Karaya gum is a complex carbohydrate that manufacturers use as a thickening or stabilizing agent in foods. The only source of karaya is the sterculia tree which grows in India. To obtain the gum, trees are tapped, causing the extremely viscous gum to exude slowly out of the wound. Tear-shaped masses of gum, which weigh up to five pounds, are harvested from the tree trunks. In 1982 American companies imported 8.9 million pounds of karaya.

Manufacturers use karaya gum to prevent oil from separating out of whipped products and salad dressing and to prevent fat from separating from meat and juices in sausages. It improves the texture of manufactured ice cream and sherbet by preventing large ice crystals from forming. Karaya is proving to be a cheap substitute for tragacanth gum.

What distinguishes karaya from other natural gums is its exceptional proclivity for water, in which it can expand to one hundred times its original volume. This property makes it an effective bulk-type laxative. The stickiness of karaya solutions enables it to be used in hair wave-set products. Considerably more karaya is used in pharmaceuticals and cosmetics than in foods.

Good long-term feeding studies need to be done, with particular attention paid to the effect of karaya on the absorption of nutrients. The ability to function as a laxative indicates that very little of this gum is digested and absorbed, but the fact that some persons are allergic to karaya indicates that some is absorbed. The metabolism of karaya should be thoroughly investigated. An official committee of the European Economic Community recommended in 1979 that this additive be phased out of use unless several key studies were conducted.

Ref.: FAO (46A)-102; *J. Nutr. 36,* 27 (1948); *J. Am. Med. Assoc. 114,* 747 (1950); *Food Chem. News,* p. 6 (Aug. 6, 1979); *21* CFR 184.1349.

Lactic Acid (calcium lactate)   Safe

The significance of lactic acid for animals and plants has been nicely described by Dr. Myron Brin, professor of nutrition at the University of California at Davis:

> To a biologist, lactic acid is consonant with life, since the presence of this acid is a hallmark for energy metabolism for virtually every living organism . . . It is ubiquitous in distribution, being found wherever life persists.

Lactic acid is also found where many food industries persist. Food manufacturers use the acidic properties of lactic acid to inhibit the spoilage of Spanish-type olives, to adjust the acidity in cheese-making, and to add a note of tartness to frozen desserts, carbonated fruit beverages, and other foods. Calcium lactate, a non-acidic salt of lactic acid, inhibits the discoloration of fruits and vegetables and improves the properties of dry milk powders and condensed milk.

As a consequence of its chemical structure, lactic acid exists in two forms: L-lactic acid, which is the form normally encountered in nature, and D-lactic acid, which is the mirror image of the first form (like right-handed and left-handed gloves). Commercial lactic acid is a 50-50 mixture of the two forms. Animals are able to metabolize D-lactic acid, though not so readily as the L form. Unmetabolized lactic acid is excreted in the urine. The FAO/WHO Expert Committee on Food Additives recommends that because the metabolism of D-lactic acid has not been studied in infants, it should not be used in baby foods. (It is not used in infant formula in the United States.)

Ref.: FAO (40A)-144; M. Brin in *Ann. N.Y. Acad. Sci. 119,* 108 (1965) (whole issue on lactic acid); *Fed. Reg. 48,* 8086 (1983); *21* CFR 182.1061.

Lactose   Blacks, Orientals: ?
                                             Most others: **Safe**

Lactose, a carbohydrate that is found only in milk, is Nature's way of delivering calories to infant mammals. Human milk contains about 7 percent lactose, and cow's milk contains 5 percent. Milk turns sour when bacteria convert lactose to lactic acid.

Food manufacturers use lactose in whipped topping mix, fortified breakfast pastry (toaster tarts), and other foods as a slightly sweet source of carbohydrate. Lactose is one sixth as sweet as table sugar.

The intestine secretes an enzyme that splits lactose into glucose and galactose, two sugars that the body absorbs and metabolizes. The only persons who may be seriously harmed by lactose are the rare—perhaps one out of twenty thousand—individuals who suffer from galactosemia, a genetic disease. Galactosemics lack the enzyme that metabolizes galactose. In the absence of the enzyme, the galactose that forms from lactose accumulates in the blood and causes enlargement of the liver, cataracts, and mental retardation. Proper treatment for this disease entails simply the avoidance of milk. Interestingly, galactosemia is mainly a childhood disease. The reason for this is that children have only one enzyme that metabolizes galactose, and this enzyme is missing in galactosemics; adults develop a second enzyme that puts the galactose to good use.

Less serious, but far more common, than galactosemia is "lactose intolerance." While virtually all infants can digest lactose, most adults around the globe cannot absorb and digest lactose well. The undigested lactose passes through the small intestine, where absorption would normally take place, and into the large intestine. The compound may be metabolized by bacteria, in which case it would produce gas, bloating, and flatulence. Or, if not digested by bacteria, it would bind water and lead to diarrhea. In either case, the uncomfortable effects discourage sufferers from drinking milk or other foods that contain substantial amounts of lactose.

The great majority of Orientals and most people of black African heritage cannot tolerate much lactose after early childhood. In these cultures, milk is often converted into yogurt and similar fermented foods. The bacteria in these foods help digest the lactose. On the other hand, most Northern Europeans and certain tribes whose cultures developed over many thousands of years with milk as a common food have adapted so as to be able to digest lactose.

The underlying cause of lactose intolerance is the absence in the walls of the small intestine of the enzyme lactase, which breaks down lactose. To make up for the missing lactase, at least one company is selling purified lactase obtained from yeast. The lactase can be added to milk to predigest the lactose. Others are marketing "sweet acidophilus milk," which contains bacteria that metabolize lactose after the milk is consumed.

Nutritionists and antihunger advocates, after numerous mishaps, are well aware of lactose intolerance. Many black Americans cannot tolerate much lactose, so alternatives to milk should be available in school lunchrooms. Overseas, many Third World recipients of well-intended powdered milk used it as whitewash on their houses or threw it down the drain, because drinking it made them sick.

Over on the other side of town, lactose is sometimes used to dilute heroin.

Ref.: Scientific American, October 1972, page 71; *New Engl. J. Med. 310,* 1 (1984).

Lecithin   Safe

Lecithin occurs in nearly all animal and plant tissues and is an important constituent of the human body. The average person consumes one to five grams (up to one sixth of an ounce) of lecithin in his or her daily diet. Food manufacturers use about 100 million pounds of lecithin annually in various processed foods.

Pure lecithin is an important source of one nutrient, choline, but the lecithin that is sold commercially contains many valuable "impurities," including vitamins B_1, B_2, E, inositol, niacin, and biotin, as well as soybean oil and other compounds.

The lecithin used as a food additive is obtained almost exclusively from the soybean, as it has ever since that versatile plant was introduced into the United States in the 1920s. Prior to that time it was obtained from egg yolk. In an era of sky-high prices, soy lecithin is inexpensive, because it is a waste product of the soybean industry. Before shipowners will transport soy oil, they require that the lecithin be removed, because it absorbs moisture and forms difficult-to-remove deposits in oceangoing tankers.

In living animals and plants, lecithin protects polyunsaturated fats from attack by oxygen and helps maintain biological membranes. The food industry takes advantage of the antioxidant action and adds up to 0.5 percent lecithin to margarine, shortenings, and oils to retard spoilage and rancidity. Lecithin is a weaker antioxidant than the synthetic compounds BHA, BHT, and propyl gallate, but it is certainly safer.

Lecithin serves as an emulsifier in margarine, chocolate, ice cream, and baked goods to promote the mixing of oil (or fat) and water. It is one of the few natural, edible substances that has a strong emulsifying effect. Like other emulsifiers, lecithin works by lowering the surface tension of water.

In baked goods lecithin helps the shortening mix with the other dough ingredients, retards the crystallization of starch, and stabilizes air bubbles in cake batter. The end result is bread and rolls that are more tender and stay fresh longer and fluffier cakes.

Adding 0.2 percent lecithin to chocolate enables manufacturers to reduce the cocoa butter content slightly. Most manufacturers employ this trick because cocoa butter is the most expensive ingredient in chocolate. The Hershey Foods Corporation says that its consumer tests prove that this substitution has no effect on the taste of the chocolate.

The lecithin in egg yolk serves as a natural emulsifier in many foods. In mayonnaise, for instance, it stabilizes the vinegar-vegetable oil mixture, preventing these ingredients from separating into two layers. The fact that egg lecithin is associated with protein makes egg yolk an even more powerful emulsifier than pure lecithin.

The only safety question associated with lecithin is from the hydrogen peroxide that is used to bleach 80 percent of lecithin used in the United States. Small residues of the peroxide may contaminate the lecithin. The FDA reviewed this matter in 1982 after learning of a Japanese study associating large amounts of peroxide with cancer of the small intestine. FDA scientists concluded that the evidence on peroxide was inconclusive and that people consume very little lecithin, which in turn contains only trace amounts of peroxide. If you buy lecithin as a nutrient supplement, you would be slightly better off with unbleached lecithin, but I would certainly not make this a high priority worry.

The most interesting question about lecithin is not whether it poses a risk, but whether it offers great benefits. In the 1940s and 1950s, several doctors did small studies on patients suffering from heart disease. The patients were given between one and six teaspoons of lecithin a day. The lecithin appeared to reduce their cholesterol levels significantly. These studies were not well controlled and must be considered with skepticism. However, they do raise the possibility that lecithin may be a safe aid to treating heart disease and deserve well-designed follow-up work.

Ref.: FAO (35)-151; *ECT 12,* 343; West, E. S., and Todd, W. R., *Textbook of Biochemistry,* Macmillan, N.Y., p. 147 (1961); *Geriatrics* p. 12, Jan. 1958; Central Soya, Ft. Wayne, Ind.; *Fed. Reg. 47,* 34161 (Aug. 6, 1982); *21* CFR 182.1400.

Locust Bean Gum   Safe
(Carob seed gum, St. John's bread)

Locust bean gum, or St. John's bread as it is sometimes called, is obtained from the endosperm of the bean of the carob tree, a Mediterranean species. In ancient Egypt the gum was used as an adhesive in mummy bindings. Today it serves as a stabilizer in foods and, when taken in greater quantity, as a gentle laxative. Spain, Portugal, Italy, and Greece fill America's demand for this gum (4 million pounds in 1982).

Locust bean gum is used to improve the texture and freeze-melt characteristics of ice cream; thicken salad dressing, pie filling, and barbecue sauce; make softer, more resilient cakes and biscuits when used as a dough additive; and increase the palatability of carrageenan gels by decreasing their brittleness and melting temperature.

That locust bean gum as a laxative action indicates that it is not absorbed to any great extent by the body. When tested on several species of pregnant animals, this gum did not cause birth defects. Good, lifetime animal feeding studies have indicated that this additive is safe.

Ref.: FAO (46A)-99; *Am. J. Dig. Dis. 18,* 24 (1951); WHO(8)-32; *Fd. Chem. Toxicol. 21,* 305 (1983); *21* CFR 184.1343.

Magnesium compounds   Safe
(magnesium carbonate, magnesium chloride, magnesium hydroxide, magnesium phosphate, magnesium stearate, magnesium sulfate, and other magnesium-containing salts)

Magnesium is a mineral that is essential to health. It is a crucial component of many enzymes and plays a unique role in muscle contraction. Magnesium occurs in virtually all foods, but is especially abundant in nuts, peanuts, beans, whole grains, blackstrap molasses, and dairy products. Used as an additive, magnesium salts serve numerous purposes: anticaking agent (carbonate, stearate), alkali (carbonate, hydroxide), nutrient (any magnesium compound), and water corrective (sulfate). Magnesium-containing additives are safe.

Despite the widespread occurrence of magnesium in foods, some Americans may not be consuming enough. According to the Department of Agriculture, the average American consumes only about 250 milligrams of magnesium a day. Two out of five individuals ingest less than 70 percent of the recommended dietary allowance. The recommended intake is 350 milligrams for adult men and 300 milligrams for adult women, with pregnant and lactating women and teenaged boys needing more. Frank deficiencies are rare, but some animal studies have indicated that diets lacking adequate magnesium can promote hardening of the arteries, stiffness of joints, and nervous symptoms. Getting more of this mineral is one reason why most people should be trying to eat a more nutritious diet (grains, vegetables, dairy, poultry, fish, and meat all provide magnesium).

The only deaths related to a magnesium additive occurred in a most unusual way. Warner-Lambert Company used magnesium stearate, an explosive, as a lubricant in the production of Freshen-Up gum. The factory was not kept clean and the powdery chemical silently accumulated. On November 21, 1976, an errant spark met up with the chemical. Six workers died in the explosion.

Ref.: The Washington *Post,* p. D19, Jan. 29, 1976; Aug. 19, 1977; *Recommended Dietary Allowances,* 9th Ed., National Research Council (National Academy of Sciences, Washington, D.C., 1980); *Fed. Reg. 50,* 13557 (April 5, 1985); *21* CFR 184.1425–184.1443, 182.5431–182.5443.

Malic Acid

Infants: **?**
Others: **Safe**

Malic acid sometimes goes by the name "apple acid," because large amounts occur in apples (0.4 to 0.7 percent in apple juice). Other fruits contain smaller amounts of this tart acid. The change in flavor that occurs as a fruit ripens is due partly to a decrease in the malic acid content and to an increase in the sugar content. Malic acid is an important metabolite and is present in all living cells.

The food industry has used malic acid for over forty years as an acidulant and flavoring agent in fruit-flavored drinks, candy, lemon-flavored ice-tea mix, ice cream, and preserves.

Because of its chemical structure, two mirror-image forms of malic acid exist: the D form and the L form. L-malic acid, the form that occurs in natural products, is metabolized routinely. Commercial malic acid, however, is a mixture of the D and L forms. While adults can probably utilize the D-malic acid, it is not known whether infants can. Therefore, it is important that synthetic malic acid not be added to baby food.

Ref.: FAO (40A)-149; C&EN-117; CUFP-44, 144; *Fd. Cos. Tox.* 7, 103 (1969); *21* CFR 184.1069.

Maltol, Ethyl Maltol

Safe

Food manufacturers use maltol and ethyl maltol to enhance the flavor and aroma of fruit-, vanilla-, and chocolate-flavored foods and beverages the way they use MSG to bring out the flavor of meat. Small amounts of maltol occur naturally in bread crust, coffee, and chicory and as a degradation product in heated milk, cellulose, and starch. It has been available commercially since 1942.

Chemical manufacturers frequently synthesize families of compounds that are closely related to substances that they already manufacture. The purpose of creating these new substances is to learn whether a close relative of a widely used compound might have greater potency, stability, or safety, or lower cost. Using this technique, one manufacturer synthesized ethyl maltol and discovered that it was four to six times as strong a flavor enhancer as its close relative, maltol.

Maltol and ethyl maltol are used in gelatin desserts, soft drinks, ice cream, and other foods that are high in carbohydrate. Levels used range from 15 to 250 parts per million for maltol and 1 to 50 ppm for ethyl maltol. Ethyl maltol can be used in diet foods to mask saccharin's bitter aftertaste and in ordinary foods to permit a lower sugar content.

In studies on rats, ethyl maltol did not cause tumors, impair growth, or cause reproductive problems. Additional tests of shorter duration on dogs also indicated safety. Ethyl maltol is completely absorbed by the body; following absorption, it is metabolized in the liver and then excreted in the urine.

Ref.: FAO (44A)-56; FAO (54); *Tox. Appl. Pharm. 15,* 604 (1969); Chas. Pfizer & Co. Data Sheet No. 635; *21* CFR 172.515.

Manganese   Safe

Manganese is a necessary nutrient that occurs in a wide variety of natural foods. It is used as an additive in infant formula and vitamin/mineral supplements. Modest amounts pose no problem.

Ref.: Fed. Reg. 47, 56513 (Dec. 17, 1982); *21* CFR 182.5446–182.5464.

Mannitol   Safe

Sweetness, disdain for moisture, poor absorption by the body, and diuretic action are some of the properties that make mannitol an interesting and useful chemical. This versatile substance occurs naturally in the manna ash tree, in which it helps to close wounds, and in seaweed and microorganisms. Commercial quantities of mannitol are made from sugar.

Perhaps the most familiar use of mannitol is as the "dust" on chewing gum. The dust prevents gum from absorbing moisture and becoming sticky. Mannitol's sweetness—it is two thirds as sweet as sugar—is an added bonus.

Although mannitol is chemically quite similar to sugar, few organisms are well adapted to use it as a source of energy. The human digestive tract, for instance, absorbs only about two thirds of a given dose of mannitol, and even some of that is excreted unchanged in the urine. Approximately 50 percent is used by the body, which means that mannitol provides only half as many calories as an equal weight of sugar. Thus, mannitol may be used as a sweetener in reduced calorie foods.

Mannitol is frequently used as the sweetening agent in noncariogenic (sugarless) chewing gum, because bacteria in the mouth have an even harder time digesting it than do humans. Tooth decay is caused by acid produced by oral bacteria as they metabolize sugar.

Physicians sometimes call upon mannitol to help clean out the body's plumbing. Moderate amounts (about one or two ounces) have a laxative effect because it is poorly absorbed. When mannitol is injected or fed intravenously, it is totally eliminated by the kidneys and has a powerful diuretic effect. The increased production of urine helps eliminate poisons circulating in the bloodstream. The diuretic effect also helps prevent kidney shutdown in patients undergoing certain major operations; this technique has saved many lives.

Some people may have discovered accidentally to their regret and inconvenience that mannitol, as well as its close chemical relative sorbitol, can cause diarrhea. To forewarn consumers, the Food and Drug Administration requires label notices on all foods which might result in the daily ingestion of 20 grams of mannitol or 50 grams of sorbitol. The notice reads: "Excess consumption may have a laxative effect."

Mannitol has been used for decades to "cut" heroin. According to a Justice Department spokesman, a typical bag of heroin purchased in New York City contains eight times as much mannitol (mannite) as heroin. (Most heroin also contains a dash of quinine, which mimics some of heroin's physiological effects and also adds to the bitterness of the dope. This twofold effect leads addicts to believe that they are using high quality heroin.)

People have used mannitol for centuries as a sweetening agent without adverse effect. The body converts mannitol to a sugar, which in turn is converted to energy. These considerations, plus a variety of short-term tests and one recent chronic feeding study on both rats and mice, indicate that mannitol is safe.

Ref.: FAO (40A)-160; CRC-Ch. 11; Atlas Chemical Company's "Atlas Products for the Food and Beverage Industry"; *Chemical & Engineering News,* January 17, 1972, page 13; *Fd. Chem. Tox. 21,* 259 (1983); *21* CFR 180.25.

Meat Tenderizer   Safe

The average life span of medieval magicians would probably have been increased greatly had they spent less time trying to turn lead into gold and more time trying to make tough meat more tender.

The best procedure that butchers, if not magicians, developed to improve the texture of meat was to age it. Scientists have discovered that during aging, natural protein-digesting enzymes (proteases) in the meat gently loosen up muscle fibers that had contracted in rigor mortis.

Food technologists took a cue from nature and found that meat could be artificially tenderized simply by treating it with proteases, which are readily purified from plants, animals, or microorganisms. This trick was discovered ages ago by natives of Mexico, South America, and the South Sea Islands who traditionally tenderized meat by wrapping it in papaya leaves, a rich source of proteases.

Family cooks tenderize steak by sprinkling a small amount of tenderizer on it shortly before cooking. A more efficient method that some meatpackers use is to inject proteases into a steer's bloodstream shortly before the animal is slaughtered. The blood carries the enzymes to all parts of the animal, resulting in a better job than the superficial tenderizing at home. Federal regulations require that meat treated in this way be appropriately labeled. In practice, however, only the carcass is stamped "tenderized"; individual steaks will probably not be labeled.

Meat tenderizing proteases are extracted from plants or microorganisms. The ones derived from plants—bromelain (pineapple*), papain (papaya), ficin (fig)—act most effectively on gristle (connective tissue composed of collagen and elastin), although they also tenderize the muscle portion of the meat. Bacterial and fungal proteases (from *Aspergillus* and *B. subtilis)* have the opposite priorities.

While I could not recommend eating spoonfuls of meat tenderizer straight from the jar, it is normally harmless. The enzymes are destroyed when the meat is cooked and even if they were not destroyed, our mouth and throat are amply protected by saliva and mucus.

Meat tenderizer preparations consist mostly of seasoning; a small amount of edible fat, such as calcium stearate, is added to prevent caking and to keep down the dust.

Ref.: CRC-62, 87; *Enzymes in Food Processing,* G. Reed, Academic Press, N.Y., 1966; pers. comm. from Swift & Co., Chicago, and Adolph's Food Products Mfg. Co., Burbank, Calif.; *21* CFR 182.1585.

Mono- and Diglycerides and related substances   Safe

The words "mono- and diglycerides" are familiar to every red-blooded, label-reading American. This chemical additive makes bread softer and prevents staling (by preventing the starch from crystallizing), improves the stability and taste of margarine, makes cakes fluffier (by helping generate and trap air bubbles), decreases the stickiness of caramels, prevents the oil in peanut butter from separating out . . . the list goes on and on. The average American consumes over a half pound of mono- and diglycerides as food additives annually.

Mono- and diglycerides are safe. In fact, they comprise about 1 percent of normal food fat and are part of our normal diet. Moreover, the bulk of normal food fats and oils is composed of triglycerides, which cooking and our body's digestive system convert to mono- and diglycerides. The mono- and diglycerides derived from either food fat or food additives are absorbed into intestinal

---

* Fresh pineapple cannot be used in gelatin desserts because the bromelain dissolves the gel, which is made of protein (gelatin).

cells where they are largely converted to triglycerides. The triglycerides then pass into the bloodstream.

While mono- and diglycerides are completely harmless from a toxicological point of view, they may displace more nutritious or desirable ingredients from some foods. Thus, "modern" peanut butter contains several percent mono- and diglycerides to keep the oil from separating, which means that it is several percent less nutritious than "old-fashioned" peanut butter made solely from peanuts.

Food technologists have synthesized useful new substances by reacting mono- and diglycerides with other compounds. Bakers use one of these, ethoxylated mono- and diglycerides as a dough conditioner to improve the baking characteristics and texture of yeast-raised bakery goods. Judging from reports on file at the FDA of rat and dog studies, none of which studies lasted longer than ninety days, this substance is partially digested and absorbed into the blood. Ethoxylated mono- and diglycerides should be studied in a complete battery of tests on mice, rats, and dogs.

A second derivative is sodium sulfoacetate mono- and diglycerides. This chemical was developed as a synthetic substitute for lecithin and, like the more nutritious lecithin, is used as an antispattering agent and emulsifier in margarine. As far as could be determined this chemical has not been adequately tested. If this additive is better technologically than lecithin, the difference is probably marginal. Most margarine manufacturers find lecithin perfectly adequate.

Acetylated mono- and diglycerides is one of the more unusual derivatives of the parent compound. Unlike its greasy relatives, this substance is a highly flexible and waxlike solid at room temperature. You are likely to encounter it in the coatings on jelly beans and chocolate-covered ice cream bars. It is completely digestible and harmless.

Three other harmless derivatives are the lactylated, citrated, and succinylated mono- and diglycerides. All of these normally serve as emulsifiers, although the citrate derivative also retards spoilage of oils (see citric acid).

Oxystearin is a modified fatty acid that manufacturers add in amounts up to 0.125 percent to vegetable oils to prevent them from clouding up in the refrigerator. Procter & Gamble has sponsored lifetime feeding, metabolic and reproduction studies on animals that indicate that oxystearin is safe.

The final derivative, diacetyl tartaric acid ester of mono- and diglycerides, is used by the baking industry. When this emulsifier was introduced, about 1950, only small-scale feeding experiments had been conducted. These studies are crude and incomplete by today's standards and need to be updated so that we can be certain that this synthetic compound does not cause cancer, birth defects, or other harm.

Ref.: Mono- and diglycerides: C&EN-120; CUFP-22; NAS-NRC Pub. No. 1271; CRC-Ch. 10; FAO (35)-145-151; *21* CFR 182.4505.

Ethoxylated mono- and diglycerides: pers. comm. from FDA; *21* CFR 172.834.

Sodium sulfoacetate mono- and diglycerides: *ECT 12,* 359; FAO/WHO Expert Committee on Food Additives, tentative specifications.

Acetylated mono- and diglycerides: FAO (40A)-71; *J. Am. Oil Chem. Soc. 29,* 11 (1952); *J. Nutr. 58,* 113, *59,* 277 (1956); *21* CFR 172.828.

Diacetyl tartaric acid ester of mono- and diglycerides: FAO (40A)-90; *J. Am. Pharm. Asso., sci. ed. 39,* 275 (1950); *21* CFR 182.4101.

Oxystearin: FAO (46A)-155; *21* CFR 172.818.

Other derivatives: FAO (40A); *21* CFR 172.830, 172.832.

Monosodium Glutamate (MSG) ?

Monosodium glutamate is the sodium salt of glutamic acid, an amino acid, and is one of the building blocks of which protein molecules are made. It is present in all proteins and many foods. When it is consumed as part of protein, it does not pose any problems or provide any special gustatorial benefits. MSG's benefits and risks arise when it is consumed in a free form as a condiment.

MSG was just another amino acid until 1908. In that year Dr. Kikunae Ikeda, a chemist at Tokyo University, discovered that MSG could intensify the flavor of protein-containing foods and was the active component of soy sauce and sea tangle, traditional oriental condiments. Japanese chemical firms soon began producing MSG commercially, selling it to both food manufacturers and consumers. Persons all around the world now use MSG to enhance the flavor of meat, soup, seafood, poultry, cheese, and sauces. Manufacturers use MSG to accentuate the meatiness of a food (and to reduce the amount of expensive meat or meat extract in a food). Significant amounts of free glutamate occur naturally in Parmesan and Camembert cheeses, peas, and other foods.

In 1982 Americans consumed about 48 million pounds of MSG, most of which was imported from Japan. Chemical companies produce MSG primarily by the bacterial fermentation of sugar; they obtain the remainder from plant proteins rich in glutamic acid.

The first indication that MSG did anything but improve the flavor of food came in 1968 when a doctor of Chinese extraction, Ho Man Kwok, discovered what he dubbed "Chinese Restaurant Syndrome (CRS)." Approximately twenty to thirty minutes after beginning a meal at a Chinese restaurant, Dr. Kwok experienced a burning sensation in the back of his neck and in his forearms, tightness of the chest and headaches. With exemplary scientific vigor, several New York doctors followed up Kwok's observations by eating three meals a day, sampling a wide variety of dishes, at their favorite Chinese restaurant. Many meals later they traced the cause of CRS to the soups. Back in the kitchen they discovered that the cook routinely added great quantities of MSG to the soup. Subsequent experiments confirmed the existence and cause of CRS and showed that some persons were ten or more times as sensitive as others. Chinese Restaurant Syndrome is readily produced by intravenous injection of small amounts of MSG. Recent research has indicated that people sensitive to MSG have borderline deficiencies of vitamin B_6.

Many foods besides soups in Chinese restaurants contain MSG, but due to a curious combination of circumstances few others cause CRS. Chinese soups that contain large amounts of MSG are so potent because persons frequently go to restaurants on empty stomachs, and because soup is the first course of a meal. These factors ensure that a large amount of MSG is rapidly and completely absorbed into the blood, which carries it to nerve endings where it probably exerts its effects.

Chinese Restaurant Syndrome normally causes only temporary discomfort, though there have been occasional unproven reports that MSG may be responsible for more severe reactions. Dr. Liane Reif-Lehrer of Harvard Medical School, who has studied the effects of MSG on the retina, says:

> It seems unlikely, for example, that MSG even in large doses is overtly harmful to normal adult individuals. The more interesting question, are there subgroups of individuals for whom glutamate is not safe or at least not advisable, has not, as yet, been adequately explored.

She testified at an FDA hearing that:

> Because . . . an appreciable number of people do perhaps react adversely to ingestion of elevated levels of glutamate, it would seem the better part of wisdom not to have unrestricted use of this material until further research has been done . . .

In 1969, Dr. John Olney of the Washington University School of Medicine in St. Louis reported that feeding large amounts of MSG to infant mice destroyed nerve cells in the hypothalamus, the region of the brain that controls appetite, body temperature, and other important functions. The identical effect was seen when MSG was injected under the skin of mice and of a monkey. When massive brain damage occurred, the baby mice grew up to be short and fat, and their coats, livers, uteri, and ovaries were visibly affected. The nature of the effects on the infant monkey, Dr. Olney wrote:

> . . . when a small percentage of its brain cells were being destroyed is evidence of a subtle process of brain damage in the developmental period which could easily go unrecognized were it to occur in the human infant under routine circumstances.

A second effect of feeding large amounts of MSG to newborn rats and mice was injury to the retina of the eye. Fortunately, though, the human eye is further developed at the time of birth than is the rodent eye and, therefore, is less susceptible to injury.

Baby food manufacturers in the United States had been adding MSG to their meat- and vegetable-containing products for many years. The companies admitted that the function of MSG was to make baby food more palatable to mothers, and not to make the product more nutritious or tastier for the infant. But they maintained that there was too little of the compound in a jar to harm a baby. Olney's experiments, however, suggested that a toxic amount of MSG might be contained in as few as four jars of food—a margin of safety too small for most parents' comfort. Moreover, viral infections, retarded development of enzyme systems, an empty stomach, and metabolic variations might cause many babies to be supersensitive. It took massive public pressure and the glare of publicity, but the baby food companies stopped adding MSG to their products in 1969.

Lifetime feeding tests on rats and mice confirmed the expectation that MSG, an important metabolite and dietary element, does not cause tumors.

Persons who must restrict their intake of sodium, but want to use a flavor enhancer should use monoammonium or monopotassium glutamate. They have the same gustatory and biological effects as MSG.

Ref.: FDA Report on Monosodium Glutamate (November 17, 1969); NAS-NRC Food Protection Committee Report (July 1970), "Safety and Suitability of Monosodium Glutamate for Use in Baby Foods"; *Nut. Rev. 28,* 124, 158 (1970); *Science 163,* 826 (1969); *170,* 549 (1970); *Nature 227,* 609 (1970); *New Engl. J. Med. 293,* 1204 (1975); *Food Tech.,* p. 49 (Oct. 1980); *Biochem. Biophys. Res. Commun. 100,* 972 (1981); L. Reif-Lehrer in *Proc.,* Wenner-Gren Excitotoxin Symp., Stockholm, August 1982; *21* CFR 182.1045–182.1047, 182.1500–182.1516.

Niacin   Safe

Niacin (or niacinamide) is vitamin B_3. It is safe. Niacin is added to many fortified and enriched foods. People who consume inadequate amounts of niacin (virtually all Americans consume enough) suffer from the disease pellagra, which is characterized by severe mental disturbances and ultimately death. Pellagra was wiped out in the United States in the 1930s and 1940s by restoring the niacin that was lost during the refining of flour and by an improved standard of living that enabled people to eat more adequate diets. Niacin is now added to many processed foods, such as breakfast cereals, to enable producers to make extravagant nutritional claims.

Spurred, in part, by knowing that niacin deficiencies could affect the mind, a number of doctors have attempted to cure schizophrenia and certain other mental problems by administering megadoses of niacin to their patients. The doctors have reported mixed results. The use of vitamins as drugs is likely to be one of the most exciting fields of biomedical research in the 1980s.

Ref.: Nutrition Foundation, *Present Knowledge in Nutrition*, p. 162 (1976); *Fed. Reg. 48,* 52032 (Nov. 16, 1983); *21* CFR 182.5530–182.5535.

Nitrous Oxide (N$_2$O)   Safe

Nitrous oxide is often used as the propellant to drive foods out of pressurized containers. It is better known as laughing gas and is safe.

Ref.: 21 CFR 182.1545.

Pantothenic Acid (and sodium pantothenate)   Safe

This substance is one of the water-soluble B vitamins. Human deficiencies have never been observed.

Ref.: Nutrition Foundation, *Present Knowledge in Nutrition,* 226 (1976); *21* CFR 172.330–335.

Papain   Safe

Papain is a harmless enzyme obtained from papaya. See meat tenderizer for a discussion of how it is used.

Parabens   ?

Parabens is the nickname for the methyl, propyl, and heptyl esters of para-hydroxybenzoic acid. These dreadful sounding chemicals are used as preservatives and are closely related to sodium benzoate. Parabens are more versatile than benzoate because they can prevent bacteria and mold from growing in almost all foods; benzoate is effective only in acidic foods. Parabens have also been used for many years in pharmaceutical products, where their relatively high cost is acceptable.

The most commonly used parabens, the methyl and propyl compounds, have been fairly well tested in rats, but should also be tested on mice. The body absorbs parabens and converts them to para-hydroxybenzoic acid, which is coupled to another substance (glucuronic acid, sulfate or glycine) and then excreted. Dr. C. Matthews and his colleagues at Emory University did not detect any adverse effects on the growth, life span, or internal organs of rats that ate food containing 2 or 8 percent parabens for ninety-six weeks. An experiment conducted by Swedish biologists showed that parabens do not cause birth defects.

Heptyl paraben acts as a preservative in beer (12 ppm), noncarbonated soft drinks, and fruit-based beverages. It does not appear to cause cancer or interfere with the reproduction of rats, but it needs to be tested on mice and in the presence of alcohol.

Ref.: FAO (31)-30-37; FAO (40A)-22-27; CRC-142-151; *Acta. Paediat. Scand.* 54, 43 (1965); *J. Am. Pharm. Asso., sci. ed.* 45, 260, 268 (1956); pers. comm. from FDA; GRAS (up to 0.1 percent); *21* CFR 172.145, 184.1490, 184.1670.

Pectin (and sodium pectinate)   Safe

Pectin is a carbohydrate that strengthens cell walls in citrus fruits, apples, beets, carrots, and other fruits and vegetables. Fruits get soft as they ripen because the pectin breaks down to a soluble form.

Pectin forms gels that are the basis of fruit jellies. Jelly manufacturers add purified pectin to their products when the fruits contain too little natural pectin to form good gels. You may also find it used to thicken barbecue sauce, cranberry sauce, canned frosting, and yogurt.

Ref.: ECT *14* 636; *Fed. Reg.* 47, 35243 (Aug. 13, 1982); *21* CFR 184.1775.

Phosphoric Acid   Safe

Phosphoric acid is most widely used as the acid and flavoring in colas and other soft drinks. It is also used to provide acidity in making processed cheeses, to increase the effectiveness of antioxidants in fats and oils, and to provide nutrient phosphorus for yeast in baked goods. At least two dozen different salts of phosphorus, such as sodium phosphate and potassium phosphate, serve hundreds of different purposes in food.

Phosphorus, the key element in phosphoric acid and phosphate salts, is an extremely important mineral. Calcium phosphate is the basic substance of which bone is formed. Phosphate is present in blood, enzymes, and several vitamins.

According to the National Research Council's committee on recommended dietary allowances, "Phosphorus is present in nearly all foods, and dietary deficiency is extremely unlikely to occur in man." According to the U.S. Department of Agriculture's 1977–78 nutrition survey, only 8 percent of the population consumes less than 70 percent of the recommended intake. The recommended daily allowance for adults of phosphorus is 800 milligrams per day, though average intake is 1,159 milligrams. Natural foods generally provide most of the dietary phosphorus, but soda pop and other phosphorus-containing processed foods may provide hefty amounts of extra phosphorus for many consumers. Four cans of Coke, not an unusual amount for millions of soft drink addicts, provide 280 milligrams.

Nutritionists recommend that people consume at least as much calcium as phosphorus, but meat-eating and cola-drinking Americans actually consume about fifty percent more phosphorus than calcium. Researchers are investigating whether modest excesses of phosphorus, coupled with deficits of calcium, increase the risk of osteoporosis or other health problems. Dr. Linda Massey, of Washington State University, has expressed concern that people who replace calcium-rich milk with soda pop are increasing their risk of bone loss and diarrhea.

Ref.: Recommended Dietary Allowances, National Research Council (National Academy of Sciences, Washington, 1980); *J. Am. Diet. Asso. 80,* 581 (1982); Stauffer Chemical Company (Westport, Conn.); FAO (26)-13; *21* CFR 182.1073.

Polydextrose   Safe

Artificial sweeteners like aspartame may taste like real sugar, but because such tiny amounts replace large amounts of sugar, they do not provide the bulk that sugar provides. If artificial sweeteners were used by themselves, soda pops would taste watery, cookies would not be moist, and cakes would come out like pancakes. Not to worry though. Another miracle in the chemistry labs has produced polydextrose, a substance similar to cellulose. It is low in calories (one fourth the calories of sugar), without taste, but virtuous in bulk. It is one of a series of new food additives that are designed to be absorbed poorly or not at all by the body.

Pfizer, Inc., which developed this fabulous chemical, advertises that "Polydextrose fattens up your profits without fattening up your customers. The lite market is booming, with customers willing to pay up to 30% more for reduced calorie treats!"

Polydextrose was first approved in 1981 and is slowly working its way into frozen desserts, baked goods, hard candies, instant puddings, and other processed foods. It can be used as a replacement for sugar, starch, and fat.

Polydextrose is a polymer made up primarily of dextrose (corn sugar, glucose) molecules, plus about 10 percent sorbitol and 1 percent citric acid.

One little problem with polydextrose is that large amounts of the additive can have a laxative effect or cause flatulence. For adults, these effects start showing up at doses of about two or three ounces. Smaller amounts would cause the same problems in children. When a serving of food contains one-half ounce or more of polydextrose, FDA requires a label notice, "Sensitive individuals may experience a laxative effect from excessive consumption of this product." With constipation such a problem for millions of Americans, the laxative effect may be deemed more a benefit than a problem by many.

A second problem is that foods in which polydextrose replaced some or all of the sugar or fat do not taste as good as their normal counterparts, according to Pfizer's own carefully done tests. However, the polydextrose-containing foods do taste about the same as other reduced-calorie foods.

Polydextrose does not seem to interfere with the absorption of essential nutrients. Neither does it cause dental caries, reproductive problems, mutations, or cancer.

Ref.: FAO (24)-21; *Food Engineering,* p. 140 (June 1981); *Food Tech.,* p. 58 (July 1981); Washington *Post,* p. E1 (May 12, 1982); FDA files; *21* CFR 172.841.

Polysorbate 60, 65, 80 — Safe

Manufacturers have been adding polysorbate emulsifiers to processed foods since the 1940s. Like other emulsifiers, the main effect of polysorbates is to enable oil to remain dispersed in water. This action improves the texture and promotes "dryness" in frozen desserts, makes bread, rolls, and doughnuts more tender and keeps them from going stale, prevents oil from separating out of artificial whipped cream, helps nondairy coffee creamers dissolve in coffee, keeps dill oil dissolved in bottles of dill pickles, and keeps flavor oils dissolved in candy, ice cream, and beverages. The polysorbates are often used in combination with sorbitan monostearate. This mouth-watering combination may make up as much as 1 percent of a food product. In most of their functions, polysorbates are considerably more potent (on a weight basis) than fat or mono- and diglycerides.

The three different polysorbates are made by reacting different amounts of oleic or stearic acids first with sorbitol and then with ethylene oxide. The full chemical names of these additives are polyoxyethylene-(20)-sorbitan monostearate, tristearate, and monooleate. Our national diet contains about 1.5 million pounds of polysorbate 60; 96,000 pounds of polysorbate 65; and 550,000 pounds of polysorbate 80 annually, according to FDA figures.

During the 1950s there was considerable controversy about the safety of the polysorbates. In some experiments, rats and hamsters whose diets contained 25 percent polysorbate developed bladder stones, died prematurely, lost their tails, and suffered sundry other side effects. When hamsters ate food containing 5 percent polysorbates, they suffered diarrhea, early death, changes in the kidney, liver, and large intestine, and retardation of growth.

The FAO/WHO Expert Committee on Food Additives examined the experiments casting doubt on the polysorbates and ascribed most of the adverse effects to inadequate laboratory diets and to the chronic diarrhea (and resulting water imbalance) caused by the enormous intakes of polysorbates. The Committee questioned "the validity of using levels above 10 percent in the assessment of the toxicological hazard of a food additive." Subsequent, but small, experiments on well-fed rats, hamsters, and dogs bore out the Committee's contentions. Levels of 5 percent and below were harmless, while greater amounts caused diarrhea and changes in some organs. More up-to-date tests are needed, especially on the lesser used polysorbates 65 and 80.

The polysorbates did not appear to be carcinogenic or otherwise harmful in several tests. Tumors did not develop when scientists fed polysorbate 60 to several species of rodents. A four-generation study on rats showed that the emulsifiers do not affect reproduction.

The fact that polysorbates appeared safe in tests turned out to be more an indication of the insensitivity of animal studies than of the absolute harmlessness of the chemicals. In 1978, Thomas Birkel, an FDA scientist, discovered that polysorbates were contaminated with 1,4-dioxane, a known carcinogen. Depending upon the manufacturer, up to 700 parts per million of dioxane contaminated the popular additive. That amount of dioxane was apparently too little to cause tumors in the animal tests of polysorbates, but dioxane itself caused cancer in both rats and mice. FDA now limits dioxane to 10 parts per million. This level is twenty times higher than what some FDA scientists wanted.

The way the body digests polysorbates is well understood. The fatty acid portion (stearate, oleate) of the molecule is absorbed in the intestine and readily metabolized. The remainder of the molecule—polyoxyethylene sorbitan—is absorbed to the extent of 5 percent and subsequently excreted in the urine. The rest (95 percent) of the polyoxyethylene sorbitan is eliminated in the stools.

Doctors have fed polysorbates to patients suffering from certain diseases to help them absorb fat in food into the bloodstream.

Ref.: FAO (35)-127-145; *J. Nutr. 61*, 149, 235 (1957); *J. Fd. Sci. 31*, 253 (1966); *Tox. Appl. Pharm. 16*, 321 (1970); *J. Assoc. Off. Anal. Chem. 62*, 981 (1979); *21* CFR 172.836–840.

Potassium compounds (potassium bicarbonate, potassium hydroxide, potassium phosphate, potassium sulfate, and other potassium salts)

Potassium is an essential mineral that is widely distributed in foods and occurs in dozens of different additives. Potassium is not only safe, but helps counteract sodium's ability to raise blood pressure.

Several specific potassium-containing additives are described following; for other additives, look up the corresponding sodium salt (for example, sodium nitrate).

Potassium Bromate, Calcium Bromate   Safe

Millers and bakers have used potassium bromate since 1916 to artificially age and improve the baking properties of flour. Bromate is used at levels of 5 to 75 parts per million. Baking converts bromate (BrO_3^-) to bromide (Br^-), which is absorbed by the body when bread is digested. The bromide circulates in the blood and is slowly excreted in the urine. Calcium bromate is sometimes used in place of potassium bromate.

In 1982, Y. Kurokawa and other scientists at the Japanese National Institute of Hygienic Sciences reported that potassium bromate caused tumors in rats, when the animals consumed large amounts of the chemical in their drinking water. FDA scientists pointed out, though, that this study was not relevant, because baking converts all the bromate to bromide. Animal tests involving baked, bromated flour did not suggest any problems. Nevertheless, if I had my druthers, I would choose baked goods that did not contain this flour treatment agent, just because it is so chemically reactive. It is probably perfectly harmless, but it won't do anything good for you.

Ref.: J. Sci. Fd. Agric. 25, 1471 (1974); *Fd. Chem. Tox. 21,* No. 4 (1983); FAO (35)-164; FDA files; *21* CFR 172.730, 182.1613–182.1631.

Potassium Chloride   Safe

As more and more people are learning that sodium promotes high blood pressure, makers of processed foods are switching from sodium salts to potassium salts. Some salt substitutes, such as No-Salt, consist entirely of potassium chloride, while others, such as Morton's Lite Salt, are half potassium, half sodium chloride.

Very large amounts of potassium can be harmful to people with kidney disease and certain heart conditions, as well as those using "potassium-sparing" diuretics. Check with your doctor before using a potassium-containing salt substitute, if you think you are one of these people. Some of us are protected from consuming too much potassium chloride by its extremely unpleasant taste when consumed to excess.

Ref.: 21 CFR 182.5622.

Potassium Iodide, Cuprous Iodide   ?
Potassium or Calcium Iodate

Iodine is one of the trace elements, small amounts of which are needed for a person's proper growth, development, and health. In the early nineteenth century it was discovered that a deficiency of iodine in the diet causes goiter, the disease in which the thyroid gland grows to many times its normal size in a vain attempt to produce the iodine-containing hormone thyroxine. News of the miraculous effect of iodine spread like wildfire among sufferers of goiter, who quickly made iodine-rich seaweed a standard part of their diet. Ironically, seaweed contains so much iodine that while most people were cured, a few suffered from iodine-*excess* goiter.

In the 1910s and '20s, large-scale experiments proved that routine consumption of iodine could eradicate goiter in whole populations. Public health experts agreed that simply adding iodine to table salt would be the best, least expensive solution to an age-old problem. Salt manufacturers use 0.01 percent potassium iodide or cuprous iodide to supply the iodine.

Despite our thorough understanding of goiter and its virtual disappearance in the 1930s and '40s, this disease is now having a mild resurgence in the United States. The new cases of goiter are probably due to iodine excess rather than deficiency. The FDA has analyzed the iodine content of average diets and discovered that an adult is likely to be consuming three to six times the recommended daily intake (RDA). Many infants and toddlers are ingesting ten or twelve times the recommended amount. In two startling examples, FDA scientists found almost three times the RDA in a typical meal at McDonald's (a Big Mac, french fries, milkshake) and almost twenty-nine times the RDA in a single frozen fried chicken dinner!

The tremendous amount of iodine in our food comes from several sources. Dairy foods provide 56 percent of the iodine, which comes from dietary supplements added to the cows' food and from disinfectants used to clean udders and milking machines. FDA has urged farmers to use less iodine.

Baked goods provide the next largest share of iodine, 16 percent, much of it coming from dough conditioners that facilitate quicker baking. Still more iodine derives from Red No. 3 food dye, the use of which has risen greatly since other red dyes were banned; processed foods contaminated with disinfectants and processing aids; iodized salt; and naturally occurring iodine.

The health risks of very high intakes of iodine are relatively unknown, though the American Thyroid Association has expressed concern. Very high levels could precipitate goiter and other thyroid diseases. FDA has acknowledged that "rising iodine intakes may also be responsible for decreased remissions in the treatment of hyperthyroidism with anti-thyroid agents." The rate of success has dipped from 60 to 17 percent. While further research is being done to evaluate the effects of moderately high iodine intakes, FDA should clamp down on iodine use by food producers.

Ref.: FAO (40)-15; FAO (40A)-112, 113; *Bull. World Health Org. 9,* 211, 293 (1953); *New Engl. J. Med. 280,* 1431 (1969); "Iodine Nutriture in the United States," Food and Nutrition Board, Nat. Acad. Sci. (summary of a conference, Oct. 31, 1970); "FDA Consumer," p. 15 (April 1981); *J. Am. Diet. Asso. 79,* 17 (1981); *21* CFR 172.375; 184.1634–184.1635.

Potassium metabisulfite—*see* Sulfiting Agents

Potassium nitrate and potassium nitrite—*see* Sodium Nitrate, Sodium Nitrite

Propyl Gallate   Avoid

Since 1948 manufacturers have added propyl gallate to foods to retard the spoilage of fats and oils and thereby increase slightly their shelf life. Propyl gallate is used at levels up to 0.02 percent (of the fat or oil content) in animal fat, vegetable oil, meat products, potato sticks, and chicken soup base, and up to 0.1 percent in chewing gum. It is sometimes added to food packaging material, in which case it migrates as a vapor onto the food (breakfast cereals, potato flakes).

You will often find propyl gallate used in combination with BHT or BHA because of the synergistic effect these three food additives have in preventing fats from going rancid. The synergism permits a reduction of the total concentration of antioxidants. Another reason for using propyl gallate in combination with other antioxidants is that high levels of propyl gallate produce an undesirable blue or green color in foods that contain minute amounts of iron or copper and moisture.

Rats—and presumably humans—have little trouble disposing of propyl gallate. (Ready for a little biochemistry?) The preservative is hydrolyzed to release gallic acid, which is converted in the liver to 4-methyl gallic acid. The latter is either directly excreted in the urine or coupled with another chemical (glucuronic acid) and then excreted. Gallic acid is also produced when rats metabolize tannic acid, which is found in tea, coffee, and cocoa. Metabolic studies need to be conducted in humans.

The best, and virtually only, long-term feeding study that evaluated the cancer risk associated with propyl gallate was initiated by the National Cancer Institute and completed in 1981. The study was peppered with suggestions of cancer: brain tumors in female rats, malignant lymphomas in male mice, and liver adenomas in female mice, all at statistically significant levels. However, in each case the reviewers of the study managed to find some excuse to diminish the significance of the tumors. In one case, rats ingesting 6,000 parts per million of the preservative developed rare brain tumors, whereas rats consuming twice as much did not develop such tumors. Usually, higher doses of a chemical cause more tumors. In other cases, the current results were compared to previous experiments to explain away the tumors. The review committee concluded:

> . . . propyl gallate was not considered to be carcinogenic in F344 rats, although there was evidence of an increased number of male rats with . . . tumors . . . Propyl gallate was not considered carcinogenic for B6C3F1 mice of either sex, but an increased number of malignant lymphomas in male mice may have been related to the administration of the test compounds.

Companies concerned about its customers would not use this unnecessary preservative, and a government concerned about health would not allow it at all. A tumor is far too high a price to pay for a few extra months' shelf life for some processed foods.

Ref.: CRC-219, 704; *Fd. Cos. Tox. 3,* 457 (1965), *6,* 25 (1968); *J. Food Hyg. Soc. 20,* 378 (1979); Dept. Health & Human Services Pub. No. 82-1796 (National Toxicology Program); Nat. Toxicol. Prog., Board of Scientific Counselors, *Summary Minutes,* meeting of June 16, 1982; *21* CFR 181.24; 184.1660.

Propylene Glycol — Safe
Propylene Glycol Mono- and Diesters — Safe

Propylene glycol is one of several additives (glycerol and sorbitol are two others) that are used in foods to help maintain the desired moisture content and texture. Manufacturers add between 0.03 and 5 percent propylene glycol to candy, baked goods, icings, shredded coconut, and moist pet foods. This additive also serves as a carrier for oily flavorings and helps them dissolve in soft drinks and other water-based foods. It is also used in many cosmetics and drugs (including K-Y lubricating jelly).

The human body converts propylene glycol to either chemical building blocks or to energy.

In a chronic feeding study done by FDA biologists, rats that ate food containing 4.9 percent propylene glycol suffered no ill effects. Shorter tests on dogs also indicated that this substance is safe. Several medical reports have demonstrated that some people are allergic to propylene glycol. They develop a severe, itchy rash that can last weeks or even months.

Propylene glycol is closely related to glycerol and, like glycerol, can be chemically reacted with fatty acids. The propylene glycol mono- and diesters that form are analogous to mono- and diglycerides and natural fats and oils. Enzymes in the intestine convert the mono- and diesters back to propylene glycol and fatty acids, which are then absorbed and metabolized. Propylene glycol monostearate and similar compounds are used in shortening to help make lighter, fluffier cakes.

Ref.: FAO (40A)-102; CRC-Ch. 11; *Arch. Biochem.* 29, 231 (1950), 77, 428 (1958); *Poult. Sci.* 48, 608 (1969); *Arch. Dermatol.* 115, 1451 (1979); *21* CFR 172.856, 184.1666.

Propylene Glycol Alginate   Safe

"Propylene glycol alginate, the additive that made our beer famous." You've never seen that slogan in an advertisement, but I can imagine that the producers of propylene glycol alginate might use it to publicize the additive's value to the brewing industry. Some brewers add the additive to their products to stabilize the foamy head. According to *American Brewer,* a beer industry magazine:

> When beer was made with more malts and hops than is the practice today, stability of foam was rarely a problem. Today's lighter-type lagers and ales, however, made with higher percentages of adjuncts and only mildly hopped, require assistance in maintaining an expected head of foam.

The next time you see a beer's foamy head touted in a television commercial, remember the chemical additive that may deserve the credit.

Propylene glycol alginate serves as an emulsifier, thickener, or stabilizer in a wide variety of products, including puddings, ice milk, frostings, cheeses, and baked goods. It may comprise as much as 1 percent of the finished product.

This scrumptious-sounding additive is made by reacting alginic acid, which is extracted from seaweed and used as an additive itself (see alginates), with propylene oxide. The advantage that propylene glycol alginate has over plain alginates is that it is stable in acidic solutions, such as soda pop and salad dressings. Alginates precipitate out of such foods.

Ref.: Am. Brewer, p. 22 (Dec. 1963); *Fed. Reg.* 47, 29946 (July 9, 1982); *21* CFR 172.858.

Pyridoxine (or pyridoxine hydrochloride)   Safe

The importance of pyridoxine, or vitamin B_6, was highlighted in 1951, when a number of infants developed convulsions. Some medical detective work determined that the babies' infant formula contained almost no vitamin B_6. Once the babies were given some B_6, their symptoms disappeared promptly.

Breast-feeding advocates point to this kind of problem as a reason to give babies the "perfect food."

Vitamin B_6 serves a variety of functions in the body and performs a central role in amino acid metabolism. Wheat germ, brown rice, and yeast are especially good sources of this vitamin.

In recent years, doctors have been testing the ability of huge amounts (megadoses) of B_6 to treat mental disorders. One small, but well-controlled, study by Dr. Bernard Rimland indicated that some autistic children respond favorably to B_6. Also, some women say that large doses of vitamin B_6 ameliorate premenstrual tension. One should be very cautious, though, when taking megadoses of this (or any) vitamin. A 1983 study traced nervous system problems of seven individuals to the enormous doses of vitamin B_6 that they had been consuming for two to forty months. Doses one thousand to three thousand times higher than the recommended daily allowance caused numb feet, loss of tendon reflexes, and an unstable gait. Biopsies showed degeneration of nerve cells.

Vitamin B_6 is added to many breakfast cereals and "health food candy bars" (an oxymoron, if there ever was one) as an advertising gimmick.

Ref.: Recommended Dietary Allowances, Nat. Acad. Sci., Washington, D.C. (1980); *Am. J. Psych. 135,* 472 (1978); *Fed. Reg. 48,* 51614 (Nov. 10, 1983); *New Engl. J. Med. 309,* 445 (1983); *21* CFR 182.8676.

Quillaia   ?

Quillaia is extracted from the soapbark tree and permitted for use as a natural flavoring. While quillaia does not appear to have been tested, the FDA says it has no record of it being used.

Ref.: Food Chem. Tox. 20, 15 (1982); FDA files; *21* CFR 172.510.

Quinine   Pregnant women: **Avoid**
                                        Others: ?

In the early 1600s Jesuit priests living in Peru discovered that a substance in the bark of a local tree could cure malaria, the deadly, mosquito-borne disease. The miracle drug came to be called quinine. The sole natural source of quinine is the cinchona tree, a species indigenous to the mile-high eastern slopes of the Andes Mountains.

Large amounts of quinine were shipped from South America to Europe from 1650 to 1850, during which time little attention was paid to the dwindling population of cinchona trees. To prevent the extinction of the species and avert disaster, the Dutch began to cultivate the valuable tree in Java. A similar venture by the British in Madras, India, which state had the world's highest incidence of malaria, was a tragic failure. Fortunately cinchona flourished in Java and that island became the major supplier of the alkaloid. Quinine's heyday ended when Japan's capture of the Dutch East Indies in World War II forced the Allies to develop synthetic antimalarial drugs. These drugs have proved to be cheaper and more effective than quinine.

Aside from preventing the growth of the parasite that causes malaria, quinine has been used to induce abortions. It is also a nonspecific remedy for pain and fever (it reduces fever by dilating small blood vessels of the skin, thereby facilitating loss of body heat).

The sole use of quinine in foods is as a bitter flavoring in quinine water, tonic water, bitter lemon, and similar drinks. These beverages may contain quinine at levels up to 83 parts per million. A total of about 18,000 pounds per year is consumed in the United States.

Reports in medical journals dating back to 1870 document quinine's ability to cause deafness in developing human and animal fetuses. A number of pregnant women who took quinine either to treat malaria or in unsuccessful attempts to abort their babies in the early months of pregnancy gave birth to deaf children. The quantities of quinine involved ranged from 600 milligrams to several grams. In a laboratory experiment, the auditory nerves of rabbit fetuses were damaged when the mothers consumed moderate dosages of quinine. This study was conducted in the 1930s and does not appear to have been followed up by further studies involving lower dosages or additional species. The sensitivity of the auditory apparatus to quinine is further indicated by the temporary hearing impairments that adults often experience when they are treated with quinine for malaria.

Tonic water and similar beverages contain approximately thirty milligrams of the drug quinine per twelve-ounce serving. This level of drug in one or two gin and tonics a day would certainly not cause deafness in a human fetus, but could conceivably cause a temporary or more subtle effect. Decreases of 1, 5, or 10 percent in hearing ability would never be spotted by pediatricians or parents, but such a side effect of a food additive would certainly be undesirable. Prudence would dictate that pregnant women avoid quinine.

Quinine water is definitely known to have at least one occasional deleterious effect. As few as five ounces of the beverage have caused purpura, a disease in which blood escapes from vessels near the skin, causing the victim to turn purple. More than fifty cases of this sensitivity to quinine have been reported.

The ability of quinine to cause cancer, mutations, or birth defects must be investigated before this additive can be considered safe.

Ref.: Encyclopedia Brittanica ("quinine," "cinchona," "malaria"); *Ann. Int. Med. 66*, 583 (1967); *Pediatrica 32*, 115 (1963); *Am. J. Obs. Gyn. 36*, 241 (1930), *Munchen med. Wchnschr. 108*, 2293 (1966); *J. Egypt. Med. Asso. 58*, 144–57 (1975); *21* CFR 172.575.

Riboflavin (or riboflavin-5 phosphate)   Safe

This fancy-sounding additive is simply vitamin B_2. Riboflavin plays a crucial role in activating numerous enzymes. It is safe.

Riboflavin is added to enriched flour, many breakfast cereals, and other "vitamin-fortified" foods. Because riboflavin deficiency (fissuring at the corners of the mouth, swelling of the tongue, and other skin problems) is essentially nonexistent in the United States, one must conclude that companies add this and other inexpensive nutrients to food more as an excuse to make lofty claims ("New! Fortified with 10 vitamins!") than to promote health. Riboflavin may occasionally be used as a yellow coloring.

For additional information, please refer to the *Nutrition Scoreboard* section of this book (page 92).

Ref.: 21 CFR 73.450, 182.5695–182.5697.

Saccharin   Avoid

Controversy over the artificial sweetener saccharin was the biggest food additive story of the past decade. Newspaper headlines from 1970 to 1983 alternated between reassurances of safety and new evidence of hazard. Consumers, accustomed to eating artificially sweetened foods and confused beyond belief by the endless debate, ended up ignoring the whole matter and sipped diet sodas that had the word "cancer" on their labels. The case of saccharin, like nothing else before, focused public attention on food safety and spurred the food industry to lobby for weaker laws.

First, the chemical. Saccharin is about 350 times sweeter than sugar. About half of all saccharin consumed is in soda pop, 20 percent in tabletop sweetener (such as Sweet'N Low), and the rest in canned fruit, chewing gum, toothpaste, drugs, and other products. Americans have consumed six to eight million pounds of saccharin annually, though that amount is declining rapidly as more and more companies are switching to aspartame. Because the body does not convert saccharin to glucose, persons suffering from diabetes can use saccharin to sweeten their foods. Saccharin is also safe for teeth.

The way in which saccharin was discovered illustrates well the phenomenon of scientific serendipity (or, how sloppy, but intelligent, scientists make the most of their blunders). In 1879 Constantin Fahlberg, a graduate student in chemistry at Johns Hopkins University, ate a piece of bread that tasted unexpectedly sweet. Believing that he had accidentally contaminated his food with a chemical, Fahlberg returned to the laboratory and tasted some of the coal tar derivatives that he had synthesized. Sure enough, one of them was incredibly sweet. The chemical was given the name saccharin and since about 1900 has been sold commercially. Incidentally, Fahlberg obtained a patent on saccharin and made a good deal of money from his accidental discovery. He also incurred the lifelong wrath of his professor, Ira Remsen, who claimed codiscovery of the chemical.

The large amounts of sugar normally present in soft drinks, preserves, and other heavily sweetened foods add "body" or thickness to the foods as well as sweetness. When comparatively small amounts of saccharin replace sugar, the sweetness is there but not the body. Because of this, diet drinks and other products are frequently artificially thickened with vegetable gums, such as gum arabic or carboxymethylcellulose (cellulose gum).

Saccharin's major gustatory shortcoming is its disagreeably bitter aftertaste. This problem enabled cyclamate, following its discovery in 1944, to capture a large share of the artificial sweetener market. After cyclamate was banned in 1970, manufacturers devised ways of masking saccharin's aftertaste. Most commonly, they add about 0.2 percent glycine, a natural amino acid, to the food.

Artificial sweeteners are touted for their ability to aid dieters and diabetics. The Calorie Control Council, a trade association of manufacturers and suppliers of foods for dieters, claims "Saccharin . . . a benefit to millions." Officials of the American Diabetes Association and the American Cancer Society have defended saccharin on the grounds that its ability to control obesity and prevent diabetes outweighed its "theoretical" ability to cause cancer. The producer of Sweet'N Low bragged in an ad in the *Journal of the American Medical Association* that "Sweet'N Low has saved more diets and eliminated more excess sugar usage than any other sugar substitute."

In fact, saccharin is not a magic cure for obesity, and there is little scientific evidence that saccharin aids dieting. In a 1971 study on mice, researchers at New York University School of Medicine found that substituting no-calorie beverages for drinks containing sugar did not result in weight loss. Other studies, on humans, mice, and rats showed that saccharin actually lowered blood sugar levels. This hypoglycemic effect would induce hunger. Thus, eating saccharin might make it even harder for people to lose weight! Overweight individuals should certainly avoid refined sugar, but that doesn't mean they need to eat saccharin.

Controversy over saccharin goes back to the early years of the century. In 1908, Harvey Wiley, the first director of America's food protection agency, believed that all chemicals related to benzoic acid, including saccharin, impaired kidney function. President Theodore Roosevelt, a daily consumer of saccharin, dismissed the health problem summarily, saying, "Anybody who says saccharin is injurious is an idiot." A review committee—they even had them back then—conducted new studies (ones that were hopelessly crude by today's standards) and found no problem. The chemical continued to be used by a narrow segment of the population.

The real battles over saccharin began forty years later. A 1951 study on rats by FDA scientists provided a hint that the sweet chemical might promote cancer. This study and several others conducted in the 1950s and 1960s were intriguing, but flawed in several regards.

The fireworks began going off in 1970 when University of Wisconsin scientists implanted little pellets of saccharin mixed with cholesterol in urinary bladders of mice. They found that the saccharin caused a fourfold increase in the number of tumors compared to mice implanted with cholesterol but no saccharin. In 1971 preliminary results of a feeding study also indicated that saccharin could cause bladder tumors in rats. This new evidence spurred FDA to remove saccharin from the list of "Generally Recognized As Safe" (GRAS) food additives.

During the next decade dozens of scientific studies and official review committees evaluated saccharin. SACCHARIN CAUSED CANCER. SACCHARIN RISK DEBUNKED. The headlines reflected the ups and downs of the saccharin battles. After it was clear that the studies were indeed indicating cancer, scientists discovered an impurity (ortho-toluene sulfonamide) in the sweetener and suggested that maybe the intruder rather than saccharin itself was responsible for the tumors. So back to the labs they went to do more studies. In early 1977 the results of the new tests emerged from a Canadian government lab. The results were unequivocal: the impurity did not cause cancer; saccharin caused malignant bladder tumors. On March 9, 1977, FDA announced that it would ban saccharin.

FDA's decision lit a firestorm of opposition. Part of the fire was fueled by FDA's spokesperson, acting Commissioner Sherwin Gardner, who emphasized the large amount of saccharin fed to the rats, adding that there was no evidence that saccharin ever harmed humans. (Gardner later left FDA to work for the Grocery Manufacturers of America, a major food industry lobby.) The Calorie Control Council immediately began publishing full-page ads in major newspapers around the country to save saccharin. Thousands of consumers wrote to the FDA and their congresspersons, urging, sometimes pleading, that saccharin be permitted. FDA backed off a little, proposing in April that saccharin would be allowed as a nonprescription drug, if—and this was a big if—manufacturers could "demonstrate it is effective in medical uses such as the management of diabetes or in weight control programs." The almost unprecedented grassroots and industrial pressure (if only public ire could be aroused by more substantial social issues!), however, would not be satisfied with compromise and soon won passage of a law that postponed any ban for at least eighteen months while an official review was conducted by the National Research Council. The law also required companies to print a warning notice on foods containing saccharin:

> Use of this product may be hazardous to your health. This product contains saccharin which has been determined to cause cancer in laboratory animals.

Grocery stores that sold saccharin-containing foods had to post signs with similar wording. Food processors complied with the law, but sometimes printed the warning notice in tiny, virtually illegible type, often in a color that blended into the background. Many grocery stores soon removed the required signs, knowing that FDA would not enforce this aspect of the law. Meanwhile, FDA's new Commissioner, Donald Kennedy, proved to be an extraordinarily articulate critic of saccharin. Kennedy argued that "we should not allow even weak carcinogens in the environment if we can help it. Our systems may already be overloaded."

As it became clearer that saccharin caused cancer in rodents, supporters of saccharin began arguing that animal studies were inherently unreliable and that human studies should be done before FDA and Congress decided saccharin's fate.

While the human studies were being designed, a special panel of the National Research Council reviewed the existing studies on saccharin. The committee's conclusions were unequivocal:

> In rats saccharin is a carcinogen of low potency relative to other carcinogens . . . In addition to acting by itself, saccharin promotes the cancer-causing effects of some other carcinogenic compounds in rats . . . Saccharin must be viewed as a potential carcinogen in humans, but one of low potency in comparison to other carcinogens. Although saccharin would be expected to be of low potency in humans, even low risks applied to a large number of exposed persons may lead to public health concerns . . . Essentially, there is no scientific support for the health benefits of saccharin.

The expert committee tried to estimate the number of cancers that saccharin might cause. It discovered, though, that the techniques for extrapolating from animal studies to human risks were rather imprecise. The best the committee could do was say that, depending upon the mathematical model used, saccharin would cause anywhere from 0.0007 to 3,640 cases of bladder cancer in the 50 million consumers of saccharin.

Identifying human cancers caused by saccharin is virtually impossible. First, saccharin and cyclamate were almost always used in combination. Furthermore, humans who ingested saccharin also were exposed to any number of cancer-causing agents in the form of drugs, cigarettes, pollutants, and other chemicals. Nevertheless, several studies were undertaken to correlate the incidence of bladder cancer with consumption of artificial sweeteners (not distinguishing between cyclamate and saccharin).

The largest and most sensitive study was cosponsored by the National Cancer Institute and the Food and Drug Administration. It compared the dietary, smoking, and other habits of more than three thousand bladder cancer patients to the habits of almost six thousand people from the general population who did not have cancer, but who were similar in age and sex. This careful study concluded that "heavy users of artificial sweeteners, particularly those who consumed both diet beverages and sugar substitutes, showed a 60 percent increased risk of bladder cancer. Heavy use was defined as six or more servings a day of sugar substitutes or two or more eight-ounce diet beverages a day." Nonsmoking women who consumed artificial sweeteners twice or more a day also had a 60 percent increased risk of cancer. Judging from animal studies, the higher cancer risk could well have been due to a direct effect of saccharin, with some enhancement from cyclamate, which may increase the potency of cancer-causing chemicals. In other, smaller studies, researchers at Harvard School of Public Health and the American Health Foundation failed to link artificial sweeteners to cancer.

The NCI-FDA study was the culmination of a long series of studies on which scientists spent hundreds of person-years and government and industry spent tens of millions of dollars. The animal studies provided substantial evidence that saccharin could cause cancer in animals and presumably in people. The large human study added the final piece to the puzzle. Despite this mass of evidence, despite the nastiness of cancer, saccharin was still not banned.

If saccharin's benefits are dubious, if saccharin might increase the risk of cancer even by a tiny amount, why have both consumers and producers fought so hard for its continued use? It may be that using saccharin and eating diet foods gives overweight people the comfort of thinking they are really doing something for their obesity. Drinking a diet soda is certainly easier and more comfortable than jogging a mile or eating nothing. Never mind that the hundred calories avoided may be ingested enthusiastically later that day in the form of several bites of meat. In other words, saccharin offers the pretense of dieting without apparent sacrifice.

One need not resort to psychological theories to understand the food industry's love of saccharin. First, one goal of processors is to grab as much supermarket shelf space as possible; the more shelf space a company garners, the more food it is likely to sell. Making low-calorie versions of soda pop, canned fruit, and chewing gum can instantaneously double the shelf space.

Furthermore, saccharin costs only one twentieth as much as sugar for equivalent sweetening power. Diet soda and regular soda usually cost the same, but diet soda is much cheaper to produce. Consumers have paid several hundred million dollars a year extra, because of this overcharge for diet sodas. As long as companies can get people to pay sugar prices for a cheaper substitute, they will fight like the dickens to keep the impostor on the market.

Americans perceived the risk of cancer from diet foods to be trivial, despite the periodic recommendations from government officials and label warnings. Total saccharin consumption dipped briefly, if at all. By 1985 saccharin's "temporary" exemption from the Delaney Clause's prohibition had been renewed several times by Congress. But saccharin was tolerated primarily because it was the only artificial sweetener on the market, and it is still the only one that can be used in certain foods. As safe substitutes are developed, they will displace saccharin. The first partial replacement was aspartame, a better-tasting sweetener marketed under the brand names Equal and NutraSweet. It began replacing some uses of saccharin in late 1982, even though it is much more expensive. By 1984 the trickle of aspartame-sweetened products had turned into a flood, and saccharin sales slumped. Aspartame and possibly other artificial sweeteners will gradually erase saccharin from our food supply, making a ban feasible or unnecessary.

Avoid saccharin, because it both increases slightly the risk of cancer and is used primarily in foods with little or no nutritional merit.

Ref.: Proc. Soc. Exp. Biol. Med. 66, 175 (1947); *Science 168,* 1238 (1970); *Fed. Reg. 42,* 19996 (Apr. 15, 1977); Public Law 95-203 (Nov. 23, 1977); "Saccharin: Technical Assessment of Risks and Benefits," Nat. Acad. Sci., (1978); "Progress Report to the FDA from the NCI Concerning the National Bladder Cancer Study," (Dec. 1979); *Lancet i,* 377 (1980); Hearing: Senate Committee on Labor and Human Resources, April 2, 1985; *21* CFR 180.37.

Silicates (Aluminum calcium silicate, magnesium silicate, calcium silicate, sodium alumino silicate, sodium calcium alumino silicate, tricalcium silicate) Silicon Dioxide

Safe

Most of us have been annoyed at one time or another by lumpy salt that just would not come out of the shaker. The problem arises when moisture adheres to grains of salt, enabling them to melt together; lumps form when hundreds of particles get into the act. Many persons put a few grains of rice into salt shakers to absorb the moisture. To save the consumer that effort, manufacturers add 2 percent silicates or silicon dioxide to salt. The additive coats the salt grains, keeping them from becoming damp and melting together. You will also find silicate anticaking agents in powdered coffee whitener, vanilla powder, baking powder, dried egg yolk, and seasoning salts.

Silicon dioxide, or silica as it is often called, is the principal component of 95 percent of the earth's rocks. Combinations of silica with other minerals are termed silicates, also major constituents of the earth's crust. Thus, these additives are simply finely pulverized rock dust.

Silica occurs naturally at very low levels in all living organisms (10–200 mg/100g dry weight of human tissue). Silica in food is absorbed in the intestines to a limited extent and then excreted in the urine and stools. Humans eliminate 10–30 milligrams of silica per day in the urine. Negligible amounts remain in the body. However, industrial workers who inhale and ingest relatively large amounts of silicates and other finely powdered crystalline chemicals might encounter problems after years of exposure.

Rats and rabbits have been fed diets containing 1 percent silica for ninety days. There was no effect on growth, survival, reproduction, blood, urine, and several internal organs. Humans have eaten 5–10 grams of silica a day for several weeks without apparent effect. The FAO/WHO Expert Committee on Food Additives has given silica and silicates a clean bill of health.

Ref.: FAO (46)-18; FAO (46A)-143; CUFP-269; *Am. J. Cardiology 17,* 269 (1966); *21* CFR 172.410, 172.480, 182.2122–182.2906.

Smoke Flavoring ?

Humans have probably been smoking food for thousands of years. Not only does smoking add a distinctive flavor, but it also preserves food. Traditional smoking processes for meat and fish are losing favor, because the smoke contains significant amounts of carcinogenic chemicals (polycyclic aromatic hydrocarbons). An occasional smoked food doesn't pose much of a risk, but among cultures whose traditional foods are often smoked (as in Finland, for instance), an appreciable number of gastrointestinal cancers are probably due to the contaminants in smoke.

For people who like the flavor of smoke, but would just as soon do without the contaminants, smoke flavoring is a distinct improvement. Smoke from real wood is trapped and then partially purified. In 1975, the Joint FAO/WHO Expert Committee on Food Additives refrained from endorsing the safety of liquid smoke, because there is virtually no information about this additive.

The U.S. Department of Agriculture has devised a hairsplitting regulation that determines whether a food should be labeled "naturally smoked," "smoked," or "smoke flavoring added."

Ref.: FAO (55); Nat. Acad. Sci., *Diet, Nutrition, and Cancer* (1982); USDA (Food Safety and Insp. Serv.) policy memo 058 (March 22, 1983).

Sodium compounds

Dozens of different sodium-containing chemicals serve a multitude of purposes in foods. The most important sodium additive is sodium chloride, ordinary table salt, which comprises 90 percent of all sodium added to foods. Monosodium glutamate, sodium benzoate, sodium propionate, and others are discussed separately in these pages. The problem with all of these chemicals is that they add sodium to our diets. Diets high in sodium all too often lead to or worsen high blood pressure. This condition, in turn, greatly increases the risk of heart attack and stroke. About the only way to avoid all sodium-containing additives is to avoid processed foods.

Some of the sodium-containing additives, many discussed elsewhere in *Eater's Digest*, are:

Monosodium glutamate	flavor enhancer
Sodium aluminum phosphate	acid in baking powder
Sodium benzoate	preservative
Sodium bicarbonate	baking soda
Sodium bisulfite	preservative
Sodium carbonate	alkali
Sodium gluconate	sequestrant (traps unwanted metal ions)
Sodium hexametaphosphate	sequestrant
Sodium metaphosphate	sequestrant
Sodium phosphate (mono-, di- and tribasic)	sequestrant
Sodium pyrophosphate	sequestrant
Sodium pyrophosphate (tetra)	sequestrant
Sodium thiosulfate	antioxidant, sequestrant
Sodium tripolyphosphate	sequestrant

Other than adding sodium, these additives do not pose any significant health risk (with the exception of sodium bisulfite—see discussion under sulfiting agents).

Sodium Benzoate (benzoate of soda, benzoic acid)   Safe

Food manufacturers have used sodium benzoate as a preservative for over seventy years. Although it can prevent the growth of almost all microorganisms (bacteria, fungi, and yeast), it is effective only under acidic conditions. Thus, its use is limited to such foods as fruit juices, carbonated drinks, pickles, salad dressing, and preserves. It is used at levels of 0.05 to 0.1 percent. Sodium benzoate occurs naturally in many fruits and vegetables, notably cranberries (0.05 to 0.09 percent) and prunes, and so is no stranger to the human body. Moreover, in 1954 Dr. W. H. Stein reported in the *Journal of the American Chemical Society* that benzoate is a natural metabolite in our body.

Benzoate has been tested in lifetime and short-term feeding experiments in man, dogs, and rats. In an experiment conducted in Germany, four generations of rats were continuously exposed to 0.5 or 1 percent sodium benzoate in their diet. Scientists did not observe any harmful effects on growth, life span, or internal organs; no tumors were detected. All the evidence indicates that sodium benzoate is quite safe, except, possibly, for occasional allergic reactions.

In the United States, food may contain up to 0.1 percent sodium benzoate. Some nations permit as much as 1.25 percent benzoate in certain foods.

Ref.: FAO (31)-27; *J. Am. Chem. Soc. 76,* 2848 (1954); *Tox. Appl. Pharmacol. 19,* 373 (1971); *Lancet ii,* 1055 (1981); *21* CFR 184.1021, 184.1733.

Sodium Bisulfite—*see* sulfiting agents

Sodium Erythorbate, Safe
Erythorbic Acid, Sodium Isoascorbate

According to Chas. Pfizer & Co. sodium erythorbate assures "a more appetizing red 'showcase' color in processed meats . . . When sprayed on presliced ham and bacon, sodium erythorbate retards color fading and preserves eye appeal." According to some consumers the use of erythorbate on meat is a deceptive practice because the additive helps make the meat look better than it really is.

Sodium erythorbate is a close but nonnutritive relative of vitamin C (ascorbic acid). Its most important use is in processed meats. Occasionally, it is used as an antioxidant in beverages, baked goods, and potato salad. Erythorbate is sometimes called isoascorbate.

Erythorbate is not a vitamin, despite its structural similarity to vitamin C. But because oxygen reacts slightly more readily with erythorbate than with ascorbate, erythorbate helps protect the vitamin in certain foods.

Sodium erythorbate has not been extensively tested. In experiments on animals and man, biochemists found that this chemical does not replace vitamin C in the body and that it is fairly rapidly excreted, but only one chronic feeding study has been reported. That study, done in the early 1940s on rats by FDA scientists, did not reveal any problems. Thorough long-term feeding, genetic, and teratogenic experiments should be conducted. Meanwhile, meat packers should switch to sodium ascorbate, which is certainly safe, and adds to the nutritional value of the food.

Ref.: FAO (31)-23; *Food Tech. 12* (6) (1958), *19,* 1719 (1965); *J. Nutr. 81,* 163 (1963); Chas. Pfizer & Co. "Pfizer and Food" (1965); Ziegler, P. T., *The Meat We Eat,* Interstate Printers and Publishers, Decatur, Ill., 1966; *21* CFR 182.3041.

Sodium Nitrate, Sodium Nitrite (NaNO₃, NaNO₂) Avoid

No food additive has been more controversial in the past decade than sodium nitrite. And no food additive is more complex in a scientific sense, also. Cancer, poisonings, corporate pressures, and governmental credibility have all been part of the debate.

Sodium nitrite is added to approximately 9 billion pounds of cured meat and fish each year in the United States. In fact, approximately 7 percent of our entire food supply is treated with the agent. Bacon, bologna, ham, hot dogs, salami, liverwurst, Spam, and a multitude of similar foods contain sodium nitrite.

Nitrite serves several purposes. Most obviously, it creates the pinkish color that is characteristic of cured meats. It also contributes to the flavor. Finally, it can inhibit the growth of bacteria that might otherwise cause spoilage.

Nitrate and nitrite are chemically quite similar, just one oxygen atom different. Nitrate, itself, is safe, except for the fact that it slowly converts to nitrite. Nitrite, as discussed later, is the chemical to watch out for. The sodium salts of nitrite and nitrate are most widely used by industry, but occasionally potassium nitrite and nitrate are used. Except for the extra sodium added to the diet by the sodium form of these additives, there is no practical difference between the sodium and potassium versions.

The value of nitrate and nitrite in curing meat was probably discovered accidentally. Legend has it that salt-preserved meat, which is brown, frequently had isolated bright red patches that resembled fresh meat. A little investigating revealed that the red patches were due to nitrate impurities in the salt. From then on merchants intentionally added nitrate to curing solutions to maintain or create an appearance of freshness in meat.

In 1899 scientists discovered that nitrate itself is not the active curing agent, but that it serves as a source of nitrite. Shortly thereafter scientists learned that the nitrite decomposes to nitric oxide, which reacts with the red or brown iron-containing pigments (heme) in muscle and blood. The reaction converts the pigments to stable, bright red or pink compounds, nitrosylmyoglobin and nitrosohemoglobin. Nitrate is rarely used anymore, except in a few dried, cured meats.

For many years the primary concern about nitrite was that large amounts are toxic. Dozens of persons have died from nitrite poisoning and countless others have been incapacitated. This toxicity is due to nitrite's ability to disable hemoglobin, the molecule in red blood cells that transports life-giving oxygen. The nitrite converts hemoglobin to methemoglobin, which cannot carry oxygen. Human blood normally contains about 1 percent methemoglobin and 99 percent normal hemoglobin. However, if nitrite is present and raises the percentage of methemoglobin to above 10 or 20 percent, the blood's ability to carry oxygen is severely impaired. This condition is known as methemoglobinemia. Victims discolor and have difficulty breathing. Death may result when the methemoglobin level exceeds 70 percent.

Infants are much more susceptible to methemoglobinemia than adults. This special sensitivity is due to several interesting factors:

- infant blood contains less hemoglobin than adult blood;
- all hemoglobin is not the same: as much as 60 percent of infant hemoglobin is of a type that is more sensitive to nitrite than adult hemoglobin;
- the fluid intake of infants is ten times that of adults when adjusted for body weight, so nitrate and nitrite in the water supply present special hazards to infants;
- an enzyme that converts methemoglobin back to hemoglobin is in short supply in infants;
- the less acidic environment in the stomach and small intestine of infants favors the multiplication of nitrite-producing bacteria.

All of these factors disappear within the first year of life.

Nitrate and nitrite have caused deaths when people, especially infants, drank contaminated well water in rural areas. The use of nitrogen fertilizer adds to the hazard posed by the natural nitrate content of soil.

Adults occasionally fall victim to nitrite poisoning, because of human carelessness. In one well-publicized incident in 1971, a jar that was supposed to contain Spice of Life Meat Tenderizer was accidentally filled with pure sodium nitrite. A Washington, D.C., man sprinkled the innocent-looking white powder on his dinner and died hours later. Other fatal mishaps have resulted from the substitution of nitrite for table salt in a restaurant's salt shakers and from the overcuring of homemade sausages. Fortunately, these accidents are exceptionally rare.

The nitrite controversy began in earnest in 1969 when scientists discovered that nitrite could react with other chemicals, called secondary amines, in foods to form nitrosamines. Extremely tiny amounts of many different nitrosamines cause cancer in laboratory animals. Nitrosamines are among the most potent causes of cancer yet discovered. When government scientists analyzed cured foods, they discovered significant levels of nitrosamines in cooked sausage, cured pork, dried beef, bacon, and fish. Bacon, because it is so thin and is fried at a high temperature, contained the highest levels of nitrosamines. The nitrite may also form nitrosamines when it encounters secondary amines in the stomach. Secondary amines occur naturally in protein-containing foods and are present in some drugs.

The processed meat industry, which had used nitrate or nitrite for as long as anyone could remember, was severely shaken by the blossoming nitrite controversy. The industry's immediate reaction was to deny that any problem existed. The industry contended that not only was nitrite safe, but that the chemical actually improved the safety of the food supply, because it inhibited the growth of bacteria that could cause botulism. This contention immediately became the focus of the nitrite controversy: even if nitrite and nitrosamines did pose a slight cancer risk, did the benefits outweigh the risks? Meanwhile, processed meat sales slid.

Nitrite *can* prevent the growth of *Clostridium botulinum,* the botulism-causing bacterium, but whether it actually *does* so and is vitally necessary in cured meats is another matter. Actual meat industry practices suggest that the risk of botulism is smaller than industry spokespersons would lead one to believe. For instance, nitrite-free brands of certain foods, such as chicken bologna, are available and placed right next to nitrite-containing counterparts in supermarket display cases. Some companies produce frozen, nitrite-free bacon and frankfurters; the freezing prevents any bacterial growth. Some food stores did offer refrigerated nitrite-free bacon and discovered that putrefactive (smell-producing) bacteria rendered the product inedible long before botulism posed a threat.

I believe that the meat industry exaggerates the deadly specter of botulism in order to continue to take advantage of the coloring and flavoring properties of nitrite. The industry fears that people would buy less processed meat if it tasted and looked just a little bit different.

As the debate over nitrite progressed, the plot thickened when scientists discovered that most of the nitrite in the body is actually produced from naturally occurring nitrate found in certain vegetables, especially celery, beets, radishes, and leafy vegetables. Now the meat industry argued that only a small percentage, perhaps less than 10 percent, of the nitrite we are exposed to comes from nitrite intentionally added to processed foods. Of course, while the nitrite in vegetables is largely unavoidable (though changes in farming practices might reduce levels somewhat), it would be simple to stop adding *extra* nitrite to our diet. Furthermore, it is unclear whether the nitrite that derives from produce actually forms nitrosamines in the body, whereas it is certain that cooking causes nitrosamines to form in bacon and other processed foods.

Citizens groups, including Center for Science in the Public Interest and Ralph Nader's Center for Study of Responsive Law (you are forgiven if you can't keep these unwieldy names straight in your mind!), petitioned the U.S. Department of Agriculture in 1972 to ban unnecessary uses of sodium nitrite and to establish an expert committee to determine whether nitrite was really necessary and irreplaceable. USDA—under the directorship of Nixon-appointee Earl Butz—ignored the petition for a while, but the growing controversy forced the agency to appoint an advisory committee in 1973 to investigate the problem. Initially, the advisory committee was stacked in favor of industry, but four years later, when the Carter Administration came into office, a new Secretary of Agriculture added several new members, including the author. The committee's ultimate advice was pretty weak, emphasizing the need for research, for restricting excessive levels that were found in some foods, and for developing ways of reducing the formation of nitrosamines, either by using a completely different additive or by adding chemicals—such as vitamin C—that inhibit nitrosamine formation.

Nitrite hit the front page of the news on August 11, 1978, when the Department of Health and Human Services and the Department of Agriculture revealed new research findings. The research indicated that nitrite itself—not the nitrosamines—causes cancer of the lymph system in rats. A joint announcement from the two departments stated:

> . . . the use of nitrite as a deliberate additive to food may pose a hazard to human health. However, nitrite also protects against the formation of botulinum toxin, a deadly food poison. We thus are presented with a difficult *balance* of *risks* . . . In the past we have moved without hesitation to ban outright a number of food additives when they pose a hazard to human health . . . In this case the need to balance two kinds of health risks—one by taking nitrite out of food and the other by leaving it in—creates a difficult challenge.

Because of the tenuousness of the one study and the billions of dollars involved, FDA contracted with an independent team of cancer specialists to review the new study, microscope slide by microscope slide, animal by animal. After many months, the committee concluded that the original investigator, Prof. Paul Newberne, a highly respected scientist at M.I.T., misjudged numerous tissue samples, calling them cancerous when, in fact, they were not. The government canceled any intention to ban nitrite and suffered a great deal of embarrassment. Nevertheless, FDA Commissioner Jere Goyan stated that, "nitrites are not home free by any means. There are still questions, and I'm sure they will eventually be phased out of the food supply because of the nitrosamine problem."

Though the M.I.T. animal study was invalidated, researchers continued to investigate the possibility that nitrite is causing human cancer. In 1983, Professor Philip Hartman, of the Johns Hopkins University, compared the amount of nitrite various population groups consumed with their incidence of stomach cancer. He discovered a striking correlation between nitrite intake and cancer. The Japanese consume quite large amounts of nitrite and have the world's highest incidence of stomach cancer. By contrast, in the U.S., the rate of stomach cancer has declined steadily for more than 50 years. Hartman dredged up old figures on nitrite and nitrate intake and found that Americans are eating less and less of the questionable compounds. This research provides interesting evidence, but not proof, that nitrite has been causing human cancer deaths.

The great nitrite debates ultimately yielded real benefits for the public. Nitrite is now listed on the label of every food in which it is used: this was not the case before 1973. Companies are using less nitrite: the legal limit in bacon was lowered from 200 to 120 parts per million (ppm), and the amount and frequency of nitrosamine contamination decreased significantly. Recently, the American Meat Institute has urged, and in 1985 USDA has proposed, that the limit be reduced to 100 ppm. Also, the Department of Agriculture requires that ascorbic acid (vitamin C) or similar chemical be added to cured meats to reduce nitrosamine formation. Finally, nitrite-free meats are somewhat more available than they had been.

The ideal solution to the nitrite problem would be a chemical that served all the functions that nitrite does—coloring, flavoring, preservative—but is completely safe. Second best would be a replacement for nitrite's preservative function, using other additives for coloring and flavoring. Salt is an effective preservative, but it, unfortunately, promotes high blood pressure. Cured meats already contain too much sodium.

In 1984 USDA-sponsored studies proved that a solution might be near at hand. The Food Research Institute at Madison, Wisconsin, developed a commercially feasible method for producing bacon with little or no nitrite. The clever process involves injecting bacon with sugar and harmless bacteria. If the bacon is left at room temperature, the bacteria begin to multiply and gradually release lactic acid. The acid prevents any botulinal bacteria that may be present from growing. According to USDA, without any nitrite, the process provides "botulinal protection . . . equal to that of control bacon." When the lab tested bacon with 40 ppm nitrite, "the antibotulinal protection . . . was far superior to that of control bacon." The flavor was claimed to be as good or better than normally produced bacon (120 ppm), but the bacon did not look quite as attractive. Low-nitrite bacon should be available in late 1985 or 1986.

After a decade of controversy, of hearing first that nitrite is dangerous, then that it is safe, then that it really is dangerous, many consumers are still trying to answer the original question: "Is it safe to eat nitrite-containing foods?" I believe that nitrite-treated meats are problems in two regards: they increase slightly the risk of cancer, and they are generally loaded with saturated fat and salt. For these two reasons, I suggest that you eat salami, bologna, hot dogs, and especially bacon rarely or not at all.

Ref.: Hearings, House Comm. on Gov. Oper., (March 1971); *J. Nat. Can. Inst. 48*, 1687 (1972); *Meat Curing Principles and Modern Practice*, Koch Supplies, Inc., Kansas City, Mo. (1973); *Fed. Reg. 42*, 44376 (Sept. 2, 1977), *43*, 20992 (May 16, 1978), *45*, 43447 (1980), *50*, 14711 (1985); "Final Report on Nitrites and Nitrosamines," Expert Panel on Nitrites and Nitrosamines, U.S. Dept. of Agric. (Feb. 1978); U.S. Department of Health and Human Services press releases, Aug.

11, 1978, Aug. 19, 1980; *Science 200,* 1487 (1978), *209,* 1100 (1980); GAO Report HRD-80-46, Jan. 31, 1980; "The Health Effects of Nitrate, Nitrite, and *N*-Nitroso Compounds," Nat. Acad. Sci. (1981); *Environ. Mutagen.* 5 (1) (1983); *Lancet i,* 629 (1983); USDA Memo by R. W. Johnston (June 21, 1984); *21* CFR 172.160–172.177, 181.33–181.34; *9* CFR 318.7, 381.147.

Sorbic Acid, Potassium Sorbate   Safe

Food manufacturers have been using sorbic acid and potassium sorbate since the 1950s to prevent the growth of molds and fungi. You will find it added to cheese, syrup, jelly, cake, mayonnaise, soft drinks, wine, dried fruits, margarine, and canned frosting at levels up to 0.3 percent. Much higher levels are sometimes used in soft candy. Sorbic acid occurs naturally in some plants and was first isolated in 1859 from the berries of the mountain ash tree.

Sorbic acid is an effective preservative over a broad range of acidities (up to pH 6.5) and therefore more appropriate in many foods than sodium benzoate, which is effective only in quite acidic foods. Moreover, the human body treats this virtually odorless, tasteless additive as a food instead of as an unwanted foreign chemical. Sorbic acid cannot be used in foods that are pasteurized, because it breaks down at high temperatures.

The sorbates are potent inhibitors of mold and fungi, but only marginally effective against bacteria. This specificity makes them perfect for use in cheeses, because the fermentative action of bacteria may proceed while mold growth is prevented.

Sorbic acid is chemically similar to fat (caproic acid, to be specific) and is metabolized by the body just as if it were a natural fat. Thus, our bodies use it as a food and source of energy. Sorbic acid can also be metabolized by microorganisms when there is a small quantity of sorbic acid and a large number of microbes. However, when a small number of microbes is confronted with a relatively massive amount of sorbic acid—as is the case in treated foods—one or more of the microbes' enzymes is inhibited and growth stops. A few strains of mold are resistant to even high concentrations of sorbic acid, and these strains may contaminate treated foods.

Experiments on rats and mice have shown that sorbic acid does not cause cancer or birth defects. In a lifetime feeding study conducted by German scientists, rats suffered no ill effects when their food contained 5 percent sorbic acid. In fact, the male rats even enjoyed a 15 percent increase in their life span, which was possibly due to the chemical having prevented the growth of germs.

Hints that potassium sorbate might not be totally benign came in the mid-1970s. Food scientists had suggested that adding this chemical to processed meat might allow the use of lower levels of the cancer-promoting preservative sodium nitrite. One problem was quickly detected when people tasted samples of the sorbate-treated meat. It had chemical-like flavors and an unusual smell and also caused marked prickly mouth sensations, characteristics that would not boost sales. Other scientists discovered that nitrite and sorbate could react to form mutagenic compounds, though vitamin C, which is generally added to cured meat, could prevent this reaction. These unexpected problems dashed the hopes of sorbate manufacturers that their product would be added to billions of pounds of processed meats each year.

Ref.: Arzneimittel-forschung 10, 997 (1962); FASEB Report No. 57 (1975); *Fd. Cosmet. Toxicol. 13,* 31 (1975); Hartman, P. in *Environ. Mut. 5* (2) (1983); *21* CFR 182.3089, 182.3225, 182.3640, 182.3795.

Sorbitan Monostearate   Safe

Sorbitan monostearate serves as an emulsifier in cakes, cake icing, whipped vegetable oil toppings, frozen pudding, coconut spread, and many other foods. It is used at levels up to 1 percent, often in combination with one of the polysorbate emulsifiers.

Judging from several studies, sorbitan monostearate is safe. In chronic feeding studies conducted by FDA, rats and dogs were not harmed by a diet containing 5 percent sorbitan monostearate. In a study conducted by a private testing laboratory, four generations of rats ate food containing 20 percent sorbitan monostearate; their growth, reproduction, lactation, metabolism, behavior, mortality, and tissues appeared normal. Although this additive is composed of two chemicals (stearic acid and sorbitol) that the body can ordinarily use as sources of energy, it is less nutritious, because the body absorbs only 50 to 75 percent of it from the intestine.

Persons suffering from certain diseases use sorbitan monostearate to help their bodies absorb fat from food.

Ref.: FAO (35)-107; *J. Nutr. 61,* 235 (1957); *Tox. Appl. Pharm. 1,* 315 (1959); CUFP-26; CRC-442; *21* CFR 172.842.

Sorbitol   Safe

Sorbitol is a close relative of the sugars and mannitol and, like them, has a pleasant sweet taste. It is about 60 percent as sweet as sugar. One manufacturer claims that "sorbitol is one of the 'miracle' products of modern chemistry— long known as a nutritive ingredient of many fruits, berries, and plants." If not exactly a "miracle," sorbitol does serve an interesting variety of purposes.

After we ingest it, sorbitol is absorbed into the bloodstream and converted to sugar, thereby providing calories. But because sorbitol is absorbed slowly and incompletely, blood sugar levels rise only slightly. This feature made sorbitol useful in the treatment of diabetes prior to the use of insulin. Foods sweetened with sorbitol instead of sugar provided diabetics with a relatively safe source of sweetness and energy and allowed them to decrease their intake of fats.

Chewing gums and candy sweetened by sorbitol do not promote tooth decay, because bacteria in the mouth metabolize sorbitol slowly or not at all. (Tooth decay is caused by acid produced by bacteria in the mouth.)

Soft, sugar-based candy retains its "as made" firmness and chewing properties when it is "doctored" with 1 to 3 percent sorbitol; also shelf life is extended because the sorbitol inhibits the crystallization of sugar. In shredded coconut and other foods sorbitol acts as a sweetener and helps maintain the proper moisture levels.

Moderately large amounts of sorbitol have a laxative effect, and as more foods are made with this sweetener, diarrhea may replace constipation as Americans' main gastrointestinal malady. One report in the *Journal of the American Medical Association* described a case of diarrhea in a twenty-nine-year-old man who consumed 50–55 grams (about two ounces) of sorbitol per day by eating two packs of dietetic gum, two rolls of dietetic mints, two dietetic candy bars, and two dietetic wafers. In a study on two-to-three-year-old children, one package of dietetic mints, containing 9.3 grams (one-third ounce) of sorbitol, caused diarrhea.

The Food and Drug Administration requires label warnings on foods that might provide 50 grams or more (about 1¾ ounces) of sorbitol in a day. The label notice reads: "Excess consumption may have a laxative effect." Of course, you may get 50 grams of sorbitol from two different foods, neither of which would have that notice. Something to ponder while you sit on the john.

Other than having a mild laxative effect, sorbitol is safe.

Ref.: FAO (35)-96; CRC-Ch. 11; *Physiol. Rev. 42,* 181 (1962); Atlas Chemical Ind. Bulletin "Atlas Products for the Food and Beverage Industry"; *Treatment of Diabetes Mellitis,* Joslin, E. P., Lea and Fabiger, Philadelphia, Pa. (1959); *J. Am. Med. Asso. 244,* 270 (1980); *21* CFR 184.1835.

Stannous Chloride   Safe

Food manufacturers sometimes use stannous chloride (tin chloride) as an antioxidant in soft drinks (15 ppm) and bottled asparagus (20 ppm). Stannous chloride reacts readily with oxygen, thereby preventing the oxygen from combining with chemicals in food and causing discoloration and offensive odors.

Food additives contribute relatively little to our daily intake of tin. Toothpaste containing stannous fluoride and canned goods are more important sources. (The FAO/WHO committee on food additives recommends that food not be stored in opened tin-coated cans.)

Studies on the biological effects of tin are progressing from two directions. Toxicologists are seeking to determine whether chronic ingestion of tin compounds has any adverse effects. They have found that stannous chloride and other tin compounds are poorly absorbed by the body and do not accumulate to any great extent. Thus, tin appears to be harmless.

On the other hand, nutritionists are interested in learning whether tin is a necessary ingredient in our diet. In an experiment reported in 1970, one group of rats ate food which contained all the known essential nutrients and trace elements, but from which tin was rigidly excluded. Another group of rats ate the same food plus a dose of tin. The rats whose diet contained tin grew significantly faster than those deprived of tin. This result means that small amounts of tin may be essential for normal growth.

Ref.: FAO (26)-32; FAO (43)-16; *Fd. Cos. Tox. 3*, 271, 277 (1965); *J. Nutr. 96*, 37 (1968); *Bio. Bio. Res. Comm. 40*, 22 (1970); L. Friberg et al., ed., *Handbook on the Toxicology of Metals*, Elsevier, (1979). *21* CFR 172.180, 184.1845.

Starch   Safe

Starch is the major component of wheat flour, potatoes, and corn and is normally thought of as a food, not a food additive. However, because starch can absorb large amounts of water, manufacturers and individuals use it to thicken soup, gravy, and other foods.

Ref.: *21* CFR 184.1847.

Starch, Modified   ?

Natural starch is an effective, wholesome, and inexpensive thickening agent, but it has several technical limitations. It does not dissolve in cold water, solutions are not stable in the presence of acids, and it separates from water on standing. Food technologists have found that these and other limitations can be overcome by treating starch (usually cornstarch, less often potato starch) with any of a variety of chemicals.

Treating starch lightly with an oxidizing agent (oxygen, chlorine, potassium permanganate) bleaches the colored impurities (xanthophylls), but does not affect any other physical properties. Manufacturers add the ultra-white product to confectioners sugar and baking powder to absorb moisture and prevent caking.

Treating starch with acid (hydrochloric or sulfuric) or alkali (sodium hydroxide) breaks the large starch molecules into smaller pieces. The pieces, called dextrin, are a normal component of the diet and perfectly safe. Dextrin solutions are much thinner than solutions containing an equal weight of untreated starch. (See separate discussion of dextrin.)

Amylose

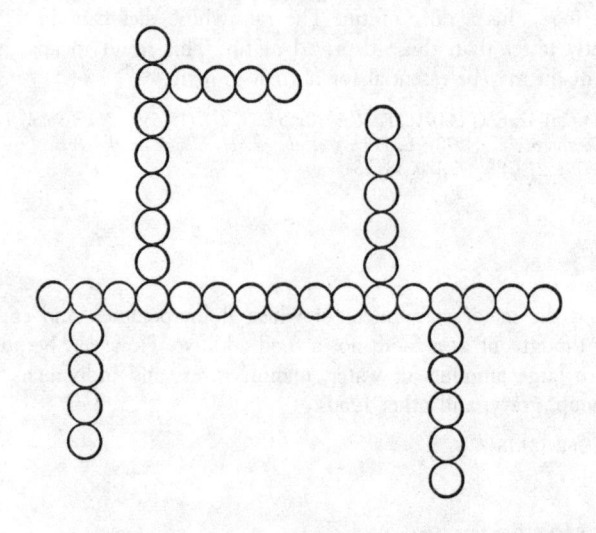

Amylopectin

Other kinds of modification make greater changes in the physical and chemical properties of starch. To understand these modifications and their effects, we must first examine the chemical structure of starch. Starch molecules are long, thin chains composed of hundreds or thousands of glucose (a sugar) molecules linked end to end like the cars in a long train. Linear chains are called amylose, branched chains amylopectin.

In one class of modified starches, chemicals are used to tie chains together (whether the chains are linear or branched is irrelevant). These are called cross-linked starches.

A very small number of bridges (one per 500 to 1,000 glucose units) stabilizes starch solutions against the effects of acids and strong agitation. Cross-linking increases the thickening ability of starch, thereby decreasing the amount needed in a food. In 1978 a government advisory committee expressed concern about certain cross-linked starches, because the cross-linking agent, epichlorohydrin, can cause mutations and possibly cancer. The Special Com-

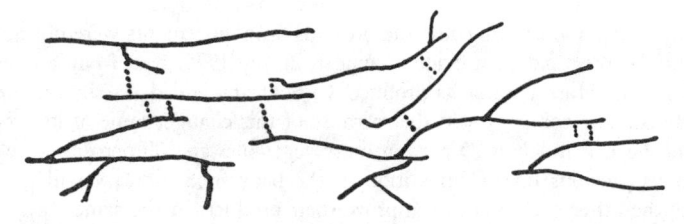

Cross-linked starch

mittee on GRAS Substances stated, ". . . it would be prudent to discontinue use of such cross-linked starches in foods until animal feeding experiments with graded levels of epichlorohydrin have been carried out." The food industry complied with this recommendation.

Starch can also be modified by the addition of chemical side chains. A representation of a molecule of derivatized starch is shown in the following figure:

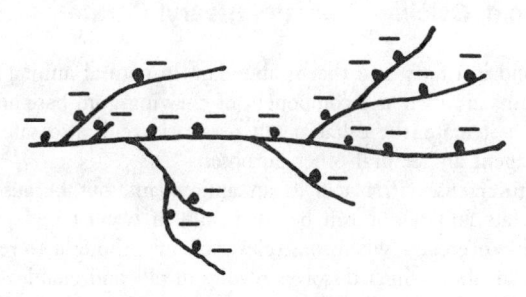

Derivatized starch

Side chains that carry a negative electrical charge, such as acetate, succinate, or phosphate, cause starch molecules to repel one another. The repulsion prevents molecules from clumping together or crystallizing, which normally causes starch to separate out of solution or to gel. Solutions of derivatized starch have increased viscosity and clarity. You are most likely to encounter derivatized starch in frozen foods, in which they serve as thickening agents.

Baby food manufacturers have traditionally used modified starches to improve the consistency of their bottled products. The starches comprise as much as 6 percent of the entire product, replacing nutritious fruit, meat, or vegetable in the process. For many years, companies maintained that it was impossible to produce baby foods with chemically modified starches; and normal starch, they said, would coagulate and form a starch product "plug" that is unusable by the consumer. Demonstrating that the previous pronouncements were not quite as definite as they had been made to appear, in mid-1985, Beech-Nut announced that it was reformulating its products without any added starches, natural or modified. The company said that because of this change, some of its products would have as much as 25 percent more vegetables and 50 percent more meat than its previous line. Competition in the baby food industry will probably force the other companies to improve their products in the same way.

Any treatment that adds side chains to or cross-links starch molecules could introduce a hazard and, therefore, modified starches should be evaluated in appropriate scientific studies. Most modified starches have been studied only in ninety-day experiments, rather than in lifetime feeding studies.

Ref.: FAO (26)-29; FAO (46), (46A), (599); *ECT 18,* 685; CRC-Ch. 9; Whistler, R. L., and Paschall, E. F., *Starch: Chemistry and Technology, Vol. 2,* Academic Press, New York (1967); NAS-NRC Report, "Safety and Suitability of Modified Starches for Use in Baby Foods" (September 1970); *Fd. Cosmetic Toxicol. 12,* 201 (1974); FASEB-SCOGS, "Evaluation of the Health Aspects of Starch and Modified Starches as Food Ingredients," (1980); *21* CFR 172.892.

Stearic Acid, Calcium Stearate, Stearyl Citrate   Safe

Stearic acid is a fatty acid that is abundant in natural animal fat. It is safe. Small amounts are used as a component of chewing gum base and as a flavoring. Calcium stearate, the calcium salt of stearic acid, also safe, serves as an anticaking agent and several other purposes.

Manufacturers use citric acid as an antioxidant, but because it does not dissolve in fats and oils it can be used only in water-based products. This limitation was overcome when some clever chemist thought to react citric acid with stearyl alcohol, which dissolves readily in oils and enables citrate to dissolve in oil. The compound that forms, stearyl citrate protects oils by trapping metal ions that might otherwise catalyze oxidative reactions and cause rancidity. Stearyl citrate is used in margarine (up to 0.15 percent).

Stearyl citrate was last tested on animals over twenty years ago. Lifetime feeding studies, which encompassed four generations of rats, showed that diets containing up to 10 percent of the additive did not affect growth, tumor incidence, health, or reproduction. The body converts stearyl citrate to citrate and stearyl alcohol, which are digestible and harmless.

Ref.: FAO (31)-51; FAO (40A)-54; FAO (46A)-112; *Food Res. 16,* 258, 294 (1951); *Fed. Reg. 48,* 4486, 52444 (Feb. 1; Nov. 18, 1983); *21* CFR 182.6851, 184.1090, 184.1229.

Succistearin   Safe

Succistearin is an emulsifier used to a limited extent in shortening to help make baked goods more tender. The full, mind-boggling name of this food additive is stearoyl propylene glycol hydrogen succinate.

Biochemists have shown that succistearin is metabolized well by rats (and presumably humans). The body converts the additive to succinic acid, stearic acid, and propylene glycol, all of which may be used as sources of energy.

Ref.: Tox. Appl. Pharm. 17, 519 (1970); *21* CFR 172.765.

Sucrose   Moderate amounts: Safe
                                             Large amounts: Avoid

Sucrose, ordinary table sugar, is the most widely distributed sugar and is present in all plants. Sugar cane, the tropical plant that supplies two thirds of our sugar, grows in many parts of the world, but it originated in northeastern India. Traders carried it westward to Egypt and eastward to China about fifteen hundred years ago. A thousand years later, in 1494, Christopher Columbus brought the valuable plant to the West Indies. Other sources of sugar are sugar beets, maple trees, honey, sorghum, pineapple and other ripe fruits.

Americans consume enormous amounts of sugar—approximately 75 pounds of sucrose per person per year, plus another 50 pounds of corn syrup and other refined sugars. The sugar we get from soft drinks, cakes and cookies, preserves, presweetened breakfast cereals, desserts, and the sugar bowl contributes greatly to this nation's incredible toll of tooth decay and, presumably (the evidence is limited), diabetes and obesity. (Americans spend about $6 billion a year repairing decayed teeth.) Some breakfast "cereals" are more than 50 percent sugar, and a few baby food desserts derive 20–45 percent of their calories from added sugar. Of the average diet 10 to 20 percent is refined sugar.

Pure, white, granulated sugar, unfortunately, is as pure as its makers claim. The refining process removes every last trace of vitamins, minerals, and protein. Sugar that has been extracted from cane but not yet refined is called raw sugar. It contains minuscule amounts of trace minerals in addition to the sucrose, but it still makes you fat and rots your teeth.

There is no denying that sugar and sweetened foods taste good and supply energy. However, Americans have gone overboard in their affection for sugar. Except for those who enjoy large dentist bills and large girths, most of us should decrease our consumption of sugar.

For further information, please refer to the discussion of sugar in the *Nutrition Scoreboard* section of this book (page 41).

Ref.: Sugars in Nutrition, Sipple, H. L. and K. W. McNutt, Academic Press, New York (1974); *Consumer Reports,* p. 136 (March 1978).

Sucrose Polyester (SPE)   Safe

Not only will we be wearing polyester, we may soon be eating it. Chemists have discovered that they can make a substance that looks, smells, and tastes like ordinary cooking oil, but is not absorbed by the body. The substance can be used to make salad dressings, milk shakes, baked goods, and margarine that are remarkably low in calories. For instance, the calorie count of a milk shake can be reduced from 235 to 95. The miracle chemical is called sucrose polyester. It is made by reacting sucrose (table sugar) with fatty acids.

So far, the FDA has approved sucrose polyester, or SPE to the in-crowd, for use as a protective coating on fruit. But as food technologists, toxicologists, and advertising agencies understand SPE better, you can be sure that food manufacturers will be asking FDA for permission to use it in a variety of diet foods.

Dr. Charles Glueck, of the University of Cincinnati, has been testing SPE as a weight-loss aid on obese patients with remarkable results. Though they had free access to between-meal snacks, Glueck's patients lost an average of 0.4 pounds per day. They also enjoyed 10 percent lower cholesterol levels.

So far, SPE appears safe, though its effect on the availability of fat-soluble vitamins will have to be monitored carefully.

Ref.: Am. J. Clin. Nutr. 35, 1352 (1982); *Fed. Reg. 47,* 55475 (Dec. 10, 1982); *21* CFR 172.859.

Sulfiting Agents   Asthmatics: **Avoid**
                                                                               Others: **?**
Sulfur dioxide (SO_2), potassium metabisulfite ($K_2S_2O_5$), sodium bisulfite ($NaHSO_3$), sodium metabisulfite ($Na_2S_2O_5$), sodium sulfite (Na_2SO_3)

On October 17, 1982, James Sapanaro and his family were eating at a restaurant at the racetrack in Phoenix, Arizona. The thirty-year-old man was eating a salad, when he experienced a tremendous difficulty breathing. He died within minutes.

On November 10, 1982, Gideon Lawhon had a medical checkup and then, celebrating his doctor's verdict, went with his family for lunch at a local Tempe, Arizona, restaurant. After eating the meal, and while waiting for the check, Lawhon turned red in the face, had difficulty breathing, and collapsed on the floor. An ambulance was called, and the paramedic on the scene injected Lawhon with epinephrine and dopamine to help him breathe. The fifty-three-year-old man died shortly after being admitted to the hospital.

In March 1983, Jo Valone, of Garden Grove, California, went with her husband to eat at a local restaurant. She asked the waitress if any of the foods contained a preservative and was assured that they did not. She went into a three-week-long coma after eating the potatoes. It turned out that the supply house which provided the potatoes used a preservative, but did not tell the restaurant.

On August 5, 1984, Susan Trapnell and her husband went for brunch at a cafeteria at the Naval Air Base in Corpus Christi, Texas. Shortly after eating salads containing cherries and apples, Susan Trapnell began gagging and lapsed into a coma for five days. She died at the hospital.

On September 11, 1984, Murray Lertzman was eating processed potatoes at a restaurant in Tarzana, California. He felt difficulty breathing and rushed out to his car to use an inhalator. He died before he could use it.

On February 20, 1985, 10-year-old Medaya McPike was eating with her family at a Mexican restaurant in Salem, Oregon. After downing a good-sized portion of guacamole, she had trouble breathing. Her parents rushed her to the hospital, but she died within hours.

All six victims were asthmatics. They did not know that they were among the 5 to 10 percent of asthmatics who are sensitive to a group of food and drug preservatives called sulfiting agents. Fortunate ones have mild asthmatic attacks and recover quickly, especially if they use a breath-assisting inhalator. Unfortunate ones have near-fatal or, like little Medaya McPike, fatal reactions. Subsequent tests indicated that all the restaurants at which the victims had their fateful meals used sulfiting agents. The "lifesaving" drugs administered to Lawhon on the way to the hospital also contained sulfiting agents and probably contributed to his death.

How many other people have been killed by sulfiting agents is unknown. I suspect that the list of victims runs into the dozens, if not hundreds, with other deaths mistakenly classified as choking or "unknown cause."

Sulfites have a long history of use, dating back, by some accounts, thousands of years. Food processors treat foods and beverages with these sulfur-containing agents to prevent discoloration and inhibit the growth of bacteria. Sulfiting agents are often used to prevent discoloration, bacterial growth, and fermentation in wine; to control "black spot" in freshly caught shrimp; to prevent discoloration of lettuce, potatoes, and other vegetables at restaurants; to prevent darkening of dried apricots, raisins, and other dried fruit; to strengthen baking dough; and to prevent bacterial growth in some drugs. Maraschino cherries are bleached with this additive before they are dyed red or green.

Sulfur dioxide is a gas or, below 20 degrees centigrade, a liquid. The other sulfiting agents, such as potassium metabisulfite, sodium sulfite, sodium bisulfite, and sodium metabisulfite, are solids. When added to food or dissolved in water, they all lead to the formation of bisulfite (HSO_3^-), which is the active component.

Bisulfite is a very reactive chemical, a property that defines its uses and its dangers. Bisulfite protects foods from discoloration by combining with sugars and other chemicals (aldehydes and ketones), as well as with enzymes and oxygen. In the absence of bisulfite, sugars tend to react with other chemicals to form colored compounds, while enzymes catalyze reactions that also generate colored compounds.

Bisulfite destroys vitamin B_1 (thiamin) and therefore has been banned from foods rich in this vitamin. However, the FDA never enforced this section of the law with any vigor. Potatoes and salads, which do contain significant amounts of thiamin, have often been treated with sulfiting agents.

Unscrupulous butchers can use bisulfite to restore a "fresh-red" color to old or spoiled meat, a practice that is specifically prohibited by law. Once in a great while, though, government inspectors catch someone using this old trick.

The reaction that many asthmatics and occasional nonasthmatics have is the clearest indication that these additives are not benign. Nonfatal reactions include weakness, tightness in the chest, shortness of breath, hives, severe wheezing, and loss of consciousness. That bisulfite could cause acute reactions was first recognized in 1976. Drs. Bruce Prenner and John Stevens, both allergists at the University of California, San Diego, School of Medicine, had a fifty-year-old male patient who "experienced a systemic allergic reaction minutes after eating lunch in a local restaurant." The unfortunate restaurant-goer developed hives, swelling of his tongue, and a tightness in his chest, and had difficulty breathing. The allergists traced his troubles to a salad that had been treated with sodium bisulfite. Prenner and Stevens urged "more complete labeling of the contents of food products, including all their chemical additives."

Doctors Ronald Simon and Donald Stevenson at the Scripps Clinic and Research Foundation in La Jolla, California, have done the most extensive work on the sensitivity of asthmatics to bisulfite. In July 1981, they described five patients who were highly sensitive to bisulfites. The reactions usually occurred after eating certain restaurant foods or, less often, wine. On the basis of their research, these doctors wrote that "it seems very likely that metabisulfite sensitivity is not as rare as one might initially conclude." Based on their routine screening of asthmatics, they calculated that upward of half a million of the nation's 8.9 million asthmatics are sensitive to sulfiting agents.

Carolyn Knight, one of Dr. Simon's patients, describes vividly the problems that sulfiting agents can cause:

> I have had nine life-threatening bouts with anaphylactic shock and have endured the daily heartache of chronic asthma for more than ten years. Besides living with the day-to-day shortness of breath which deprives me of leading a normally active

life, I live with the fear that I will accidentally encounter the substance that can, within ten minutes, snuff out my life if I do not receive immediate help.

Besides the effect on asthmatics, there are other reasons why we should not add sulfiting agents to food. First, they can cause genetic mutations in microorganisms, though they have not yet been shown to cause mutations in mammals. Second, in a study on rats, sulfur dioxide interacted with another chemical to increase the incidence of tumors. Among fifteen rats exposed to sulfur dioxide, no tumors occurred; only one tumor occurred in another group of rats exposed to benzopyrene. However, nine tumors developed in forty-six rats that were exposed to both substances.

Dr. Simon's most sensitive patient reacted to as little as one milligram of sulfur dioxide. Using that level as a benchmark, consider the amounts that may be present in various foods: green salad: 160 milligrams; three ounces of dried apricots: 175 milligrams; four-ounce glass of wine: 40 milligrams. The World Health Organization has recommended that human exposure be limited to 0.7 milligrams of sulfite per kilogram of body weight per day. That translates into 42 milligrams for a 132-pound person. The FDA has estimated that up to half of the U.S. population could be exceeding that level.

The least controlled uses of sulfiting agents are on shrimp boats and in restaurants. Dangerously large amounts can easily be applied by an inexperienced employee. Since restaurants are simply using the chemicals to deceive customers into thinking that slightly aged lettuce and other foods are really fresh, this use should be the very first one banned. Food processors that sell food to restaurants should also be prohibited from using sulfiting agents. Shrimpers, too, can use the additive to mask spoilage and should not be allowed to use it. Sulfiting agents should either be sharply restricted in, or banned entirely from, wine and dried fruits, two other major sources.

In July 1982, the Food and Drug Administration, oblivious to the evidence that sulfiting agents cause hypersensitivity reactions in hundreds of thousands of consumers, proposed that they be declared "generally recognized as safe" (GRAS). The following October, the Center for Science in the Public Interest, along with Dr. Simon, Arizona State University food scientist Woodrow Monte, and several sulfite victims, formally petitioned FDA to ban or severely curtail the use of the additives. If they ever are used, the petitioners urged that they be clearly labeled.

Two years later, the FDA was still suffering from a severe case of bureaucratic inertia and had done essentially nothing but appoint an unnecessary committee to examine the studies and urge restaurants that use sulfites to post signs to that effect. FDA had taken no regulatory action that would lead to a phaseout of sulfites from restaurant food, packaged foods, shrimp, or wine. However the National Restaurant Association urged its members not to use sulfiting agents and informed allergists of the possibility of sulfite reactions in restaurants. Also, the Bureau of Alcohol, Tobacco and Firearms (BATF) has proposed that sulfite levels in wine be reduced from 350 ppm to between 125 and 175 parts per million for dry wines and 275 parts per million for sweeter wines.

In early 1985, the logjam began to break, spurred by the tragic death of Medaya McPike. Senator Albert Gore, Jr. (Democrat, Tennessee) and Representative Ron Wyden (Democrat, Oregon) sponsored legislation to ban restaurant uses of sulfites. In March, Representative John Dingell, chairman of the House Committee on Energy and Commerce, presided over a dramatic hearing that exposed FDA's ineffectiveness and BATF's ineptness. FDA Commissioner Frank Young admitted that his agency's failure to act resulted in unnecessary deaths. Dingell discovered that the limited steps that the safety agency had initially proposed—requiring warning labels on drugs and ingredient labeling on foods—were rejected by the Secretary of Health and Human Services and the White House. But just days after the hearing, FDA's superiors relented and allowed FDA to propose a rule that would require foods containing any detectable level of sulfites to be labeled. BATF proposed a similar rule for alcoholic beverages. (Proposing and actually adopting a rule are two different things; at the very least, adoption takes many months, if it occurs at all.) FDA again began exploring the possibility of banning restaurant uses of the preservative. And, moving more quickly than federal agencies, California, Washington, Chicago, and other local governments either banned the use of sulfites by restaurants or required warning signs when sulfites were added in foods.

Sulfiting agents are the only food additives now in use that have caused known human deaths. Asthmatics and any others who have reason to believe they are sensitive should avoid sulfites.

Ref.: Sulfur Dioxide, L. Schroeter, Pergamon, New York (1966); *Ann. Allergy 37,* 180 (1976); *Mutat. Res. 39,* 149 (1977); *J. Allergy Clin. Immunol. 68,* 26 (1981); *Food Cosmet. Toxicol. 19,* 667 (1981); *Fed. Reg. 47,* 29956 (July 9, 1982), *49,* 44217 (1984); CSPI petition to FDA (Oct. 28, 1982); *Food Chem. News,* p. 4 (March 21, 1983); *Hearing,* House Committee on Energy and Commerce, Subcommittee on Oversight and Investigations, March 27, 1985; *21* CFR 182.3616, 182.3637, 182.3739, 182.3766, 182.3798, 182.3862.

Sulfur Dioxide—see Sulfiting Agents

Tannin, Tannic Acid   ?

Tannin, or tannic acid as it is also called, is a mixture of chemicals obtained from the bark, leaves, and galls of a wide variety of shrubs and trees. We ingest significant amounts of tannin (100 to 500 milligrams) with every cup of tea, coffee, and cocoa that we drink. The name tannin is derived from the traditional and major use of this substance, the tanning of leather.

Food manufacturers take advantage of tannin's taste and chemical properties. They use tannin as a flavoring in baked goods, alcoholic beverages, frozen dairy desserts, and candies, as well as an ingredient in butter, caramel, fruit, brandy, maple, and nut artificial flavorings. They employ tannin's ability to form insoluble complexes with proteins and other substances to remove undesired material from beer, wine, and oils. After tannin is added to these products, the tannin-protein complexes are filtered out.

In the 1930s doctors used tannin as a burn ointment. They sprayed it over the burnt area, where it formed an artificial scab that alleviated the pain and enhanced the healing process. This treatment was discontinued when physicians discovered that tannin sometimes entered the bloodstream and damaged the liver.

The most serious concern about tannin comes not from its rather meager use as a food additive, but from its presence in tea. Several studies have shown that injecting tannin under the skin of rats and mice caused tumors to develop at both the site of injection and in the liver. The injection-site tumors are not considered significant, but the liver tumors justify concern.

The evidence from human studies is shaky, but interesting. "Esophageal cancer is one of the most pitiful and hopeless of human afflictions . . ." is the first sentence of Julia Morton's fascinating account of the evidence linking human esophageal cancer with tannin. Morton, a botanist at the University of Miami, began her fieldwork by identifying popular folk remedies in the Netherlands Antilles, where esophageal cancer was relatively widespread. She identified twenty-two plant species that were frequently consumed as teas by cancer victims. The National Cancer Institute injected preparations made from those plants into rats and found that three caused cancer at the injection site in 100 percent of the animals. Morton discovered that tannin is present not only in those plants, but also in the betel nut—which has been linked to oral and esophageal cancer in Asia and Africa.

Once Morton had evidence that tannin was the culprit, she switched her thread of inquiry from folk remedies to products containing tannin. This thread led to:

- Honan, China, where the incidence of esophageal cancer is the highest in the world . . . and where a tannin-rich sorghum is used extensively in food and wine;
- Western Kenya, where a sorghum-using tribe has a high incidence of esophageal cancer;
- Holland, where esophageal cancer was common until the early 1800s, when the Dutch switched from tea to coffee;

- England, where esophageal cancer was rare, possibly because the British Medical Association warned people to add milk to tea to bind the tannin and make it insoluble;
- Miami, where a fifty-three-year-old lawyer died of esophageal cancer after drinking three or four or more glasses of iced tea daily, without added milk, for twenty-seven years.

Would you care for a little milk in your tea?

Ref.: FAO (40)-13; CUFP-193, 270; *Cancer Res. 19,* 501 (1959); *Prog. Exp. Tumor Res. 2,* 245 (1961); *Fd. Cos. Tox. 7,* 364 (1969); J. F. Morton, in *Toxicology and Occupational Medicine,* W. B. Deichmann, *ed.,* Elsevier, North Holland, New York (1979); *21* CFR 184.1097.

Tartaric Acid, Potassium Acid Tartrate, Sodium Potassium Tartrate, Sodium Tartrate   Safe

Tartaric acid occurs naturally in grapes, other fruits, and coffee beans. It is made commercially from waste products of wine production. It was once more widely used than it is today, but American industry began to replace tartaric acid with other acids, especially fumaric, when World War II wreaked havoc with its price and supply. Tartaric acid, as one might guess from its name, has an extremely tart, acidic taste.

Tartaric acid is a constituent of grape and other artificial flavors that are used in beverages, candy, ice cream, baked goods, yogurt, and gelatin desserts. It also serves as the acid in some baking powders. Wineries sometimes have to add tartaric acid to wine to "correct natural deficiencies" in grapes. Most of the tartaric acid we ingest is digested by bacteria in the intestines. The 20 percent that is absorbed into the bloodstream is rapidly excreted in the urine. Guinea pigs and humans metabolize this additive identically, but rabbits, dogs, and rats go to the trouble of absorbing, then excreting, the entire dose. Figure that one out!

People have consumed large amounts of tartaric acid as a laxative without apparent harm. In 1947 Drs. Fitzhugh and Nelson, FDA biologists, published the results of lifetime feeding studies on rats; they concluded that dietary levels as high as 1.2 percent were harmless.

The salts of tartaric acid are also widely used and safe. Potassium acid tartrate, sometimes called cream of tartar, serves as a leavening agent, anticaking agent, and other functions in baked goods and other processed foods. Sodium tartrate and sodium potassium tartrate (Rochelle salt) are sometimes used as emulsifiers and to control the acidity of foods. They are used in cheeses, fats, jams, and jellies.

Ref.: FAO (31)-96; CRC-261-3; *Fed. Reg. 47,* 35772 (Aug. 17, 1982), *48,* 52445 (Nov. 18, 1983); FAO/WHO (21)-13; *21* CFR 182.1077, 182.1099, 182.1804, 182.6099.

TBHQ (tertiary butylhydroquinone) ?

Watch out BHA and BHT! There's a new antioxidant on the scene. In 1972, FDA approved the use of TBHQ, which is chemically very similar to BHA. It retards rancidity in some processed foods that contain oils.

The tests that have been done on TBHQ did not indicate any problem. However, only one—not the recommended two—rodent species was tested, and even this test used a suboptimal number of rats and lasted only twenty instead of twenty-four or more months. Considering that the more extensive tests recently conducted on BHA and BHT have raised the possibility of carcinogenesis and that TBHQ differs from BHA only by one methyl group, the FDA should demand much more exhaustive studies.

Ref.: J. Am. Oil Chem. Soc. 43, 683 (1966); WHO (8) p. 65; FDA files; *21* CFR 172.185.

Textured Vegetable Protein (TVP)   Safe
Isolated Soy Protein

Isolated soy protein and textured vegetable protein are being used in a growing number of manufactured foods. Isolated soy protein is simply protein purified from soybeans. Textured vegetable protein is soy protein that has been combined with chemical additives and processed into granules, chunks, or strips that resemble meat.

Soy protein was originally developed to help solve the protein shortage and hunger problems in underdeveloped nations, but its versatility and low cost could make imitation meat products popular in the United States. The composition of products made from soy protein can be selected arbitrarily by the manufacturer. A typical dehydrated item may contain 35 to 50 percent protein, 20 to 30 percent carbohydrate, and 1 to 20 percent fat. The natural flavor of soy-based products is bland and nutlike, but seasonings and flavorings can make it taste remarkably like chicken, pork, ham, bacon, pepperoni, fruit, nut, or other flavors. Soy-based imitation meats are often eaten by persons who do not eat meat for religious reasons.

The major ways in which we will be consuming textured soy protein in the coming years were described in one company's promotional brochure. We are advised that:

> TVP enhances nourishment, so it is well suited for institutional feeding, restaurants, and drive-ins . . . It is an excellent protein ingredient for casseroles, pat-

ties, meatballs, pizza toppings, sandwich fillings, stews, salads, snacks, and convenience foods. TVP is especially applicable to dietary foods whose vegetable origin and control of fat content are of prime importance.

Initially, restaurants, hospitals, and other institutions will be the big market for imitation meat products partly because they do not have to tell their patrons the ingredients of the food.

Products based on soy protein are undeniably nutritious, because the biological value of soy protein is similar to that of meat protein. However, imitation meat products could lack the generous amounts of vitamins and minerals contained in the real thing. To prevent this from happening, the FDA requires imitation meat products to be fortified with numerous nutrients.

Imitation meat is seasoned, held together, and colored with a flock of flavor enhancers, thickening agents, emulsifiers, artificial colorings, and flavorings. One recipe for artificial bacon includes soy protein, hydrolyzed yeast protein, salt, spices, monosodium glutamate, vegetable gum stabilizer, yeast, corn oil, artificial coloring, and water. The wholesomeness of the food depends on the nature of each of the additives. Obviously, these new products do not relieve shoppers of the eye-straining job of scrutinizing labels.

Ref.: Protein Food Supplements, Noyes, Robert, Noyes Development Corp., Park Ridge, N.J.; Archer-Daniels-Midland Co. Brochure "TVP/A fabulous new food"; *The Wall Street Journal,* October 2, 1969.

Thiamin mononitrate, thiamin hydrochloride — Safe

Thiamin is the technical name for vitamin B_1, which is abundant in yeast, pork, wheat germ, and peas. It is added in the form of a nitrate or hydrochloride salt to replace nutrients lost during processing or to increase the nutritional value of foods. It is added to all enriched white flour and to fortified breakfast cereals. Doses even several hundred times the required intake are safe.

Severe thiamin deficiency leads to the disease beriberi, which affects the nervous system. Male volunteers who were deprived of thiamin (anything for science!) developed nausea, vomiting, loss of appetite, impaired coordination, and general weakness. All these symptoms disappeared when thiamin was added to their diets. Thiamin is the key portion of many important enzymes and is present throughout the body.

Don't worry about the "nitrate" part of thiamin. Nitrate is much less of a potential danger than nitrite, and we get a thousand times more nitrate from natural foods than from vitamin B_1 supplementation.

Ref.: Recommended Dietary Allowances, Nat. Acad. Sci. (Washington, D.C.), 1980; *Fed. Reg. 47,* 47438 (Oct. 26, 1982); *21* CFR 182.5875–182.5878.

Titanium Dioxide   Safe

Titanium dioxide is a white mineral that is often used in paints and occasionally used in foods. FDA estimates that 360,000 pounds of this artificial coloring are used annually. It is inert and does not pose a risk. (Soluble forms of titanium, not used in foods, may interfere with reproduction.)

Ref.: Arch. Environ. Health 23, 102 (1971); FDA files; *21* CFR 73.575.

Tragacanth Gum   ?

Gum tragacanth exudes in the form of ribbons from the damaged bark of a small bush, astragalus, that grows wild in the Middle East. According to an importer, "The exact chemical nature of tragacanth is still not known. It is believed that the gum consists primarily of two natural polysaccharide materials." The United States imported 293,000 pounds of this gum in 1982.

The chemical exhibits a resistance to acids which is unexcelled among vegetable gums. This property makes it the ideal thickening agent for acidic foods, such as vinegar-containing salad dressings.

No good long-term feeding or biochemical studies have been conducted, so it is impossible to evaluate the safety of this additive. Some people are known to be allergic to gum tragacanth, which had been, but is no longer, used in McDonald's Big Mac sandwiches.

Ref.: FAO (46A)-104; Tragacanth Importing Corp., New York; *New Engl. J. Med. 298,* 1095 (1978); *21* CFR 184.1351.

Vanillin, Ethyl Vanillin   Safe
Vanilla

In 1520 the Aztec emperor Montezuma gave Cortés, the Spanish explorer, an unbelievably delicious drink of cocoa. It did not take the curious European long to discover that the drink's great taste was due in part to the addition of extracts of a local climbing orchid, the vanilla plant.

Cortés brought some vanilla back to spice-starved Spain, where it caused a minor sensation. Within a few years the Spaniards built factories in Spain to manufacture chocolate flavored with vanilla.

The vinelike vanilla plant is indigenous to Mexico, Central America, northern South America, and a few other scattered locations. Early attempts to cultivate vanilla plants in regions more convenient to the European market were unsuccessful. The plants would sometimes grow and flower, but they would never produce their valuable fruit. The reason for this was discovered in the 1800s: the flowers of the plant are structured in such a way that they cannot self-pollinate. In regions where vanilla was indigenous, unique varieties of hummingbirds and bees pollinated the flowers; these varieties were found nowhere else in the world. This is a classic case of different species evolving in tune with one another.

Once the pollination problem was understood, plants were pollinated by hand, and vanilla farms sprang up in several corners of the world.

Vanilla is probably the most widely used food flavoring. Manufacturers add it to ice cream, baked goods, beverages, chocolate products, gelatin desserts, and candy at concentrations ranging from 0.006 to 0.1 percent. The vanilla bean is an ingredient in many flavors—butter, root beer, fruit, chocolate, and, of course, vanilla.

The demand for vanilla outstripped the rather meager (and expensive) natural supplies years ago. The chemical industry responded to this situation by manufacturing synthetic vanillin, the major flavoring component of vanilla. Vanillin has a similar taste but is not quite as good as the real thing, because natural vanilla contains a multitude of minor constituents that modify and perfect the flavor.

Flavor chemists have synthesized a variety of derivatives of vanillin in an attempt to reproduce the exact taste of vanilla in a single chemical. So far these efforts have failed, although one of the modified molecules, ethyl vanillin, is valuable, because it comes closest to matching the desired taste and has 3.5 times the flavoring power of vanillin.

Lifetime feeding tests on rats of vanillin and ethyl vanillin did not reveal any adverse effects, but so few animals were used that the experiments should be repeated on a larger scale.

The harmlessness that was indicated for vanillin by feeding and metabolic studies and hundreds of years of use was further supported by the discovery that two hormones, adrenalin and noradrenaline, are degraded to vanillin when they are excreted by the body. The body's own production of vanillin is as much as a half milligram per day.

Ref.: FAO (44A)-39, 78; *Econ. Bot. 7,* 291 (1953); CRC-472, 746; *Cancer Res. 33,* 3069 (1973); *21* CFR 182.10, 182.20, 182.60.

Vegetable Oil   Moderate amounts: **Safe**
Large amounts: **Avoid**

Soybeans, peanuts, cottonseeds, corn, and other plant products contain large amounts of natural oils, which can be extracted and used as a food or food ingredient. The low cost, health benefits, and great versatility of some vegetable oils, as compared to butterfat, have stimulated the development of a myriad of products in which they play a key role, such as in imitation milk, powdered nondairy creamers, imitation whipped cream, margarine (imitation butter), and cooking oil. These products are useful to the general population and a boon to persons whose religion or health puts dairy products or animal fat off-limits.

A vegetable oil molecule consists of two parts, a glycerol backbone which is not too interesting, and the fatty acids which are very interesting. The body needs—but cannot itself synthesize—several fatty acids, so it is vital that we eat foods that contain them. The most important of these essential fatty acids, linoleic acid, occurs in especially high concentration in safflower and corn oils.

An important feature of fatty acids is that some are saturated, some monounsaturated, and others polyunsaturated. The chemical difference between saturated and polyunsaturated oils is based on the number of hydrogen atoms in a fat molecule. A more important difference (for consumers) is that persons who eat large amounts of saturated fats generally have high cholesterol levels in their blood. These high levels, in turn, are associated with hardening of the arteries (atherosclerosis), strokes, and heart attacks, which together kill well over half a million Americans every year. Corn, soy, and safflower oil are all high in polyunsaturates. Olive oil is rich in monounsaturated fat (oleic acid). Palm oil and coconut oil are the black sheep of vegetable oils, being even higher in saturated fat than butterfat or beef fat.

Vegetable oils are used in margarine because of their low costs. However, because most oils are liquid at room temperature, they first must be modified. The modification, which entails a reaction with hydrogen, converts some of the polyunsaturated oils primarily to monounsaturated and partly to saturated oils. This process is known as "hardening," "saturation," or "hydrogenation."

Partially hydrogenated oils are semisolid at room temperature and thus ideal for use in margarine. However, the more extensive the hydrogenation, the more of the unsaturated oils will be converted to the less desirable saturated forms. In recent years, manufacturers of margarine and shortening have been using improved methods, which result in smaller losses of polyunsaturated oils. Soft (tub-type) margarines contain more polyunsaturates than stick-type varieties.

The hydrogenation process also creates "trans" fatty acids ("trans" refers to the structure of the molecules). Though small amounts of these fatty acids occur in butterfat and meat fat, several scientists have alleged that the higher levels of "trans" fatty acids in margarine are a—or even *the*—major cause of heart disease. The studies they cite, however, have been small and unpersuasive. An FDA-appointed committee that evaluated the safety of numerous food additives concluded that the "trans" fats do not pose any special risk.

Polyunsaturated oils can react with the oxygen in air and develop a rancid odor and taste, especially in the presence of sunlight or metal ions. In living plants and animals, naturally occurring tocopherols (vitamin E) and other antioxidants prevent the oxidation. The antioxidant content of oils is reduced only slightly during commercial processing and should be sufficient to prevent the oils on supermarket and kitchen shelves from going rancid for a reasonably long period of time. Nevertheless, some manufacturers add such synthetic antioxidants as BHT, BHA, or propyl gallate to their products. The antioxidants are added either because the oils are deficient in tocopherols, out of habit, because of poor production techniques, or in order to increase slightly their shelf life. Other manufacturers produce perfectly acceptable products without adding antioxidants. As discussed in separate entries (see butylated hydroxyanisole, butylated hydroxytoluene, propyl gallate), several synthetic antioxidants may pose a slight health risk. I recommend using brands of oils and shortenings that do not contain these suspicious preservatives.

Virtually all health authorities agree that eating excessive amounts of saturated fats contributes to hardening of the arteries. In the last few years, scientists have also begun to appreciate the apparent ability of fats—regardless of type—to promote cancers of the colon, breast, and prostate. So the best advice is to *eat less of all fats,* but especially the saturated variety. For a more complete discussion of the health effects of fats, please refer to the *Nutrition Scoreboard* section of this book (page 53).

Vitamin A (palmitate) — Safe

This necessary nutrient is added to skim milk and margarine as a public health measure. More recently, vitamin A has been added to breakfast cereals, powdered breakfast drinks, and other processed foods. Additional information about this fat-soluble vitamin will be found in the discussion of beta-carotene (p. 248) and in the *Nutrition Scoreboard* section of this book (p. 91).

Vitamin D (D$_2$) Safe

Vitamin D is an essential nutrient. People who get plenty of sun do not need extra vitamin D, but many shut-ins do. The sun's ultraviolet rays activate a sterol in the deep layers of the skin, so that it is metabolized to vitamin D in the liver and kidney. Vitamin D$_2$ is produced by ultraviolet irradiation of a plant sterol, ergosterol, and seems to be equally effective in humans.

A deficiency of vitamin D debilitates calcium and phosphate metabolism, preventing normal mineralization of the bone. This results in the disease rickets in the young and osteomalacia in the adult.

Very dark skin may prevent up to 95 percent of UV light from reaching the deeper skin layers. This is protective in tropical areas where a light-skinned person could conceivably synthesize a toxic amount of the vitamin, but is a disadvantage in areas where sunlight is limited seasonally or by considerable air pollution, since energy from the sun may be insufficient for adequate formation of vitamin D in the skin.

Most commercially available milk is fortified with vitamin D, and it occurs naturally in such animal foods as fatty fish, eggs, butter, and liver. It is stable in foods and not affected by storage, processing, and cooking.

Ref.: Recommended Dietary Allowances, Nat. Acad. of Sci. (Washington, D.C.), 1980; *21* CFR 182.5950–182.5953.

Xanthan Gum Safe

Reading literature produced by its manufacturer, one might think that xanthan gum is one of the chemical finds of the twentieth century: "excellent textural quality," "pleasing mouthfeel," "lack of gumminess." This additive, developed by scientists at the Department of Agriculture's Peoria, Illinois, laboratory, serves as an emulsifier and stabilizer in salad dressings, syrups, bakery fillings, and other processed foods. Xanthan gum is said to be a truly great emulsifier, because it causes solutions to be very thick, but still eminently pourable. It is stable over a wide range of acidities and temperatures. The American population consumes about 800,000 pounds of xanthan gum each year.

This wondrous carbohydrate, a cousin of starch, is produced by a bacterium, *Xanthomonas campestris.* Not having use for xanthan gum in its own puddings or salad dressings, the bacteria use it to surround their cell wall for protection against dehydration and other adversities.

One long-term feeding study found xanthan gum to be safe; additional studies would be reassuring.

Ref.: Food Tech. 25, (5) 22 (1971); *Tox. Appl. Pharmacol. 24,* 30 (1973); "Xanthan Gum," Kelco Co. (Chicago); *21* CFR 172.695.

Xylitol   Avoid

The scientist or company that finds a safe sugar substitute that does not promote tooth decay or obesity will become very, very rich. In the 1970s, a Finnish company, Finnfoods, identified xylitol as a chemical that might do the trick. Xylitol is a natural substance found in berries, plums, mushrooms, and other foods and even in the human body. It is structurally similar, but not identical, to sugars. The Finns make xylitol from xylan, a substance in birchwood chips.

Xylitol occurs naturally in the body as a metabolite of glucose. It enters liver cells freely, not needing insulin to get in, and has little effect on blood sugar levels. For this reason, physicians in Europe and Japan sometimes recommend xylitol to diabetics.

The FDA approved xylitol in 1963, first as a substitute for sugar in dietetic jams and jellies and then for more general use. In 1977, Wrigley started marketing xylitol-sweetened Orbit gum, Life Savers used the chemical in Care*Free gum, and the following year Finnfoods began advertising its Xylitol gum as being "good news for your teeth." A two-year study showed that people who substituted xylitol for refined sugars suffered only one tenth as much tooth decay as the sugar-eaters. The picture looked rosy for gum sales, teeth, and Finland's balance of payments.

But on November 15, 1977, the bubble burst. An English study found that large amounts of xylitol increased the incidence of bladder tumors in mice and tumors of the adrenal gland in rats. All but one of the mice that had bladder tumors also had bladder stones, presumably caused by the stiff dose of xylitol. Because the stones—and the tumors—did not occur at doses below 20 percent xylitol, there was not a great deal of concern about this study. The high doses of xylitol used in the rat study may also have caused physiological changes that led to the adrenal tumors. The following February a Wrigley spokesperson said, "We . . . have no intention of stopping the use of (xylitol) in Orbit," but nine months later that company stopped using xylitol.

A July 1978 report by the Federation of American Societies for Experimental Biology (FASEB) said that until other studies are done, "It is not possible to determine with certainty the tumorigenic potential of dietary xylitol." Several months later, an FDA official, Dr. W. Gary Flamm, said, according to an agency memo, "it had to be conceded that xylitol appeared to induce tumors in a dose-related manner in both rats and mice." FDA has proposed banning xylitol, but never took final action. Finnfoods' Xylitol brand chewing gum and gumdrops are still available at candy counters.

Ref.: Acta Odont. Scand. 33 Suppl. 70, 105, 265 (1975); the New York *Times* (Nov. 16, 1977); *Science 199,* 670 (1978); "Xylitol, Summary Review," Xyrofin Ltd. (Feb. 1978); FDA memo (Oct. 27, 1978); *21* CFR 172.395.

Yellow Prussiate of Soda — Safe

Some manufacturers add yellow prussiate of soda (sodium ferrocyanide) to salt when they crystallize it. The additive generates jagged and bulky crystals, which resist caking. This mitigates the need for extra anticaking agents.

Although this additive contains cyanide, it is not toxic, because the cyanide is tightly bound to iron atoms. Individuals have attempted to commit suicide by swallowing teaspoonfuls of this dangerous-sounding chemical, but the attempts were dismal failures.

Ref.: U.S. Patent 2,642,335; *Food Cosmet. Toxicol. 7,* 409 (1969); FAO (55); *21* CFR 172.490.

VII

Food Additive Cemetery

Every few years, amid a puff of publicity, the safety of a widely used food additive is questioned. In some cases the additive is banned quickly. In other cases five or ten years may elapse, during which time additional tests are conducted, review panels convened, and congressional hearings held, before the chemical is actually banned. The period of delay is usually proportional to the importance of the additive and whether a suitable replacement is available. In still other cases, the chemical may remain in use, because the problem was considered trivial, studies were disproven or considered equivocal, suitable substitutes were not available, or industry's lobbying prevailed. Some of the chemicals whose safety has been questioned, but which were not banned, such as saccharin and sodium nitrite, were discussed earlier. The following section covers several additives that have been banned from the food supply.

Cyclamate

HEALTH HAZARD . . . BLADDER CANCER . . . MASS HUMAN EXPERIMENT . . . CYCLAMATE NIGHTMARE . . . These were some of the headlines and phrases making the news in 1969–70 when the story broke that cyclamate, a widely used sugar substitute, could cause cancer. In what was certainly a hectic period for the Food and Drug Administration, the public got rare insight into the workings of the government agency that is charged with keeping our foods free of toxic chemicals. That agency's procrastinations and evasions surfaced time and time again, in a seemingly endless stream. Fifteen years later, Abbott Laboratories was still pressing FDA to allow the use of cyclamate.

Cyclamate was originally sold in tablet form to provide a low-calorie sweetener for diabetics. Around 1960, beverage and other manufacturers began marketing "diet" foods to the general public. Industry's advertising pitch was that if you bought diet foods, you would lose weight. Sales of low-calorie drinks and foods soared. The new products opened up a whole new market, and because cyclamate could do as good a sweetening job as sugar at a lower cost, the profits were enormous. Saccharin, which is actually sweeter than cyclamate, was also available, but it had an undesirable aftertaste. Beginning in 1953, the two synthetic chemicals were used together to provide the best taste for the least money.

As the use of cyclamate increased, doctors and scientists began taking a closer look at its effectiveness in helping people lose weight and at its safety. Some claimed that the chemical really did help people lose weight; other scientists produced studies indicating that it was worthless. The general consensus appeared to be that you would not lose weight just by drinking a bottle of Fresca instead of Coke; to lose weight you had to make a strong, total diet effort to cut down on calories and had to exercise more to increase calorie expenditures.

On the safety issue, the National Academy of Sciences warned in 1954, 1955, 1962, and 1968 that artificial sweeteners should not be used by the general public. All the warnings went unheeded by industry, the government, and consumers, and in 1969 the storm broke: FDA got more and more evidence that cyclamate, or a cyclamate-saccharin mixture, caused bladder cancer, birth defects, mutations, and testicular damage in animals. While most attention addressed the possibility of cancer, some experts focused on reproductive health. They were especially concerned about rapidly growing preadolescent boys, who also happen to be some of the biggest drinkers of soda pop.

Once there was evidence that cyclamate was carcinogenic and might affect reproduction, the FDA did not comply with the law that prohibits the use in food of unsafe chemicals, particularly those that cause cancer. Instead, the FDA recommended in April 1969 that people voluntarily restrict their intake of it. After this equivocation, public pressure mounted steadily. In October, the FDA banned cyclamate totally and ruled that cyclamate-containing products could not be sold after February 1, 1970. Over the next few months, however, industry pressure took its toll. In February the FDA reversed its position and said that cyclamate could be used in food if the foods were labeled "drugs"; manufacturers had until September 1, 1970, to switch their labels. Finally, on August 14, 1970, FDA administrators succumbed to public, scientific, and congressional pressures, reversed direction again, and banned cyclamate totally. Stores were given two weeks to get the products off their shelves.

As FDA's flip-flops came to an end, industry sought to recoup some of its multimillion-dollar losses. First, companies tried dumping their products for whatever they could get. If they could sell them for a few dollars, fine; otherwise they donated them to charity to reap substantial tax savings. Carnation, for instance, saved $2 million in taxes. After September 1970, you could find the banned products wherever there were poor people. Cases of soda were piled high in thrift stores across the United States and on a ship in the Pacific, sixty thousand cases of Carnation's Slender low-calorie drink were headed for calorie-starved Laotian refugees. The shipment to Laos, at a cost of $42,000 in taxpayers' dollars for shipping fees, was conceived as a way of getting a tax break. Fortunately, Ohio Congressman Charles Vanik, calling Carnation's plan "cheap and cruel," prevented distribution of the product.

Industry's second tactic was to get the U.S. Treasury to reimburse firms for their losses. In September 1971, the House Judiciary Committee heard testimony on legislation that would do just that. The bill, which was supported by President Nixon, ultimately failed in the Senate.

The cyclamate episode gave citizens insight into how scientists think and act in a crisis situation. As one would expect, there were some heroes and some goats. Drs. Jacqueline Verrett and Marvin Legator, two conscientious FDA scientists, went public after their views had been squelched deep within the bureaucracy. Pressure from these and other scientists helped force the FDA to act.

Meanwhile, a few scientists maintained that ingesting a tiny amount of a carcinogen is OK, or that cyclamate may cause cancer in animals but because we don't know for sure if it causes cancer in humans it should not be banned. A version of the latter view was advanced by Dr. Melvin Benarde, a professor at the Hahnemann Medical College in Philadelphia, who wrote:

> Conversely, if an additive is found to be carcinogenic in animals, does it mean it will do the same in humans? *Unfortunately,* we can never learn this because the Delaney Amendment of 1958 proscribes the use of an additive for man once it is found hazardous to animals [emphasis added].

Contrast Benarde's philosophy with that of Dr. Legator and five other scientists, as expressed in a letter published in *Science* magazine:

> The decision to restrict cyclamates to the general public and to terminate a mass human experiment for which there are no demonstrable matching benefits is clearly proper. We concur that food additives be banned from products unless they have been proven safe, and either significantly improve the quality or nutritive value of the food or lower the food cost.

After the ban, Abbott Laboratories repeatedly petitioned FDA to reapprove cyclamate. In September 1980, FDA rejected an Abbott plea, saying that the "studies failed to prove that cyclamate does not cause cancer or inheritable genetic damage." Abbott Labs came back again in November 1982. This time, an FDA committee reanalyzed all the studies and concluded that the evidence was now sufficient to demonstrate that the artificial sweetener does not cause cancer.

To benefit from another opinion, the FDA asked the National Research Council (NRC) to investigate the carcinogenicity question. In June 1984 the NRC's Committee on the Evaluation of Cyclamate for Carcinogenicity commenced a yearlong study that generated both good news and bad news. The good news was that "the totality of the evidence from studies in animals does not indicate that cyclamate or its major metabolite cyclohexylamine is carcinogenic by itself." The bad news was that two studies, one each in rats and mice, "suggest that cyclamate may enhance the carcinogenic effect of other substances in the urinary bladder." The committee recommended that these studies be repeated for confirmation, a process that would take several years.

Aside from cancer, the NRC committee reminded FDA that cyclohexylamine inhibits the growth and impairs the function of testes in laboratory rats. Also, former FDA commissioner Jere Goyan, who in 1980 reaffirmed the ban on cyclamate, has noted that cyclohexylamine affects growth, reproduction, and blood pressure in rats. If usage levels were set on the basis of this research, such small quantities of cyclamate would be permitted that the artificial sweetener would be useless for diet soft drinks, the major market.

Between its toxic effects and its apparent ability to increase the potency of cancer-causing chemicals, cyclamate will not be reappearing on the market in the near future. (In Canada, cyclamate is permitted as a tabletop sweetener and in drugs.)

Ref.: Science 166, 1575 (1969); *The Wall Street Journal,* August 7, 1970; Washington *Post,* August 15, 1970; Turner, J. *The Chemical Feast,* Grossman, New York (1970); "Cyclamate Report," Appendix I, FDA (July 1970); *The Chemicals We Eat,* M. Benarde, American Heritage Press, New York (1971), pp. 126–27; "Report on Nonnutritive Sweeteners," FDA (October 16, 1971); Letter from FDA (R. J. Ronk) to Abbott Lab. (May 11, 1976); *Fed. Reg.* 45 61474-61530 (Sept. 16, 1980); "Scientific Review of the Long-term Carcinogen Bioassays Performed on the Artificial Sweetener, Cyclamate," Cancer Assessment Committee, FDA (April 1984); "Evaluation of Cyclamate for Carcinogenicity," Nat. Res. Coun., Nat. Acad. Press, Washington (1985).

Diethyl Pyrocarbonate

The FDA's final food additive headache in 1971 derived from diethyl pyrocarbonate (DEPC), a chemical that prevented microorganisms from growing in alcoholic beverages and fruit drinks. From the time it was introduced in the early 1960s, DEPC was thought to be the ideal beverage preservative, because it quickly kills microbes and then breaks down almost completely within twenty-four hours to carbon dioxide and alcohol, both of which are harmless. This preservative was developed in Germany and used more widely in Europe than in the United States.

DEPC's tragic flaw is that it is extremely reactive and can potentially combine with ammonia to form urethan, a strong carcinogen. For several years analytical chemists unsuccessfully searched for urethan in products treated with DEPC. In December 1971, however, two Swedish researchers used a sensitive technique involving the addition of radioactively labeled DEPC to orange juice, wine, and beer. They found small but significant amounts of urethan in each of the drinks. In August 1972, the FDA banned this once highly touted preservative.

Ref.: Science 174, 1248 (1971); *Washington Star* (Dec. 12, 1971); *Fed. Reg. 37,* 3060 (Feb. 11, 1972), 15426 (Aug. 2, 1972).

Red 2 (Amaranth)

In September 1971 the FDA made the startling announcement that its own study had verified the results of a Russian study indicating that Red 2 causes birth defects in animals. At the same time, the FDA announced that all other artificial colors would be tested for their effect on animal fetuses.

Red 2 was the most widely used food coloring, accounting for about one third of all colorings. More than 1.2 million pounds were certified for use in fiscal year 1971. The dye was used in soft drinks, ice cream, pistachio nuts, candy, baked goods, pet foods, sausage, breakfast cereals, and other foods.

Although scientists had been concerned since the 1962 thalidomide episode that food additives might cause birth defects, neither the FDA nor manufacturers tested colorings in this regard. The FDA was finally prodded into action in 1971 by second-rate Soviet experiments indicating that Red 2 caused birth defects and interfered with rat reproduction. The Soviet scientists also claimed, again on the basis of poor experiments, that Red 2 caused cancer in rats. However, other experiments on rats and two strains of mice seemed to support FDA's contention that Red 2 was not a cancer threat.

A committee of the National Academy of Sciences met in early February and gave the dye a clean bill of health, but this was too much of a whitewash, even for the FDA. So FDA appointed another advisory committee. This committee recommended new tests that were to delay any action for at least two years.

In 1974–75 FDA conducted a long-term feeding study to determine once and for all whether Red 2 caused cancer. The experiment was somewhat botched, but statisticians held that Red 2 increased the number of malignant tumors in female rats. FDA agreed that Red 2 could not be considered proven safe and, after four years of argument, banned the dye on January 19, 1976.

Ref.: FAO (38B)-22; *J. Pharm. Exp. Ther. 136,* 259 (1962); *J. Pharm. Pharmacol. 10,* 625 (1968); *Chem. Abst. 69,* 1366; *Vop. Pitan. 29* (2) 66, (5) 61 (1970); BIBRA (British Industrial Biological Research Association) Information Bulletin, May 1971 (review of Soviet studies); Washington *Post,* November 14, 1971; February 11, 1972; *Times Magazine,* February 29, 1976.

Red 4 (Ponceau SX)

This dye was formerly one of the most widely used, but in the early 1960s Dr. Kent Davis, of the Food and Drug Administration, found that high levels damaged the adrenal gland and urinary bladder of dogs. On the basis of these studies, FDA planned to ban the dye.

The maraschino cherry industry, however, had other ideas. The industry had persuaded itself that its very survival depended on the continued use of Red 4. Company officials convinced FDA administrators, at least temporarily, that while large amounts of dye might indeed cause part of the adrenal cortex to atrophy and produce changes in the urinary bladder, the amount of dye that one might ingest by eating artificially colored cherries was harmless. The FDA gave "provisional approval" for the use of the dye only in maraschino cherries (150 parts per million) and certain drugs and cosmetics, pending further studies.

The FDA was forced to confront the questions about Red 4 in 1976, when it was conducting its review of all food colorings. FDA advised industry several times to conduct further studies if it wanted to continue using the chemical, but industry never did those studies. On September 22, 1976, FDA banned all food uses of Red 4, though the dye is still being used in drugs and cosmetics that are applied externally but not taken orally.

Ref.: FAO (38B)-19; *J. Pharm. Pharmacol. 13,* 492 (1961); *J. Pharm. Exp. Ther. 136,* 259 (1962); *Tox. Appl. Pharm. 8,* 306 (1966); FDA press release (Sept. 20, 1976); *Food Chem. News,* p. 21 (Oct. 24, 1983).

Violet 1

The safety of Violet 1 was a question mark for many years. The dye was used to stamp the Department of Agriculture's inspection symbol on meat and also to color candy, beverages, and pet food. The FDA certified almost 67,000 pounds of this dye in 1972.

Consumers could have ingested tiny amounts of the dye when they ate a steak or roast. Workers in packinghouses were probably exposed to much greater amounts. The men who stamped USDA's mark on carcasses frequently got the dye on their hands, and occasionally large amounts dripped down their hands and arms. One Department of Agriculture meat inspector in North Carolina observed that "the dye is pretty hard to get off. Once you get it on your skin, you almost have to wear it off."

FDA expedited approval of Violet 1 as a food coloring at the behest of Malcolm Carroll, the former manager of Allied Chemical's certified color division. Carroll pleaded at a hearing that his company needed quick approval so it could gear up for the 1951 Easter egg coloring season and for fall candy orders.

Scientists conducted several chronic feeding studies on rats. The earliest two studies, using male rats only, were done by Dr. Lloyd Hazleton, then at George Washington University, and by Dr. O. Garth Fitzhugh at the FDA. Hazleton's study involved twenty rats per dosage level, while Fitzhugh's involved only fifteen. Neither study indicated any problem. The third study, published in 1962 by Dr. W. A. Mannell and his colleagues at Canada's Department of National Health and Welfare, involved more rats, rats of both sexes, and higher dosages than were used by Fitzhugh. This study indicated that the dye caused cancer. Of thirty rats (fifteen of each sex) fed 3 percent dye in their food for seventy-five weeks, five developed malignant tumors. Three of the tumors were skin tumors. Four of the five tumors occurred in females. Only one out of thirty untreated rats developed a tumor.

The FDA discounted the Canadian study because there was no proof that the Canadian dye precisely fit U.S. specifications for FD&C Violet 1. (The entire batch of dye had been used up, the manufacturer had gone out of business, and all records had been lost.) Yet the FDA had no positive evidence that the dye did, in fact, differ significantly from U.S. specifications.

At its December 1964 meeting, the Expert Committee on Food Additives, which is cosponsored by the Food and Agriculture Organization and the World Health Organization (FAO/WHO) of the United Nations, categorized Violet 1 as a dye "for which the available data are inadequate for evaluation but indicate the possibility of harmful effects." Dr. Jack Dacre, a New Zealand biochemist, wrote that this coloring "has possible harmful effects and should not be allowed to be used in food."

In early 1971, nine years after Violet 1 was first suspected of being carcinogenic, the FDA asked the National Academy of Sciences to convene a group of nongovernment scientists to evaluate all available studies. The NAS committee dismissed out of hand the Canadian study that indicated that Violet 1 caused cancer. The committee declared the dye safe, but did recommend that a lifetime feeding study be conducted on dogs. The net effect of their report would have been to postpone the permanent acceptance or banning of this coloring for at least eight years.

Immediately after the NAS released its report the Center for Science in the Public Interest petitioned FDA to ban Violet 1. It took FDA only three months to deny the petition.

In early 1973 FDA learned of a new Japanese study that proved that Violet 1 caused cancer of the breast and ear in female rats. FDA finally outlawed the dye, ending a dismal episode in that agency's record.

Ref.: FAO (38B)-107; Fed. Sec. Agency (FDA) Docket No. FDA-58 (February 1950); *J. Pharm. Pharmacol. 14,* 378 (1962); *Fd. Cos. Tox. 2,* 345 (1964); *Fed. Reg. 38,* 9077 (Apr. 10, 1973); *J. Nat. Cancer Inst. 51,* 1337 (1973).

Glossary

acids (acidulants): serve many food uses, as flavorings (citric acid—citrus; malic acid—apple; acetic acid—vinegar; tartaric acid—grape), preservatives (acidity prevents the growth of microorganisms), and antioxidants (molecules with two acidic groups, such as citric acid, can trap metal ions that might otherwise cause food to discolor or go rancid). Acids are used to adjust and stabilize the acidity of cheese and beer to optimize growing conditions for microorganisms. Carbonic acid is used to make carbonated water.

aging (maturing) agent: a chemical added to flour or dough that oxidizes the protein. Freshly milled, untreated flour makes sticky, poor-rising dough and low-quality bread and rolls. In the old days, millers aged flour by holding it in bins for several months and letting the oxygen in the air act on it. The aging causes changes in the protein in flour that make the dough elastic enough to let gas bubbles (generated by yeast) form and rigid enough to hold the bubbles in the dough. Bakers now use chemicals to age flour. Chemical aging requires much less time and space, offers little opportunity for vermin to consume or contaminate the flour, and results in batches with more consistent properties as compared to natural aging. See acetone peroxide, azodicarbonamide, chlorine, chlorine dioxide, potassium bromate, potassium iodate. Some of these agents also bleach flour.

amino acids: the subunits from which proteins are built. There are twenty major amino acids: alanine, arginine, asparagine, aspartic acid, cysteine, glutamic acid, glutamine, glycine (amino-acetic acid), histidine, *isoleucine, leucine, lysine, methionine, phenylalanine,* proline, serine, *threonine, tryptophan,* tyrosine, *valine.* The human body cannot synthesize eight of these amino acids (italicized). These are called "essential" amino acids and must be obtained from food.

anticaking compounds: chemicals that manufacturers add to powdered or granular foods to prevent them from absorbing moisture and becoming lumpy. See silicates, yellow prussiate of soda.

antioxidants: the odor, taste, and color of most foods gradually deteriorate during storage. Most of the changes are caused by reaction of oxygen in the air with fats, carbohydrates, flavorings, and colorings. This reaction is known as oxidation.

TABLE 2. Additives That Have Been Banned*

Additive	Function	Source	Last used	Reason for ban
agene (Nitrogen trichloride)	flour bleaching and aging agent	synthetic	1949	dogs that ate bread made from treated flour suffered epileptic-like fits; the toxic agent was methionine sulfoxime.
dyes	artificial coloring	synthetic		
butter yellow			1919	toxic, later found to cause liver cancer
FD&C Green 1			1965	liver cancer
FD&C Green 2			1965	insufficient economic importance to be tested
FD&C Orange 1			1956	organ damage
FD&C Orange 2			1960	organ damage
FD&C Orange B			1978†	cancer
FD&C Red 1			1961	liver cancer
FD&C Red 2			1976	possible carcinogen
FD&C Red 4			1976	high levels damaged adrenal cortex of dog; after 1965 used only in maraschino cherries and certain pills; it is still allowed in externally applied drugs and cosmetics.
FD&C Red 32			1956	damages internal organs and may be a weak carcinogen; since 1956 used under the name Citrus Red 2, to color oranges (2 ppm).
Sudan 1			1919	toxic, later found to be carcinogenic
FD&C Violet 1			1973	cancer
FD&C Yellow 1 and 2			1959	intestinal lesions at high dosages

(continued)

TABLE 2. Additives That Have Been Banned (continued)

Additive	Function	Source	Last used	Reason for ban
FD&C Yellow 3			1959	heart damage at high dosages
FD&C Yellow 4			1959	heart damage at high dosages
cinnamyl anthranilate	artificial flavoring	synthetic	1982†	liver cancer
cobalt salts	stabilize beer foam	synthetic	1966	toxic effects on heart
coumarin	flavoring	tonka bean	1954	liver poison
cyclamate	artificial sweetener	synthetic	1970	bladder cancer
diethyl pyrocarbonate (DEPC)	preservative (beverages)	synthetic	1972	combines with ammonia to form urethan, a carcinogen
dulcin (p-ethoxyphenyl urea)	artificial sweetener	synthetic	1950	liver cancer
ethylene glycol	solvent, humectant	synthetic		kidney damage
monochloroacetic acid	preservative	synthetic	1941	highly toxic
nordihydroguaiaretic acid (NDGA)	antioxidant	desert plant	1971‡	kidney damage
oil of calamus	flavoring	root of calamus	1968	intestinal cancer
polyoxyethylene-8-stearate (Myrj 45)	emulsifier (used in baked goods)	synthetic	1952	high levels caused bladder stones and tumors
safrole	flavoring (root beer)	sassafras	1960	liver cancer
thiourea	preservative	synthetic	c. 1950	liver cancer

†Ban not yet finalized.
‡NDGA was banned by the FDA in 1968, but the Department of Agriculture did not ban it until 1971.
* Ref.: 21 CFR 189; "Food Colors", Nat. Acad. Sci. Committee on Food Protection (1971); other sources.

The food constituents that deteriorate most rapidly are the unsaturated fats and oils. When these compounds react with oxygen they generate new substances that have offensive—rancid—tastes and odors.

Other substances that are unstable in the presence of oxygen include coloring matter, such as the beta-carotene in carrots and margarine, and the carbohydrates in fruits and vegetables. Carotene turns gray upon oxidation, whereas carbohydrate, such as that which is exposed when an apple or potato is peeled, turns brown.

Several means have been devised to prevent or retard oxidation and thereby extend the storage life of foods. One method is to prevent food from coming in contact with air. This can be done by using vacuum packs or by packing food in the presence of nitrogen, an inert gas. A more convenient way of eliminating food-air contact is to add to the food a chemical, such as ascorbic or isoascorbic acids or stannous chloride, that combines with oxygen and depletes the oxygen supply in a container.

The most efficient inhibitors of oxidation are the synthetic compounds BHA, BHT, TBHQ, and propyl gallate. These "primary antioxidants" can interrupt the chain reaction oxidations, which mark the deterioration of fats.* Fats going rancid might be compared to a row of falling dominoes. The more dominoes that fall, the worse the smell. BHA, BHT, TBHQ, and propyl gallate prevent oxidation much like a finger holding back a falling domino would prevent a whole row of dominoes from toppling. The tocopherols (vitamin E) and gum guaiac are natural antioxidants that function in the same way.

Another method of preventing oxidative changes in food followed from the discovery that minute amounts of metals (copper, zinc, iron, etc.) accelerate oxidation. Calcium disodium EDTA, citric acid, sodium pyrophosphate, and other chemicals trap these metal ions and curb oxidation much as a vacuum cleaner traps dirt or filters remove impurities from fluids. These chemicals are called sequestrants or chelating agents. Chemicals of this type occur naturally and help retard oxidation in living plants and animals.

The food industry, fearful that the word antioxidant has taken on a pejorative meaning, has coined several euphemisms, such as "freshness preserver."

The long shelf life of foods that contain antioxidants gives bacteria and mold more opportunity to grow. For this reason antimicrobial preservatives are oftentimes used in conjunction with antioxidants.

Antioxidants are frequently added unnecessarily to foods (see the individual sections on butylated hydroxyanisole and butylated hydroxytoluene).

baking powder: a chemical leavening system that substitutes for yeast. It consists of appropriate proportions of baking soda (sodium bicarbonate) and one or more acids. Most household baking powders are of the "double-acting type," which contain two acids, sodium aluminum phosphate [$Al_2(SO_4)_3 \cdot Na_2SO_4$] and monocalcium phosphate [$CaH_4(PO_4)_2$]. It is called double-acting because monocalcium phosphate forms gas cells during the preparation of the dough, while the other acid does not release gas until the dough is hot. The other important kind of

---

* Oxygen reacts with fats to produce peroxides, which generate free radicals; the very reactive free radicals are removed by primary antioxidants.

baking powder, said to be the more efficient, contains only baking soda and monocalcium phosphate. Starch is added to baking powder to absorb moisture and prevent the soda and acid from entering into a chemical reaction on the shelf. Flour to which baking powder has been added is called "self-rising flour."

baking soda: sodium bicarbonate ($NaHCO_3$). Carbon dioxide gas is liberated when baking soda and an acid are mixed in water. See baking powder.

bleaching agent: a chemical that makes flour white by oxidizing the colored matter (xanthophylls). See acetone peroxide, benzoyl peroxide, chlorine, chlorine dioxide. These agents destroy what little vitamin E (tocopherol) remains in white flour.

buffer: a chemical that maintains a solution or food at the desired acidity.

carcinogen: a substance that causes cancer.

cariogenic: promoting tooth decay (caries).

chelator (derived from the Greek word meaning claw): a chemical that chelates, or traps, trace amounts of metal atoms that would otherwise cause food to discolor or go rancid. See EDTA, citric acid. Same as sequestrant.

cocarcinogen: a substance that by itself does not cause cancer but increases the potency of chemicals that do cause cancer. The oil of croton seeds is a commonly used laboratory cocarcinogen. See sulfiting agents.

Delaney Clause: the sections of the 1958 Food Additive and the 1960 Color Additive amendments to the Food, Drug and Cosmetic Act that specifically prohibit in food any chemical that causes cancer when fed at any level to animals or man.

The clause is named after its chief congressional proponent, Representative James J. Delaney of New York.

detoxifying enzymes: enzymes in the liver that convert poisons into harmless chemicals, which are then excreted.

diastatic activity: ability to degrade starch to glucose and maltose; see amylases.

dough conditioner: a substance used by bakers to make dough drier (less sticky), more extensible, and easier to machine. See discussion of calcium stearoyl lactylate; see also aging agents.

emulsifiers: most liquids are either water-like or oil-like, and, as everyone knows, the two do not ordinarily mix. Both Nature and chemists, however, have developed chemicals that have both oil-like and water-like properties and that enable water and oil to mix. The mixing aids are known as emulsifiers (because they create emulsions) or surfactants (because they decrease surface tensions). They are close relatives of soaps and detergents.

Emulsifiers create emulsions, not true solutions. In other words, they stabilize and decrease the size of fat globules in water, or water globules in oil, to such an extent that the globules have little tendency to coalesce and form distinct layers.

Emulsifiers are naturally present both in foods and in the body. The major difference between mayonnaise and oil-and-vinegar dressing, for instance, is the egg in the mayonnaise. The egg protein adds body, and the egg lecithin emulsifies the vegetable oil and vinegar so that they do not separate into two layers. Bile salts, which are produced by the liver and secreted into the small intestine, emulsify fats so that they can be absorbed more readily by the body.

The most frequently used emulsifiers in foods are mono- and diglycerides, which are derived from fat or oil, and the synthetic polysorbates and sorbitan monostearate. These and other agents keep bread from going stale by preventing starch molecules from crystallizing, help powdered nondairy creamers dissolve in coffee, prevent oil from separating out of peanut butter, make cakes light and fluffy, enable oil-like colorings and flavorings to mix well with foods, serve as whipping aids in toppings, keep fat from separating out in processed meat products and pet foods, and keep butterfat in solution during the initial freezing of ice cream.

Thickening agents (stabilizers) sometimes act as emulsifiers, because they hinder the movement of oil or water globules and prevent them from forming separate layers.

Emulsifiers are rarely used to adulterate food, but their use in peanut butter may be an exception. Up to 10 percent of the peanuts may be replaced by emulsifiers to prevent peanut oil from separating out. "Ninety percent peanut butter" is considered adulterated by some consumers.

enriched: products such as bread and spaghetti to which nutrients have been added (after naturally occurring nutrients have been removed) are labeled "enriched." Enrichment does not replace all the lost nutrients.

enzymes: specialized protein molecules that facilitate the interconversion, modification, degradation, or synthesis of molecules in living organisms. Many enzyme molecules consist of protein molecules combined with a vitamin molecule or a metal atom.

epidemiology: the study of the incidence of a disease in a population. Usually, the incidence is correlated with another variable, such as body weight, geographic location, coffee consumption, etc.

essential amino acids: amino acids which the body cannot synthesize from other molecules and which must be obtained from food. Isoleucine, leucine, lysine, methionine, phenylalanine, threonine, tryptophan, valine are essential amino acids for humans.

FAO/WHO Joint Expert Committee on Food Additives: an international committee, sponsored by the Food and Agriculture Organization and the World Health Organization of the United Nations, made up of government, industry, and university scientists. The committee reviews the safety of food additives and then publishes evaluations and recommendations. The committee's work is of particular value to small nations that cannot afford to maintain extensive food safety agencies.

FDA: Food and Drug Administration, a division of the U.S. Department of Health and Human Services. The FDA was established in 1906 to protect the public from unsafe foods, drugs, and cosmetics. Its address is 5600 Fishers Lane, Rockville, Md. 20857.

fermentation: breakdown of starch, sugar, or fats, usually accompanied by the production of acids and other small molecules, by the action of bacteria, yeast, etc. The production of yogurt, bread, cheese, and beer involve fermentation. See the discussion of citric acid for a description of how fermentation can be used in the manufacture of chemicals.

firming agent: manufacturers add calcium salts (calcium chloride, calcium citrate, calcium lactate, etc.) to canned tomatoes, potatoes, lima beans, and peppers to prevent them from becoming unacceptably soft. The calcium acts like a cement by reacting with the pectin in the cell walls of fruits and vegetables.

flavor enhancer: a substance that has little or no flavor of its own but brings out the natural flavor of foods. The mechanism by which flavor enhancers operate is not known. They may sensitize taste buds, stimulate the secretion of saliva (which breaks down food and lets the flavor out), etc. See monosodium glutamate (MSG), disodium guanylate and disodium inosinate, maltol and ethyl maltol.

fortified: manufacturers sometimes add vitamins and minerals to foods, such as breakfast cereals and imitation fruit drinks, and label the products "fortified."

Because synthetic vitamins and minerals are very inexpensive, food fortification has become a highly effective, low-cost advertising gimmick. Snack foods and breakfast cereals, which many manufacturers fortify, often contain large amounts of sugar and are basically bad foods.

germs: the general name for viruses, bacteria, molds, protozoa, and other disease-causing microscopic organisms.

glycerolysis: degradation of triglycerides (fats and oils) to di- and monoglycerides.

gram: a unit of weight, approximately 1/28 of an ounce.

GRAS—Generally Recognized As Safe: a category of food additives established by the FDA. The GRAS (pronounced grass) category was created to exempt unquestionably safe chemicals, such as starch, salt, sugar, baking soda, protein, etc., from the costly toxicological tests required by the 1958 food additive law. Inevitably, though, chemicals that were once considered "unquestionably safe" turned out not to be so safe, while others that never did deserve GRAS status were put on the list.

According to the law, chemicals that were used in food prior to January 1, 1958, could be deemed GRAS without scientific testing. Chemicals introduced to the food supply after that date may not be declared GRAS unless scientific tests indicate safety. The catch is that the company that markets the additive can decide what constitutes adequate scientific testing.

GRAS chemicals differ from other food additives in three main respects:

1. GRAS chemicals are *assumed* to be safe because they have been used in food for many years; most other additives are thought to be safe because they have undergone a certain amount of scientific testing.
2. There is no limit on the levels at which most GRAS substances may be added to food; the FDA places limits on most other food additives, both as to concentration and as to the foods in which they may be used.
3. A manufacturer can declare a chemical GRAS and use it in food without consulting the FDA (the FDA can challenge a firm if it disagrees with the firm's judgment); other food additives must be tested—and the tests must be approved by the FDA—*before* they may be used in food.

Most GRAS chemicals have been used in foods for many years and are undoubtedly safe. But being on the GRAS list certainly does not guarantee safety. Cyclamate was on the list in 1969 when it was found to be carcinogenic; brominated vegetable oil (BVO) was on the list in 1970 when it was found to be toxic.

In 1971 the FDA appointed a committee to reexamine the toxicity of all GRAS compounds. After the committee submits its report on a chemical, the FDA then must decide whether to affirm the GRAS status, regulate it more tightly, or ban it altogether. That review process was still proceeding in 1985 for a number of GRAS chemicals.

hemoglobin: the oxygen-carrying protein molecule in red blood cells. The red color of blood reflects the iron content of hemoglobin.

humectant: a chemical that is incorporated into a food (marshmallows, shredded coconut, candies, etc.) to maintain the desired level of moisture. See glycerin, propylene glycol, sorbitol.

hydrolysis: the splitting of a molecule (protein, carbohydrate, etc.) by reaction with water.

in vitro experiments: experiments performed with components of living organisms (tissue slices, cultured cells, cell sap, stomach juices, etc.).

in vivo experiments: experiments done on intact, living animals.

laxative: a substance that helps move the bowels. Mineral oil and similar substances lubricate the large intestine, thereby expediting movement of stools. Karaya and carboxymethylcellulose are bulk-type laxatives. They are not absorbed in the intestine and become part of the feces. These chemicals absorb a large amount of water, expand in size, and stimulate the intestine to move the stools.

LD_{50}—Lethal Dose 50 percent: the amount of a chemical that kills 50 percent of a group of animals. The lower the LD_{50}, the more poisonous the chemical. LD_{50} is a commonly used index of a chemical's toxicity, but it says nothing about carcinogenicity, mutagenicity, cumulative effects, etc., so is often not meaningful in the context of food additives. The LD_{50} for a given chemical may vary considerably from species to species. When discussing LD_{50}s the route of administration of the chemical must be indicated (oral, subcutaneous, etc.). LD_{50}s are usually expressed in units of mg/kg (i.e., milligrams of the chemical per kilogram of the test animal's body weight).

maturing agent: see aging agent.

metabolism: the degradation, synthesis, and interconversion of molecules by living organisms.

mg/kg: dosages of a chemical used in an experiment are usually expressed in units of milligrams (mg) of the chemical per kilogram (kg) of body weight of a laboratory animal or person. One milligram is approximately 1/28,000 of an ounce; one kilogram is 2.2 pounds.

minerals: the body needs inorganic mineral nutrients such as iron, zinc, cobalt, calcium, and copper. Metal atoms in living organisms are often combined with proteins and other molecules: hemoglobin contains iron, insulin contains zinc, vitamin B_{12} contains cobalt. Calcium is a major component of teeth and bones.

mutation: an inheritable change in an organism's genetic material. The effects of mutations range from undetectably small changes in a cell, to hemophilia, to death. Mutations may be caused by radiation (X rays, cosmic rays, fallout) or certain chemicals. Agents that cause mutations are called mutagens.

myoglobin: hemoglobin-like molecules that store oxygen in muscle tissue.

nucleic acid: the molecules that contain, in chemically encoded form, the genetic information of all organisms. DNA (deoxyribonucleic acid) and RNA (ribonucleic acid) are the two kinds of nucleic acids.

pasteurization: the heat treatment of foods to kill contaminating microorganisms.

ppm: parts per million. A convenient unit used to denote how much of a chemical is present in a food or another chemical. Thus, a food may contain 200 parts (grams, ounces, pounds) of a preservative per million parts (grams, ounces, pounds) of food. Some chemicals are harmful even at levels as low as several parts per billion (ppb) in the diet.

precipitate: when a chemical comes out of solution due to chemical or physical forces, it is said to precipitate. The curdling of milk (precipitation of casein) that occurs when it is treated with acid (mix milk with vinegar or grapefruit juice) is a familiar example of precipitation.

preservative: a chemical used to increase the safety or storage life of a food. Antimicrobial preservatives inhibit the growth of microorganisms (see calcium propionate, parabens, sodium benzoate, sodium nitrate and nitrite, sulfiting agents). Antioxidant preservatives prevent rancidity and discoloration (see butylated hydroxyanisole, butylated hydroxytoluene, citric acid, EDTA, propyl gallate, stannous chloride, TBHQ).

protein: muscle, hair, nail, cartilage, and most other parts of living organisms contain protein molecules. Enzymes are proteins. Protein molecules are composed of amino acids linked end to end in a specific order.

rancidity: the offensive odor that develops as food spoils; it is caused primarily by oxygen reacting with unsaturated fats and oils. See antioxidant.

rope: a condition in bread characterized by gelatinous threads that form in the center of a loaf. Rope is caused by certain spore-forming bacteria *(Bacillus mesentericus, B. subtilis)* that may contaminate dough and survive the baking process. As the bacteria multiply they digest the bread.

sequestrant: see chelator.

stabilizer: see thickening agent.

subcutaneous: under the skin.

syndrome: the outward signs or symptoms of a disease; e.g., sneezing for hay fever; self-mutilation for Lesch-Nyhan disease; high fever, skin eruption, nasal catarrh for measles.

teratogen: a chemical that can cause birth defects (terata). *Teratos* is the Greek word for monster.

thickening agent (stabilizer)—see table following: manufacturers use thickening agents to improve the texture and consistency of ice cream, pudding, soft drinks, salad dressing, yogurt, soup, baby food and formula, and other foods. These chemicals control the formation of ice crystals in ice cream and other frozen foods. The thickness they create in salad dressing prevents the oil and vinegar from separating out into two layers. These additives are used to stabilize factory-made foods, that is, to keep the complex mixture of oils, acids, colors, salts and nutrients dissolved and at the proper consistency and texture.

Most thickening agents are natural carbohydrates (agar, carrageenan, pectin, starch, etc.) or chemically modified carbohydrates (cellulose gum, modified starch, etc.). They work by absorbing part of the water that is present in a food, thereby making the food thicker. The following table lists the source and composition of the major thickening agents.

toxic: poisonous. Mutations, cancer, blindness, liver damage, etc., are typical toxic effects that can be caused by chemicals.

toxicity tests: (a) acute toxicity tests reveal the effects of mammoth single doses of a chemical;

Thickening Agents

Substance	Source	Composition (major species of carbohydrate subunits)
agar	seaweed	D- and L-galactose (contains sulfate esters)
alginate	seaweed	D-mannuronic acid; L-guluronic acid
arabic (acacia) gum	tree exudate	L-arabinose; L-rhamnose; D-galactose; D-glucuronic acid
arabinogalactan (larch gum)	tree exudate	D-galactose; L-arabinose
carrageenan	seaweed	D-galactose; 3, 6-anhydro-D-galactose (contains sulfate esters)
cellulose, microcrystalline	plants	D-glucose
cellulose derivatives:	cellulose	D-glucose containing one or more different side chains
carboxymethylcellulose		
ethyl cellulose		
hydroxypropyl cellulose		
hydroxypropyl methyl cellulose		
methyl cellulose		
methyl ethyl cellulose		
furcelleran	seaweed	D-galactose; 3, 6-anhydro-D-galactose (contains sulfate esters)
ghatti gum	tree exudate	L-arabinose; D-xylose, galactose, mannose, glucuronic acid
guar gum	plant seed	D-mannose; D-galactose
karaya (sterculia) gum	tree exudate	D-galactose; L-rhamnose; D-galacturonic acid
locust bean (carob seed) gum	plant seed	D-mannose; D-galactose
pectin	fruits, berries	D-galacturonic acid (contains methyl esters)
propylene glycol alginate	seaweed derivative	D-mannuronic acid; L-guluronic acid; propylene glycol residues
starch	corn, potato, etc.	D-glucose
starch, modified	starch derivatives	oxidized, hydrolyzed, bleached, cross-linked, or derivatized starch molecules
tragacanth gum	tree exudate	D-galactose; D-xylose; D-glucuronic acid
xanthan gum	bacteria	D-glucose; D-mannose; D-glucuronic acid

(b) short-term toxicity tests reveal the effects of 30–180-day exposure to a substance, with special attention usually given to liver and kidney function and blood composition;

(c) long-term toxicity tests last the lifetime of an animal (two years in rats or mice and seven years in dogs). These experiments reveal whether a chemical causes cancer or chronic effects.

(d) other special tests are designed to detect interference with reproduction and causation of birth defects or mutations. The Ames test is a quick, inexpensive bacterial test that measures a chemical's ability to cause mutations. Many chemicals that cause mutations in bacteria cause cancer in animals.

vitamins: chemicals that the body needs but cannot make and therefore must obtain from foods (or vitamin pills). Not all animals require the same set of vitamins. For instance, the only animal species that cannot make vitamin C (ascorbic acid) are primates (including humans), the guinea pig, one bird species, and one species of bat.

Bibliography

REFERENCES

C&EN: "Food Additives," Sanders, H. J., *Chem. Eng. News 44*, October 10 and October 17, 1966.

CRC: Furia, T. E., ed., *Handbook of Food Additives*, Chemical Rubber Company, Cleveland, 1968.

CUFP: National Academy of Sciences–National Research Council, "Chemicals Used in Food Processing," Pub. No. 1274 (1965).

ECT: *Encyclopedia of Chemical Technology*, Interscience Publishers, New York, 2nd edition, 1963—.

FAO (17): "Procedures for the Testing of Intentional Food Additives to Establish Their Safety for Use," FAO Nutrition Meetings Report Series No. 17, WHO Tech. Rep. Series 144 (1958).

FAO (24): "Evaluation of Certain Food Additives," 24th Report of the Joint FAO/WHO Expert Committee on Food Additives, WHO Tech. Report Series No. 653 (1980).

FAO (26): "Evaluation of Certain Food Additives and Contaminants," 26th Report of the Joint FAO/WHO Expert Committee on Food Additives, WHO Tech. Report Series No. 683 (1982).

FAO (27): "Evaluation of Certain Food Additives and Contaminants," 27th Report of the Joint FAO/WHO Expert Committee on Food Additives, WHO Tech. Report Series 696 (1983).

FAO (29): "Evaluation of the Carcinogenic Hazards of Food Additives," FAO Nutrition Meetings Report Series No. 29, WHO Tech. Rep. Series 220 (1961).

FAO (31): "Evaluation of the Toxicity of a Number of Antimicrobials and Antioxidants," FAO Nutrition Meetings Report Series No. 31, WHO Tech. Rep. 228 (1962).

FAO (35): "Specifications for the Identity and Purity of Food Additives and Their Toxicological Evaluation: Emulsifiers, Stabilizers, Bleaching and Maturing Agents," FAO Nutrition Meetings Report Series No. 35, WHO Tech. Rep. Series 281 (1964).

FAO (38A): "Specifications for Identity and Purity and Toxicological Evaluation of Some Antimicrobials and Antioxidants," FAO Nutrition Meetings Report Series No. 38A (1965).

FAO (38B): "Specifications for Identity and Purity and Toxicological Evaluation of Food Colors," FAO Nutrition Meetings Report Series No. 38B (1966).

FAO (40): "Specifications for the Identity and Purity of Food Additives and Their Toxicological Evaluation: Some Antimicrobials, Antioxidants, Emulsifiers, Stabilizers, Flour-Treatment Agents, Acids and Bases," FAO Nutrition Meetings Report Series No. 40, WHO Tech. Rep. Series 339 (1966).

FAO (40A): "Toxicological Evaluation of Some Antimicrobials, Antioxidants, Emulsifiers, Stabilizers, Flour-Treatment Agents, Acids and Bases," FAO Nutrition Meetings Report Series No. 40 A, B, C (1967).

FAO (43): "Specifications for the Identity and Purity of Food Additives and Their Toxicological Evaluation: Some Emulsifiers and Stabilizers and Certain Other Substances," FAO Nutrition Meetings Report Series No. 43, WHO Tech. Rep. Series 373 (1967).

FAO (44A): "Toxicological Evaluation of Some Flavoring Substances and Non-nutritive Sweetening Agents," FAO Nutrition Meetings Report Series No. 44A (1967).

FAO (46): "Specifications for the Identity and Purity of Food Additives and Their Toxicological Evaluation: Some Food Colors, Emulsifiers, Stabilizers, Anticaking Agents, and Certain Other Substances," FAO Nutrition Meetings Report Series No. 46, WHO Tech. Rep. Series 445 (1970).

FAO (46A): "Toxicological Evaluation of Some Food Colors, Emulsifiers, Stabilizers, Anticaking Agents and Certain Other Substances," FAO Nutrition Meetings Report Series 46A (1970).

FAO (53): "Toxicological Evaluation of Some Food Additives Including Anticaking Agents, Antimicrobials, Antioxidants, Emulsifiers, and Thickening Agents," 17th Report of the Joint Expert Committee on Food Additives (1974).

FAO (54): "Evaluation of Certain Food Additives," FAO Nutrition Meetings Report Series No. 54, WHO Tech. Rep. Series 557 (1974).

FAO (55): "Evaluation of Certain Food Additives," FAO Nutrition Meetings Report Series No. 55, WHO Tech. Rep. Series 576 (1975).

FAO (599): "Evaluation of Certain Food Additives," WHO Tech. Rep. Series 599, FAO Food and Nutrition Series No. 1 (1976).

FAO/WHO (21): "Evaluation of Certain Food Additives," 21st Report of the Joint FAO/WHO Expert Committee on Food Additives, WHO Tech. Rep. Series 617 (1978).

WHO (8): "Toxicological Evaluation of Some Food Colours, Thickening Agents, and Certain Other Substances," 19th Report of the Joint FAO/WHO Expert Committee on Food Additives (1975).

RELATED READINGS

Carson, Rachel, *Silent Spring,* Houghton Mifflin, Boston, 1962.
Epstein, Samuel S., *The Politics of Cancer,* Anchor Books/Doubleday, Garden City, 1979.

Freydberg, Nicholas and Willis A. Gortner, *The Food Additives Handbook*, Bantam Books, New York, 1982.

Furia, T. E., Ed., *Handbook of Food Additives*, 2nd Ed., CRC Press, Cleveland, 1972.

Furia, T. E., Ed., *Handbook of Food Additives* Vol. II, 2nd Ed., CRC Press, Inc., Boca Raton, Fla. 1980.

Hunter, Beatrice Trum, *The Mirage of Safety: Food Additives and Federal Policy*, Stephen Greene Press, Brattleboro, Vt. 1982.

National Academy of Sciences, "Evaluating the Safety of Food Chemicals," Publication No. 1859, Washington, 1970.

Pim, Linda R., *The Invisible Additives: Environmental Contaminants in Our Food*, Doubleday & Co., Toronto, Garden City, 1981.

Publications of the
Center for Science in the Public Interest

1. *Nutri-Bytes:* This easy-to-use software package includes a data base on food additives, quizzes on food additives and nutrition, and guidance on analyzing and improving your own personal diet. Particularly appropriate for high school and college classes. $39.95 (comes with several of CSPI's colorful posters); specify Apple II, Kaypro (CP/M), Osborne (DD-80 col.), IBM-PC, Televideo (CP/M), or CP/M-8".

2. *Nutrition Express:* A computer game for ages 9 and up that guides eating habits in the low-fat, low-sugar, whole-grains direction. Includes a *Nutrition Scoreboard* poster. $39.95. Apple II computers.

3. *Chemical Cuisine:* This 18" × 24" colorful poster, based on the *Complete Eater's Digest* section of this book, is chock full of the latest information on major food additives. The additives are color-coded to tell you at a glance whether an additive is safe, unsafe, or questionable. $3.95 paper; $7.95 laminated.

4. *Nutrition Scoreboard:* This 18" × 24" poster is based on the *Nutrition Scoreboard* section of this book. The nutritional scores remind you which are the best foods and which are the worst. Posting a copy on your kitchen wall will help keep the junk out of your refrigerator . . . and stomach. $3.95 paper; $7.95 laminated.

5. *Food Scorecard:* If the *Complete Eater's Digest* is a bit hefty for your junior high school or high school child, get a copy of this handy, abbreviated booklet (5½" × 8½") containing nutritional ratings for most common foods. Perfect for classroom use. $1 per copy.

6. *Creative Food Experiences for Children:* This bestselling guide is for parents and teachers of 3–8-year-old children. The innovative activities are aimed at encouraging children to understand virtues of natural foods. 256 pages. $5.95 paperback; $12.95 hardcover.

Join CSPI! Do yourself and your neighbors a favor by joining the Center for Science in the Public Interest, a nonprofit citizens' group. You will receive information and advice ten times a year from the Center's *Nutrition Action Healthletter,* as well as a 10 percent discount on publications and free copies of the *Chemical Cuisine* and *Nutrition Scoreboard* posters. CSPI is one of the leading nutrition advocacy groups in the country.

Membership in CSPI and all of the publications listed here may be obtained from CSPI, 1501 16th St. NW, Washington, D.C. 20036. Please write for a complete list of products and more information about the Center.

Index

Abbott Laboratories, 352, 354
Abortions: quinine and, 313
Acesulfame-K, 210–11
Acetazolamide, 193
Acetic acid, 211
Acetone peroxide, 211–12
Additives. *See* Food additives
Adipic acid, 212
Advertising, 8–9, 137, 315
   budgets of major food companies for, 167
   of cereals, 146, 147
   food additive safety campaigns and, 183
   FTC policy on, 19–21
   of imitation meat, 180
Aflatoxin, 184
Agar, 212–13
Aging agents: chemical
   acetone peroxide, 211–12
   azodicarbonamide, 246–47
   chlorine, 268–69
Aging process: slowing of, 214
Agriculture, U.S. Department of (USDA), 12–13, 37, 78, 116, 125, 132, 145, 279, 293, 320, 357
   bureaucratic problems of, 199–202
   dietary guidelines committee and, 17–18
   Food Safety and Inspection Service (FSIS) of, 176
   job changes between industry and, 170–71
   nitrite controversy and, 325–27
   organic farming and, 108
   Reagan administration and, 17–18, 108
   surveys conducted by, 4–5, 98, 100, 303
Ajinomoto, 243
Alcohol, 109–11
   calorie content of, 111
   converted to acetic acid, 211
   food additives in, 196–97, 205, 311

Alginates, 213–14
Allergic reactions: BHT and, 253
Allied Chemical, 230–31
Allura Red AC (Red 40), 220, 230–32
Alpha tocopherol (vitamin E), 214
Aluminum compounds, 215–16
Amaranth (Red 2), 356
American Academy of Pediatrics, 157, 242, 278
American Brewer (magazine), 311
American Cancer Society, 19, 41, 61, 91, 96, 102, 123, 315
American Council on Science and Health (ACSH), 16
American Diabetes Association, 315
American diet, average, 11
   cholesterol in, 69–70
   diseases associated with, 5–7, 11
   fat in, 54
   protein in, 34, 35
   sugars in, 42
American Health Foundation, 267, 318
American Heart Association, 59
American Institute of Baking, 211, 269
American Meat Institute, 58, 205–6, 327
American Thyroid Association, 308
Ames, Bruce, 191
Ames test, 191, 195
Aminoacetic acid (glycine), 283
Amino acids
   in aspartame vs. food sources, 241
   cysteine, 273
   glycine, 283
Ammonia, 217
Ammonia-caramel, 263
Ammoniated glycyrrhizin, 216
Ammonium compounds, 216–17
Amylases, 217–18

INDEX

Amylopectin, 332
Amylose, 332
Anderson, James, 40
Anderson, Joseph, 70
Anderson, Richard, 106
Anderson, T. W., 95–96
Anemia, 98, 287
Animal tests, 188–90, 192–98
   artificial colorings and, 231–32
   BHT in, 252–53
   effectiveness of, 195–97
   carrageenan in, 267
   ethyl maltol in, 295
   fraud in, 197–98
   mutation studies, 194–95
   nitrites in, 326
   quinine in, 313
   Red 40 and, 230
   reform of, 207
   relevance to humans of, 193–94
   and reproduction studies, 192–95
   saccharin in, 316, 318
   sulfiting agents in, 339
   tannin in, 341
   See also Feeding studies
Annatto, 234
Anorexia, 102
Anoxomer, 198
Antacids, 215
Antibiotics, 15, 182
Antioxidants, 178, 180, 185
   ascorbic acid, 239–40
   ascorbyl palmitate, 240
   butylated hydroxyanisole (BHA), 250–51
   butylated hydroxytoluene (BHT), 251–54
   citric acid, 271, 334
   EDTA (ethylene diamine tetraacetic acid), 277–78
   gum guaiac, 284
   lecithin, 291–92
   propyl gallate, 309–10
   stannous chloride, 330–31
   synergistic, 271
   TBHQ (tertiary butylhydroquinone), 343
   unnecessary use of, 185
   in vegetable oils, 348
Appetite: serotonin's effect on, 103
Arabinogalactan (larch gum), 218–19
Arsenic, 184
Artificial colorings, 219–34, 356–59
   Blue 1 (Brilliant Blue FCF), 220, 223
   Blue 2 (indigotine), 205, 220, 224–25
   in breads, 119
   cancer and, 185, 221, 224–33, 356, 358–59
   caramel, 263
   in cereals, 145
   certified, 219–20
   Citrus Red 2, 190–91, 220, 225–26
   consumption increases for, 219–20
   FDA views on, 204
   Green 3 (Fast Green FCF), 220, 226–27
   hyperactivity and, 222
   label listing of, 21, 222–23, 232
   natural, 233–34
   Orange B, 227
   Red 2 (amaranth), 356
   Red 3 (Erythrosine), 204, 227
   Red 4 (ponceau SX), 357
   Red 40 (allura Red AC), 220, 230–32
   testing of, 186, 231–32
   unnecessary use of, 185
   uses of, 220
   violations of laws on, 221, 228–29
   Violet 1, 357–59
   Yellow 5 (Sunset Yellow FCF), 220, 233
   Yellow 6 (tartrazine), 220, 232–33
Artificial flavorings, 152, 234–39
   cinnameldehyde, 270–71
   label listing of, 21
   vanillin, 345–46
Artificial sweeteners, 240
   acesulfame-K, 210–11
   aspartame, 199, 240–46, 314, 319
   cyclamate, 352–55
   polydextrose, 304–5
   saccharin, 17, 20, 184, 199–200, 314–19, 353
   xylitol, 350–51
Ascorbic acid. *See* Vitamin C
Ascorbyl palmitate, 240
Aspartame, 199, 240–46, 314, 319
Asthmatics: sulfiting agents and, 336–40
Awake, 135
Azodicarbonamide, 246–47

Baby foods, 111–12, 285, 289
   modified starches in, 333–34
   MSG in, 185, 301
   nitrates in, 184–85
Bacteria
   agar and, 213
   mutations in, 191, 195
Baked goods
   bromated, 307
   lecithin, 291–92
   sodium content of, 120
   sweet
      fat content of, 68–69
      sodium content of, 86
   See also Breads
Balazs, Tibor, 197
Beans, 66, 116–18

Beech-Nut, 334
Beef, 20, 123–24
Beef Industry Council, 20
Beer: food additives in, 196–97, 205, 311
Behavior
  butylated hydroxytoluene (BHT) and, 253
  sugar and, 44–45
Benarde, Melvin, 354
Bennett, William, 102
Benzoyl peroxide, 247–48
Benzyl acetate, 238
Bergland, Bob, 12
Beta-carotene, 89, 90, 248
  as coloring, 234, 248
Better Business Bureau, 20
Beverages
  fat content of, 62
  juices, 132, 142–43
  nondairy, 132–36
  quinine in, 313
  sodium content of, 78–79
  sugar content of, 46–47
  See also Alcohol; Coffee; Milk; Soft drinks
BHA (butylated hydroxyanisole), 180, 185, 197, 249–51, 343
BHT (butylated hydroxytoluene), 185, 197, 205, 251–54, 343
Bile acids: high-fat diets and, 40
Bio-Dynamics, Inc., 224
Birkel, Thomas, 306
Birth defects, 133, 188, 191–94, 275
  artificial coloring and, 356
  BHT and, 252
  caffeine and, 192–93, 258–60
  food additives and, 188, 191–94
  social costs of, 192
  vitamin A and, 90
Bisulfite, 338
Biurea, 247
Blackburn, Henry, 76
Blacks
  high blood pressure in, 75
  lactose intolerance of, 290
Bladder cancer, 133, 317–18
  cyclamate and, 352–55
Block, John R., 17
Blood pressure
  calcium and, 100
  See also Hypertension
Blue 1 (Brilliant Blue FCF), 220, 223
Blue 2 (indigotine), 205, 220, 224–25
Bob Evans Farms, 20
Botulism, 157, 325
Boys' Life (magazine), 134
Brain damage
  aluminum and, 215

aspartame and, 242–43
MSG and, 300
Bran, 39
Breads, 118–22
  amylases in, 217
  artificial coloring in, 119
  ascorbic acid in, 239–40
  fat content of, 65
  food additives in, 119, 177–78, 261–63, 269
  Fresh Horizons, 264
  sodium in, 74, 79
  spreads for, 121
Breakfast: variety of foods for, 148
Breakfast cereals. *See* Cereals
Breast cancer, 5, 359
Breast disease: fibrocystic, 133
Breast feeding, 111–12
Bribes, deferred, 201
Brilliant Blue FCF (Blue 1), 220, 223
Brin, Myron, 289
British Medical Association, 342
Brominated vegetable oil (BVO), 248–49
Brooks, Philip, 260
Bulgur, 120–21
Bulimia, 102
Bureau of Alcohol, Tobacco and Firearms (BATF), 340
Burkitt, Denis P., 39, 40
Butylated hydroxyanisole (BHA), 180, 185, 197, 249–51, 343
Butylated hydroxytoluene (BHT), 185, 197, 205, 251–54, 343
Butz, Earl, 326
BVO (brominated vegetable oil), 248–49

Caffeine, 16, 254–61
  birth defects and, 192–93, 258–60
  in chocolate, 154
  in coffee, 132–34, 254–60
  content of beverages and foods, 257
  health problems linked to, 132–34, 256–60
  in soft drinks, 135, 205, 255–57
Caffeinism, 256–57
Cagan, Elizabeth, 11
Cakes
  food additives in, 261–63
  sodium content of, 86–87
  sugar content of, 47–48
Calcium, 99–101
  absorption of, 138
  osteoporosis and, 35, 99–100
  score in Nutrition Scoreboard, 166
  strontium compared to, 214
  supplements, 28
Calcium bromate, 307
Calcium compounds, 261

INDEX

Calcium disodium EDTA, 277–78
Calcium fumarate, 280–81
Calcium lactate (lactic acid), 289
Calcium propionate, 261–62
Calcium stearate, 334
Calcium stearoyl lactylates, 262–63
Califano, Joseph, 12
Calorie Control Council, 17, 315, 316
Calories, 101–3
  in alcoholic beverages, 111
  in soft drinks, 134–35
  in vegetables, 137
Cameron, Ewan, 96
Campbell Soup Company, 20
Canada, 355
  aspartame in, 245
  brominated vegetable oil in, 249
  Violet 1 study in, 358
Cancer, 188, 190–91, 195–96, 275
  acesulfame-K and, 210
  artificial coloring and, 185, 221, 224–33, 356, 358–59
  artificial flavorings and, 237, 238
  aspartame and, 243–44
  beta-carotene and, 90–91
  butylated hydroxyanisole and, 250
  butylated hydroxytoluene (BHT) and, 253
  carrageenan and, 267
  cinnamaldehyde and, 270
  coffee drinking and, 133
  cyclamate and, 352–55
  Delaney Clause and, 202–4
  diet and, 19
  fat and, 59–61, 123, 124
  food dyes and, 221–22, 224–33
  nitrite controversy and, 324–27
  obesity and, 102
  potassium sorbate and, 328–29
  propyl gallate and, 176, 309–10
  saccharin and, 184, 314–19
  selenium as protection against, 106
  sodium nitrate and, 184
  tannin and, 341–42
  vitamin C and, 95, 96
  See also specific types of cancer
Candy
  fat content of, 67–68, 154
  health food, 154
  licorice, 216
  sorbitol in, 330
  sugar content of, 48–49, 154
Candy bars
  fat content of, 154
  sodium content of, 87
  sugar content of, 49–50, 154
Canned foods

sodium content of, 74, 79–80, 85–86
sugar in, 143
See also Processed foods
Canthaxanthin, 234
Caramel, 119, 263
Carbohydrates, 36–53
  cellulose, 264–66
  cravings for, 103
  karaya gum, 288
  lactose, 289–90
  pectin, 303
  score in Nutrition Scoreboard, 164
  See also Fiber, dietary; Starch; Sugars
Carbon dioxide (carbonated water), 264
Carboxymethylcellulose (CMC, cellulose gum), 188, 264–66
Carmine, 234
Carnation, 354
Carnauba Wax, 266
Carob, 154
Carob seed gum (locust bean gum; St. John's bread), 292–93
Carrageenan, 266–67
Carroll, Malcolm, 358
Carter, Jimmy (Carter administration), 12, 326
Casein, 268
Castelli, William, 58
Catsup, 156
Cavities. *See* Tooth decay
Cellulose, 264–66
Center for Science in the Public Interest (CSPI), 15, 76, 177, 227, 230, 258, 259, 325, 339, 358
Center for Study of Responsive Law, 325
Centers for Disease Control (CDC), 244–45
Central Soya Company, 286
Cereals, 20, 144–51
  cost of, 148
  fat content of, 65
  fortified, 144, 145, 179
  how to choose, 147–48
  natural, 145–46
  sodium content of, 80–81, 84, 85
  sugar content of, 145–48, 147
  top ten selling cold, 151
Cerebral hemorrhages, 5
Certified Color Manufacturers' Association, 223, 226
Chafee, F. H., 223
Cheeses, 130–31
  food additives in, 215
  sodium content of, 82–83, 131
"Chemical Risk to Future Generations" (Crow), 194
Chemicals

in natural foods
See also Food additives
Cherry flavoring: artificial, 237
Chewing gum base, 268
Chicken, 127–28
   fat in, 66, 124–25
   hot dogs, 124
Chicken McNuggets, 125
Children
   aspartame controversy and, 241–42, 245
   hyperactivity in, 222
   interest in vegetables of, 137–38
   learning disabilities of, 229, 257
   soft drink consumption of, 134, 135
China, 107, 341
Chinese Restaurant Syndrome (CRS), 299–300
Chips
   fat content of, 62–63
   sodium content of, 82
   See also Potato chips
Chlorinated flour oil (CFO), 269
Chlorine (Cl_2), 268
Chlorine dioxide (ClO_2), 269–70
Chocolate
   caffeine in, 154
   lecithin in, 291
Cholesterol
   blood levels of, 69–72
   coffee consumption and, 134
   content of common foods, 72, 125
   dietary services of, 70
   HDL (high-density lipoprotein), 58, 110
   heart disease and, 57–59
   score in Nutrition Scoreboard, 165
Chromium, 106
Chronic (lifetime) feeding study, 189
Cinnamaldehyde, 270–71
Cinnamon, 182, 270–71
Cinnamyl anthranilate, 238
Citric acid, 271–72, 334
Citrus Red 2, 190–91, 220, 225–26
Claiborne, Craig, 78
Clapp, Neal, 253
CMC (carboxymethylcellulose), 188, 264–66
Coal tar dyes, 219
Cobalt sulfate, 197
Coca-Cola, 20
Cochineal extract, 234
Coffee, 254–60
   consumption of, 255
   decaffeinated, 133, 205
   health problems linked to, 132–34, 256–60
   See also Caffeine
Colds, vitamin C in prevention of, 95–96
Collins, Thomas F. X., 258

Colon cancer, 5, 267
   fiber and, 40–41
Colorings. *See* Artificial colorings
Colostrum, 112
Common Cause, 245
Commoner, Barry, 107–8
Community Nutrition Institute (CNI), 245
Compost, 107
Condiments, 156–59
   fat content of, 62
   sodium content of, 81
   sugar content of, 50
Congestive heart failure, 196–97, 216
Connors, C. Keith, 44, 245
Constipation: fiber and, 39, 40
Convenience foods. *See* Canned foods; Prepared dishes
Cookbooks
   for grain recipes, 121
   for low-fat eating, 60
   vegetarian, 127, 137
Cookies
   fat content of, 69
   sodium content of, 86
   sugar content of, 50
Cookware, aluminum, 215, 216
Corn-rich diets, 93
Corn syrup, 272
Coronary heart disease, 5
Cortes, Hernando, 345
Cost of food, 6
   cereals, 148
   food additives' effects on, 177–81, 318
   organic foods, 108–9
   saccharin, 318
Costs of disease, 6
   birth defects, 192
Cottage cheese, 130
Council on Agricultural Science and Technology (CAST), 15
Court of Appeals, U.S., 203
Crackers
   fat content of, 62–63
   sodium content of, 82
Cream cheese, 130–31
Cream of tartar, 342
Crosby, William, 287–88
Crow, James F., 194
Cyclamate, 352–55
Cycloheximide, 258
Cyclohexylamine, 355
Cysteine, 273

Dacre, Jack, 358
Dairy products, 128–32
   fat in, 54, 63, 129

INDEX

lactose intolerance and, 129, 130, 290
promotion of, 10
sodium in, 74, 82, 129
sugar content of, 50–51, 53, 130
Darby, William, 16
Davidson, Daniel, 224–25
Davis, Kent, 357
Deferred bribes, 201
Delaney Clause, 190, 202–4, 270, 318–19
artificial colorings and, 221–22
Delaney, James J., 190
Del Monte, 20
DEPC (diethyl pyrocarbonate), 197, 355–56
Desserts, 151–53
fat content of, 68, 152
sodium content of, 87
sugar content of, 51–52, 151–52
See also Cakes; Cookies
Deutsch, Ronald, 9
Dextrin, 217, 273, 331
Dextrose, 273–74
Diabetes, 5, 96, 102
fiber and, 40, 118
sorbitol in treatment of, 330
Diabetics, 350
"Dietary Goals for the United States" (Senate report), 12
Diet foods
sucrose polyester in, 336
See also Artificial sweeteners
Diethylpyrocarbonate (DEPC), 197, 355–56
Diet rating chart, 114
Diet-related diseases, 5–7, 11
See also specific diseases
Diet-Rite, 20
Diets
Feingold, 222
high-protein, 100
Pritikin, 11–12
sample
food faddist, 116
nutrition-conscious person, 115
See also American diet, average; Low-fat diet
Diglycerides, 297–99
Diketopiperazine (DKP), 241, 243–44
Dimethylpolysiloxane, 274–75
Dingell, John, 340
Dioctyl sodium sulfosuccinate (DSS), 275
Disodium EDTA, 277–78
Disodium guanylate (GMP), 275–77
Disodium inosinate (IMP), 275–77
Distribution systems: for organically grown food, 108–9
Diverticulitis, 40
Diverticulosis, 40

"Dominant lethal" method, 194–95
Dopamine, 229
Dough conditioners, 246–47, 298
Drugs
aluminum-containing, 215
antibiotics, 15, 182
cyclamate and, 353, 355
EDTA as, 278
quinine, 312–13
vitamins as, 301, 312
Drummon, Sir Jack Cecil, 98
"Dry eye" (xerophthalmia), 89

EDTA (ethylene diamine tetraacetic acid), 277–78
Education: nutrition, 17
Egg industry, 71
Eggs, 59
cholesterol content of, 125
cholesterol-raising effect of, 70–71
fat content of, 63, 125
lecithin in, 291–92
peas compared to, 140
Elkins, Robert, 257
Emulsifiers, 178
lecithin, 291–92
mono- and diglycerides, 298
polyoxyethylene-(40)-stearate, 196
polysorbate, 60, 65, 80, 305–6
sodium aluminum phosphate, 215
sorbitan monostearate, 329
succistearin, 335
xanthan gum, 349–50
Enriched foods. *See* Fortified foods
Enzymes
amylases, 217–18
detoxification, 192, 197, 252–53
lactase, 290
papain, 302
Epstein, Samuel, 224
Ergosterol, 278
Erythorbic acid, 322
Erythrosine (Red 3), 227
Eskimos, 126
Esophageal cancer, 341–42
Estrogen replacement therapy, 100
Ethylene diamine tetraacetic acid (EDTA), 277–78
Ethyl maltol, 294–95
European Economic Community, 284, 288
Exercise: weight control and, 102

Fahlberg, Constantin, 314–15
FAO/WHO Expert Committee on Food Additives, 225, 254, 265, 286, 289, 305–6, 320, 330, 358

Farming: organic vs. chemical, 107–9
Fast foods, 25, 26
  fat content of, 63–64, 124–26
  hamburgers in, 124
  salad bars in, 140–41
  sodium content of, 83
Fast Green FCF (Green 3), 220, 226–27
Fat(s), 53–69
  cancer and, 40–41, 59–61, 123, 124
  content of foods, 62–69, 103
    beans, 66, 117
    beverages, 62
    breads and pancakes, 65
    cereals, 65
    condiments and sauces, 62
    crackers and chips, 62–63
    dairy products, 63
    eggs, 63, 125
    fast foods, 63–64, 124–26
    fats and oils, 64, 347–48
    fish, 64, 126–27
    fruits and vegetables, 65
    grain foods, 65, 119
    meats and poultry, 66, 123–27
    nuts, 66, 117
    prepared dishes, 66–67
    seeds, 117
    soups, 67
    sweet baked goods, 68–69
    sweets and desserts, 67–68
    sweet toppings, 68
    yogurt, 63
  determining your intake of, 61
  fat content of, 64
  heart disease and, 55–59, 123, 124, 347–48
  monounsaturated, 56, 347
  polyunsaturated, 56, 347–48
  in protein-rich foods, 35
  reducing intake of, 55–56
  saturated, 56–57, 117, 123, 347–48
  score in Nutrition Scoreboard, 164–65
  sorbic acid compared to, 328
  See also Low-fat diet
Fatty acids, 347–48
  health benefits of, 126–27
FDA Papers, 220
Federal food programs, 4
Federal Trade Commission (FTC), 255
  food advertising and, 19–21
Federation of American Societies for Experimental Biology (FASEB), 207, 350
Feeding studies
  acetone peroxide in, 211–12
  adipic acid in, 212
  agar in, 213
  alginates in, 213
  azodicarbonamide or biurea in, 247
  benzoate in, 321–22
  benzoyl peroxide in, 247–48
  chlorine dioxide (ClO_2), 269
  chronic (lifetime), 189
  mannitol in, 296
  mono- and diglycerides, 298
  MSG in, 300
  propyl gallate in, 309–10
  Red 2 in, 356
  silica in, 320
  sorbic acid in, 328
  sorbitan monostearate in, 329
  stearyl citrate in, 334
  tin in, 331
  vanillin and ethyl vanillin in, 346
  Violet 1 in, 358
  weaknesses of, 195–96
  xanghan gum in, 350
Feighan, Edward, 229
Feingold, Ben, 222
Feingold Association, 222
Feingold diet, 222
Feinleib, Manning, 134
Ferric and ferrous compounds, 279
Ferrous gluconate, 279
Fertilizers: natural vs. chemical, 107
Fiber: dietary, 36–41, 117
  colon cancer and, 40–41
  constipation and, 39, 40
  content of common foods, 38–39
  diabetics and, 40, 118
  insoluble vs. soluble, 120
  types of, 39
  in weight control, 103
Fibrocystic breast disease, 133, 260
"Filet o' Fish" sandwich, 126
Finland, 59
Finnfoods, 350, 351
Fish, 126–28
  contaminants in, 127
  fat content of, 64, 126–27
  sodium content of, 83, 126
Fitzhugh, O. Garth, 342, 358
Flamm, W. Gary, 350–51
Flavor enhancers, 179–80, 275–77
  hydrolyzed vegetable protein (HVP), 285
  monosodium glutamate (MSG), 299–301
Flavor Extract Manufacturers' Association, 270
Fleiss, Paul M., 267
"Floppy baby syndrome," 157
Florida Department of Agriculture, 225
Flour
  aging of, 211, 246–47, 268–69

INDEX 383

bleaching of, 247–48, 269
bromated, 307
trace minerals in, 105–6
whole wheat
  fortification vs., 119
  phytic acid in, 120
Fluoride, 43
Flynn, Margaret, 71
Food, Drug and Cosmetic Act, 237
  See also Delaney Clause
Food additives, 104–5
  accidental contaminants as, 181–82
  in alcohol, 196–97, 205
  antioxidants. *See* Antioxidants
  artificial colorings. *See* Artificial colorings
  banned, 352–59
  birth defects and, 188, 191–94, 258–60, 356
  cancer and, 188, 190–91, 195–96, 243–44, 341–42, 356
    acesulfame-K and, 210
    Delaney Clause restrictions and, 202–4
    food dyes, 221–22, 224–33
  emulsifiers. *See* Emulsifiers
  flavor enhancers. *See* Flavor enhancers
  introduction of, 175–77
  leavening agents. *See* Leavening agents
  licensed, 206
  mutations and, 18, 191, 194–95, 339
  natural flavorings as, 181–82
  nutrients as, 178, 179
  polymer binding of, 198
  preservatives. *See* Antioxidants; Preservatives
  preventing absorption of, 198
  "prior sanction," 206
  product development and, 178, 180–81
  profit-making function of, 178–81
  reasons for use of, 177–81
  resistance to banning of, 199–200
  safety of, 176, 177, 182–207. *See also* Animal tests; Feeding studies
    aspartame controversy and, 241–46
    BHT and, 252–54
    fail-safe substitutes and, 198
    food industry view of, 183–84
    generally recognized as safe (GRAS), 186–87, 204–5, 238, 254, 316, 339
    government role and, 199–207
    to individual vs. population at large, 185–86
    labeling inadequacies and, 176
    meaning of, 209
    "Poisons in Your Pantry" view of, 183
    as relative condition, 195–97, 205
  scope of focus on, 181–82

stabilizers. *See* Stabilizers
synergism between chemicals and, 192, 197, 207, 271, 309
temporary vs. permanent approval of, 206, 207
testing of. *See* Animal tests; Feeding studies
thickening agents. *See* Thickeners
unnecessary use of, 184–85, 252
Food and Drug Administration (FDA), 18–19, 119, 135, 194, 198–207, 269, 352–55
  artificial colorings and, 221–22, 224–33, 356–59
  aspartame controversy and, 241–46
  Board of Scientific Counselors of, 224
  butylated hydroxytoluene (BHT) and, 253
  caffeine and, 255–60
  cereal quality issue and, 146
  cyclamate controversy and, 352–55
  Delaney Clause and, 202–4
  food additive testing and, 186–87, 189, 192, 197, 238, 270, 343
  infant botulism and, 157
  job changes between industry and, 168–70
  labeling and, 22–24, 330, 340
  nitrite controversy and, 326
  polysorbates and, 305–6
  reform of, 201–2
  revision of food safety laws and, 202–7
  saccharin controversy and, 316–18
  slowness to act of, 204–5, 254, 339, 352
  sodium issue and, 76–77
  studies misinterpreted by, 205–6
  sucrose polyester and, 336
  sulfiting agents and, 338–40
Food and Nutrition Board, 16–17
Food colorings, 235–36
  See also Artificial colorings
Food faddist: sample diet of, 116
Food industry (food companies)
  advertising by, 8–9
  bans on additives resisted by, 199–200, 357
  defensive strategy of, 14–15
  job changes between government and, 168–71
  testing of food additives by, 197–98
Food processors, 26
Food Research Institute, 327
Food safety laws; revision of, 202–7
Food starch; modified. *See* Starch, modified
Foreman, Carol, 12–13
Fortified foods, 101, 119, 314
  cereals, 144, 145
Framingham study, 57
Frankos, Vasilios, 193–94
Free radicals, 251

Fresh Horizons bread, 264
Frosting, canned, 175
Frozen foods: sodium content of, 84
Fructose, 279–80
Fruits, 142–44
  canned, 143, 151
  fat content of, 65
  as snacks, 153
  sodium content of, 85
  sugar content of, 51, 53, 143
Fumaric acid, 280–81
Furcelleran, 281

Galactosemia, 290
Gallic acid, 309
Gardner, Sherwin, 316
Gelatin, 152, 281–82
Gels
  agar, 212–13
  alginate, 213
  carrageenan, 267
  pectin, 303
General Foods, 135, 183
Generally recognized as safe (GRAS), 186–87, 204–5, 238, 254, 316, 339
General Mills, 145, 147, 179
Germany, Federal Republic of, 211, 249, 355
Gluconic acid, 282
Glucono delta-lactone, 282
Glucose tolerance test (GTT), 45
Glueck, Charles, 336
Glycerin (glycerol), 282
Glycine (aminoacetic acid), 283
Goiter, 308
Gore, Albert, Jr., 77, 340
Gout, 96
Government
  effectiveness of safety role of, 199–207
  food assistance programs of, 4
  job changes between industry and, 168–71
Goyan, Jere, 258–60, 326, 355
Grain foods, 118–22
  enriched or fortified, 101, 119
  fat content of, 65
  recipes for, 120–21
  unleavened vs. leavened, 120
  whole, 119–21
  See also Cereals; Flour
Grande, Francisco, 70
Gravies: sodium content of, 81
Great Britain, 211, 249, 269, 342
Greden, John G., 256
Green 3 (Fast Green FCF), 220, 226–27
Greens: nutritional rating of, 138
Grice, H. C., 249
Grocery Manufacturers of America, 316

Gross, Adrian, 230–31, 243
Gross, Mortimer D., 44
Guar gum, 283
Gum arabic (acacia gum, gum senegal), 283–84
Gum ghatti, 284
Gum guaiac, 284
Gurin, Joel, 102

Haber, G. B., 143
Hambridge, K. Michael, 106
Hartman, Philip, 326–27
Harvard School of Public Health, 318
Hatch, Orrin, 205–6
Hatch bill, 205–6
Hausman, Patricia, 140
Hayes, Arthur Hull, 18, 77, 242, 246
Hazleton, Lloyd, 358
Hazleton Laboratories, 230–31
Health and Human Services, Department of (DHHS), 12, 37, 41, 98, 201, 221, 326
  coloring law violated by, 228–29
  dietary guidelines committee and, 18
Healthy People (Surgeon General's report), 13
Heart disease, 26
  cholesterol and, 57–59
  coffee intakes and, 133, 134
  drinking and, 110
  fat intake and, 55–59, 123, 124, 347–48
  vitamin E and, 214
  See also Congestive heart failure
Hegsted, D. Mark, 12, 35, 70
Helium, 285
Hemochromatosis, 287
Hemoglobin: nitrite's effects on, 323–24
Hennekens, Charles, 106, 110
Heptyl paraben, 205
Herbs, 181–82, 233–34
Heroin: "cutting" of, 296
Hershey Foods Corporation, 291
Hesperidin, 285
High blood pressure. *See* Hypertension
High-density lipoprotein (HDL), 58, 110
High fructose corn syrup (HFCS), 272, 280
High protein diet: calcium excretion and, 100
Hillshire Farms, 20
Holland, 341
Ho Man Kwok, 299
Honey, 42, 156
Hopkins, Leon, 105
Hormones: as food additives, 182
Horowitz, Herschel, 147
Hot dogs
  food additives in, 199–200

INDEX

protein vs. fat in, 123–24
House Committee on Energy and Commerce, 340
House Committee on Government Operations, 228
House Judiciary Committee, 354
Hunger, 3
  war against, 4
Hydrogenation, 347–48
Hydrolyzed vegetable protein (HVP), 285
Hydroxylated lecithin, 286
Hyperactivity: food dyes and, 222
Hypertension (high blood pressure), 5, 18, 102
  sodium and, 75, 123
Hypoglycemia, 45–46

Ice cream, 131
Ideda, Kikunae, 299
Indigotine (Blue 2), 205, 220, 224–25
Industrial Bio-Test Laboratories, 197–98
Infant botulism, 157
Infants
  methemoglobinemia in, 324
  premature, carrageenan and, 267
Insecticides, 107, 182
Integrated pest management (IPM), 108
International Agency for Cancer Research, 190, 225
International Life Sciences Institute (ILSI), 16
Inter-Society Commission on Heart Disease Resources, 59
Invert sugar, 286
Iodine, 308–9
  excess vs. deficiency of, 229
Iron, 98–99, 105, 286–88
  bioavailability of, 287
  score in Nutrition Scoreboard, 166
Iron compounds, 286–88
Isolated soy protein, 343–44
Isopropyl citrate, 271–72
Ito, Nobuyuki, 250

Jack La Lanne's Honey-Coconut Bar, 154
Japanese, 212
  artificial protein of, 180
  butylated hydroxyanisole and, 250
  colon cancer among, 41
  hypertension among, 75
  MSG and, 299
  stomach cancer of, 326
  Violet 1 study of, 359
Japanese National Institute of Hygienic Sciences, 307
Jelly beans, 154

Jenkins, Nancy, 180
Joan's Natural Honey Bran Carob Bar, 154
Job changes between government and industry, 168–71
Joull, John, 227
Journal of the American Medical Association, 330
Juices, 132, 142–43
Justice Department, U.S., 242

Kaiser Permanente Medical Center, 110
Kamin, Henry, 18
Karaya gum, 188, 288
Kellogg Company, 147
Kennedy, Donald, 317
Kennedy, Edward, 206
Kentucky Fried Chicken, 125
Kenya, 341
Keys, Ancel, 70
Kidney problems: aluminum compounds and, 215
King, L. A., Food Products Company, 220
Kirchoff (Russian chemist), 273
Klatsky, Arthur, 110
Knight, Carolyn, 338–39
Koch, Robert, 212–13
Kodama, Sintaro, 276
Kolbye, Albert, 16
Kool-Aid, 135
Kummerow, Fred, 71
Kung people, 7
Kurokawa, Y., 307

Labeling, 21–27
  ingredient, 21–23
    artificial colors, 185, 222–23, 232
    cereals, 146–48
    food additives, 175, 176, 330, 340
    nitrites, 327
    sodium content, 18–19, 77
    spices and flavorings, 237
  nutrition, 23–27
Laboratory experiments: real life conditions vs., 196–97
Lactic acid (calcium lactate), 289
Lactose, 289–90
  intolerance of, 129, 130, 290
Lakes, 220n
Laos, 354
Lappé, Frances Moore, 35
Lawhon, Gideon, 336–37
Laxatives, 6, 295–96
  sorbitol, 330
  tartaric acid, 342
Learning disabilities in children, 229, 257
Leavening agents

ammonium compounds, 217
  sodium aluminum phosphate, 215
Lecithin, 291–92, 298
Left-handed sugar, 198
Legator, Marvin, 354
Lertzman, Murray, 337
Lettuce: romaine vs. iceberg, 138
Levy, Robert I., 18, 134
Licorice, 216
Liebman, Bonnie, 46, 73, 77, 124, 125, 154
Life expectancy, 26
  alcohol and, 110
Light: vitamins destroyed by, 89–90, 92
Liver (body organ)
  cancer of, artificial flavorings and, 237, 238
  detoxification enzymes in, 192, 197, 252–53
Liver (meat)
  cholesterol in, 125
  contaminants in, 125–26
  food additives in, 188
  riboflavin in, 92
  Vitamin A in, 89, 90
Livestock: organically raised, 108
Lockey, Stephen, 232
Locust bean gum (carob seed gum; St. John's bread), 292–93
Low-density lipoprotein (LDL), 58
Low-fat diet, 55–61
  amount of fat in, 61
  cookbooks for, 60
  government recommendations on, 59
Lung cancer: beta-carotene and, 90–91
Lymph glands, tumors in, 231
Lyng, Richard, 17

McCarron, David, 100
McDonald's, 22, 126, 140
McGovern, George, 14
MacMahon, Brian, 133
McMillan, C. W., 17
McPike, Medaya, 337, 340
Magnesium compounds, 293
Magnesium fumarate, 280–81
Magnesium gluconate, 282
Malaria, 312–13
Malic acid (apple acid), 294
Malkinson, Alvin, 252–53
Malnutrition
  types of, 3–4
  See also Nutrient deficiencies
Malt, 217
Maltol, 294–95
Maltose, 217
Manganese, 295
Mannell, W. A., 358
Mannitol, 295–96

Manufacturing Chemists Association, 183
Maraschino cherry industry, 357
March of Dimes Birth Defects Foundation, 191
Margarine, diet, 157
Margen, Sheldon, 222
Massey, Linda, 304
Matthews, C., 302
Maxwell, John C., Jr., 144
Mayonnaise: nutritional rating of, 157
Meats, 122–26
  fat content of, 66, 123–26
  imitation, 180, 343–44
  processed, 123–24, 323–25, 327–29
  sodium content of, 85
Meat tenderizer, 296–97
Megavitamin therapy (orthomolecular medicine), 27
Mellanby, Sir Edward, 269
Menopause, 100
Menstruation, 98
Mental illness
  niacin deficiency and, 93, 301
  vitamin therapy and, 312
Mental retardation: aspartame and, 241–43
Merrill, Richard, 242
Mertz, Walter, 106
Methanol, 244
Methemoglobin, 323–24
Methylene chloride, 133, 205
Methyl silicone (methyl polysilicone), 274–75
Meyer, Katherine, 224
Microcrystalline cellulose (MC), 265
Middleton, E. J., 249
Milk, 129
  breast, 111
  lactose in, 289–90
  riboflavin in, 92
  skim (or low-fat), 129, 131
    vitamin A in, 89–90
  UHT, 129
  whole
    nutrition rating of, 32, 129
    vitamin A in, 90
Miller, James C., 19–20
Miller, Sanford, 18, 221, 228
Minerals, 88, 98–101
  calcium, 99–101
  as food additives, 178, 179
  in fruit, 143
  iron, 98–99, 105
  in molasses, 157
  phosphorus, 303–4
  potassium, 306
  in refined foods, 119
  trace, 105–7, 308–9

See also specific minerals
Minton, John, 260
Moch, Ronald W., 224
Moertel, Charles, 96
Molasses, blackstrap, 157
Monoglycerides, 297–99
Monosodium glutamate (MSG), 185, 275–76, 299–301
Monsanto, 183
Monte, Woodrow, 244, 339
Morris, Cynthia, 100
Morton, Julia, 341–42
Most cereal, 144
Mother Jones (magazine), 197–98
MSG (monosodium glutamate), 185, 275–76, 299–301
Munro, Ian, 249
Mutations, 188, 194–95
  Ames test of, 191, 195
  caffeine and, 258
  sulfiting agents and, 339

Nader, Ralph, 123, 185, 201
National Academy of Sciences (NAS), 17, 100, 123, 137, 353, 356, 358
  Committee on Diet, Nutrition and Cancer of, 60–61, 91
  Food and Nutrition Board of, 119
National Cancer Institute (NCI), 19, 59–60, 123, 243, 253, 270, 309, 317–18
National Cattlemen's Association, 58
National Coffee Association, 20
National Dairy Council, 10
National Food Institute, Danish, 253
National Heart, Lung, and Blood Institute (NHLBI), 57, 71
National Institute of Dental Research (NIDR), 43
National Institute of Mental Health, 257
National Institutes of Health (NIH), 13, 99–100, 102, 144, 194, 229
National Live Stock and Meat Board, 58
National Meat Association, 58
National Nutrition Policy Study, 6–8, 12
National Pork Producers Council, 58
National Research Council (NRC), 303, 316, 317
  Committee on Diet, Nutrition and Cancer of, 96
  Committee on the Evaluation of Cyclamate for Carcinogenicity of, 355
  Food and Nutrition Board of. *See* Food and Nutrition Board
National Restaurant Association, 339–40
National Science Foundation, 107–8
National Soft Drink Association (NSDA), 9, 134, 205–6
National Toxicology Program (NTP), 228, 238
"Natural" cereals, 145–46
Natural colorings, 219, 233–34
Nelson (FDA biologist), 342
Nelson, Gaylord, 198
Nervous system problems: vitamin B_6 and, 312
Netherlands Antilles, 341
Neurotransmitters
  appetite and, 103
  blood sugar levels and, 45
  dopamine, 229
  serotonin, 45, 103, 244
Newberne, Paul, 326
New York Times, 245
New York University School of Medicine, 315
Niacin (vitamin B_3), 93–94, 301
  score in Nutrition Scoreboard, 165
Nicolich, Mark, 226
Night blindness, 89
Nitrates, 344
Nitrite. *See* Sodium nitrite
Nitrogen, 217
Nitrosamines, 324–27
Nitrous oxide (N_2O), 302
Nixon, Richard (Nixon administration), 354
  GRAS additives evaluated in, 187
Nizel, Abraham, 43
Nondairy beverages, 132–36
  See also Alcohol; Coffee; Milk; Soft drinks
Nondairy coffee creamer: ingredients in, 175
Norway, 59, 232
Novitch, Mark, 228
NutraSweet, 20
Nutrient deficiencies, 4–5
  among Americans (1977–78), 88
  See also specific vitamins and minerals
Nutrients as food additives, 178, 179
"Nutrient versus calorie rating," 103, 166
"Nutrition and Your Health: Dietary Guidelines for Americans" (government pamphlet), 13
Nutrition Education Training program (NET), 13, 17
Nutrition Foundation, 16, 222
Nutrition labeling, 23–27
Nutrition Scoreboard, 30
  beans, nuts, and seeds, 117–18
  calcium in, 101, 166
  carbohydrate score in, 164
  cereals, 149–51
  cholesterol score in, 165
  condiments, 158

dairy foods, 131–32
desserts, 152–53
fat score in, 164–65
formula for, 163–66
fruits, 143–44
grain foods, 119, 120, 122
iron, 99
iron in, 99, 166
meat, poultry, egg, and fish, 127–28
niacin (vitamin B$_3$) in, 94, 165
nondairy beverages, 135–36
nutrient vs. calorie score in, 166
protein score in, 163–64
rating method of, 31–32, 113
riboflavin (vitamin B$_2$) in, 92–93, 165
snacks, 155–56
sodium score in, 165
vegetables, 141–42
Vitamin A in, 91, 92, 165
Vitamin C in, 97, 166
Nuts, 116–18, 153
fat content of, 66

Oak Ridge National Laboratory, 253
Obesity. *See* Overweight
Office of Management and Budget (OMB), 201
Oil of calamus, 182, 237
Oils, 117, 185, 347–48
adipic acid in, 212
artificial, 336
brominated, 248–49
fat content of, 64
label listing of, 21
vitamin E in, 214
Olives: ferrous gluconate and, 279
Olney, John, 242–43, 300, 301
Olsen, Preben, 253
Olson, Robert, 18
Orange B, 227
Oregon State Department of Agriculture, 108
Organic farming, 107–9
Orthomolecular medicine (megavitamin therapy), 27
Osteoporosis, 99–100
protein and, 35
Overnutrition, 3, 5–7, 143
Overweight, 6, 102–3
fiber and, 40
grain foods and, 118–22
health problems of, 102
sugar and, 44
Oxalic acid, 138
Oxystearin, 298

Packaged dishes (prepared dishes)
fat content of, 66–67
sodium content of, 85
Packaging materials: as contaminants, 182, 203
Pancakes: fat content of, 65
Pancreatic cancer, 133, 238
Pantothenic acid, 302
Papain, 297, 302
Parabens, 302–3
Pasta, 118–22
Pauling, Linus, 26, 95–97
PCBs, 111
Peas: nutritional rating of, 140
Pectin, 303
Pellagra, 93, 301
Pepper, black, 182
PepsiCo, 20
Pert, Candace, 135
Pesticides, 107–9, 182
Peterkin, Betty B., 88
Pfizer, Inc., 304
Phenylketonuria (PKU), 241–42
Phosphoric acid, 303–4
Phosphorus, 303–4
Phytic acid, 120
Pies: sugar content of, 52
Polydextrose, 304
Polysorbate (60, 65, and 80), 305–6
Ponceau SX (Red 4), 357
Popcorn, 153–54
Pork, 124
Potassium acid tartrate, 342–43
Potassium bromate, 307
Potassium chloride, 307
Potassium compounds, 306
Potassium fumarate, 280–81
Potassium metabisulfite, 336–40
See also Sulfiting agents
Potassium sorbate, 328–29
Potato Chip Information Bureau, 9
Potato Chips
promotion of, 9
sodium in, 120
Potatoes
consumption of, 137
nutritional rating of, 138
Poultry, 127–28
fat content of, 66, 124–25
Pound cake: nutrition rating of, 33
Powdered foods: dissolving of, 275
Pregnancy
aspartame and, 242, 246
caffeine and, 258–60
quinine and, 313
vitamin and mineral consumption in, 90, 98

INDEX

Premenstrual syndrome (PMS), 27, 28
Prenner, Bruce, 338
Prepared dishes (packaged dishes)
  fat content of, 66–67
  sodium content of, 85
Preservatives, 178
  acetic acid and, 211
  BHA, 197, 249–51
  BHT, 197, 251–54
  calcium propionate, 261–62
  diethylpyrocarbonate (DEPC), 197, 355–56
  hyptyl paraben, 303
  nitrites, 323–28
  potassium sorbate, 328–29
  propyl gallate, 309–10
  pros and cons of, 184
  sodium nitrate, 234
  sodium propionate, 261–62
  sorbic acid, 328–29
  sulfiting agents, 336–37
  See also Antioxidants
Prevette, Jonquil, 259
Prices of food, 6
Pritikin, Nathan, 11–12
Pritikin Diet, 11–12
Processed foods
  iron in, 288
  meats, 123–24, 323–25, 327–29
  sodium in, 73–74, 123, 327
  See also Canned foods; Food additives
Procter & Gamble, 298
Product development: food additives and, 178, 180–81
Product 19, 144
Propylene glycol, 310–11
Propylene glycol alginate, 311
Propyl gallate, 185, 309–10
  cancer and, 176
Proteases; and meat tenderizing, 296–97
Proteins, 34–36
  artificial, 180
  carrageenan and, 266–67
  casein, 268
  isolated soy, 343–44
  score in Nutrition Scoreboard, 163–64
  textured vegetable (TVP), 343–44
  See also Amino acids; Enzymes; High protein diet
Protein Scoreboard, 35–36
Public Citizen Health Research Group (HRG), 201, 221, 224
Puddings: sodium content of, 87
Purines, 258
Purpura, 313
Pyridoxine (vitamin B$_6$), 311–12

Quillaia, 312
Quinine, 312–13

Ralston-Purina, 20
Randal, Judith, 242
Rapoport, Judith, 44, 257
Rating system. *See* Nutrition Scoreboard
Reagan, Ronald (Reagan administration), 4, 24
  Agriculture Department under, 17–18, 108
  food additive testing in, 190, 194, 204
Recipes
  grain, 120–21
  vegetable, 139–40
Red 2 (amaranth), 356
Red 3 (erythrosine), 204, 227
Red 4 (ponceau SX), 357
Red 40 (Allura Red AC), 220, 230–32
Reddy, Bandaru, 40
Reif-Lehrer, Liane, 300
Remsen, Ira, 315
Reproduction studies, 192–95
Restaurants (restaurant industry), 25
  Chinese, 299–300
  sulfiting agents and, 336–40
Retinol. *See* Vitamin A
Riboflavin (vitamin B$_2$), 92–93, 314
  score in Nutrition Scoreboard, 165
Rice, 118–22
Rice and Vegetable Nirvana, 139–40
Richmond, Julius, 12
Rickets, 144
Rimland, Bernard, 312
Ritchie, J. Murdoch, 257
Ritter, R. R., 192–93
Roosevelt, Theodore, 315
Root beer flavoring, 237
Rosenberg, Lynn, 259
Rosenthal, Benjamin, 15
Roy Rogers sandwich, 124

Saccharin, 20, 314–19, 353
  benefits vs. dangers of, 184
  Calorie Control Council's defense of, 17
  resistance to banning of, 199–200
Sacks, Frank, 71
Safrole, 237
St. John's bread, 292–93
Salad bars, 140–41
Salad dressings: sodium content of, 81–82
Salans, Lester, 18
Salt (sodium chloride), 73–87, 124, 320
  amount in foods, 78–87
  FDA policy on, 18–19
  FDA views on, 204–5
  as food additive, 104–5

hypertension and, 75–76, 123, 327
iodized, 229
potassium-containing, 307
in processed foods, 73–74, 123, 327
reducing intake of, 76–78
See also Sodium
Salts
ammonium, 216–17
of tartaric acid, 342
Sapanaro, James, 336
Sassafras, 182, 237
Sauces
fat content of, 62
sodium content of, 81
Scheuplein, Robert, 206
Schmidt, Alexander, 185, 242
Schools: food served in, 10–11, 13
Schroeder, Henry, 215
Schultz, William, 224–25
Schweigert, Bernard, 18
Science (magazine), 15, 354
Scurvy, 94, 95, 138
Searle drug company, 241, 242–44, 246
Seeds, 116–18, 153
Select Committee on GRAS Substances (SCOGS), 254
Selenium, 106–7
supplements, 28
Senility: aluminum and, 215
Serotonin, 45, 103, 244
Setpoint theory, 102
Seventh-Day Adventists, 7–8
Shai Linn, 259
Shekelle, Richard, 91
Shortening
antioxidants in, 185
Shrimp
cholesterol in, 126
Silicates, 319–20
Silicones, 274–75
Simon, Ronald, 338–39
Slater, Grant, 71
Smoke flavoring, 320
Snacks, 153–56
sodium content of, 120
sugar content of, 51–52
Snickers, 154
Sobotka, Thomas, 44
Sodium
amount in foods, 78–87
in baked goods vs. snacks, 120
hypertension and, 75–76
labeling, 77
reducing intake of, 76–78
score in Nutrition Scoreboard, 165
See also Salt

Sodium aluminum phosphate, 215
Sodium benzoate (benzoate of soda, benzoic acid), 321–22
Sodium bisulfite, 204, 336–40
safety of, 197
See also sulfiting agents
Sodium chloride. *See* Salt
Sodium citrate, 271–72
Sodium compounds, 320–21
Sodium erythorbate, 322
as dye, 185
Sodium fumarate, 280–81
Sodium gluconate, 282
Sodium isoascorbate, 322
Sodium metabisulfite, 336–40
Sodium nitrate, 234, 323–28
Sodium nitrite, 123, 124, 234, 323–28
in baby food, 184–85
benefits vs. dangers of, 184
cancer and, 324–27
as dye, 185
resistance to banning of, 199–200
toxicity of, 323–24
Sodium pantothenate, 302
Sodium pectinate, 303
Sodium potassium tartrate, 342–43
Sodium propionate, 261–62
Sodium stearoyl fumarate, 262–63
Sodium stearoyl lactylates, 262–63
Sodium sulfite, 336–40
brominated vegetable oil in, 248–49
caffeine in, 135, 205, 255
diet, 199–200, 314–15, 318–19
noncarbonated, 135
ingredients in, 175
phosphoric acid in, 303–4
promotion of, 9, 135
sodium content of, 78
Sorbic acid, 328–29
Sorbitan monostearate, 329
Sorbitol, 329–30
Soups
fat content of, 67
sodium content of, 85
Soviet Union, 356
Soy protein, 343–44
Soy sauce, 157
Special Committee on GRAS Substances, 332–33
Spices, 181–82
Spinach, 138
Spreads, 121
Sprouts, how to grow, 117
Squash, 138–39
Stabilizers, 180
agar as, 213

alginates as, 213
carrageenan, 266–67
guar gum, 283
locust bean gum, 292–93
Stanford Heart Disease Prevention Program, 125, 130
Stange Co., 227
Stannous chloride, 330–31
Starches, 37, 117, 331
　amylase digestion of, 217–18
　chemical structure of, 332
　modified, 331–34
　　cross-linked, 332–34
　　derivatized, 333–34
Stare, Frederick, 16, 18
Stearic acid, 334
Stearyl citrate, 271–72, 334
Stein, W. H., 321
Stevens, John, 338
Stevenson, Donald, 338
Stomach cancer, 326–27
　vitamin C and, 95, 96
Stools: fiber and, 39–40
Stroke, 26, 75
Strontium 90, 214
Succistearin, 335
Sucrose, 335–36
Sucrose polyester (SPE), 336
Sue Honey Association, 157
Sugar Association, The, 10
Sugars, 37, 104–5
　dextrose, 273–74
　fructose, 279–80
　invert, 286
　natural, 41, 143
　　content of foods, 53
　promotion of, 10, 146
　refined, 41–52, 103
　　behavior and, 44–45
　　in cereals, 145–48
　　condiments, 156–57
　　content of foods, 46–52
　　heart disease and, 44
　　honey, 42, 156–57
　　hypoglycemia and, 45–46
　　obesity and, 44
　　quantity consumed, 42
　　in snacks, 154–55
　　in soft drinks, 134–35
　　tooth decay and, 43, 145, 147, 155
　　trace elements lacking in, 105–6
　sucrose, 335–36
　synthetic, 198
Sulfiting agents, 336–40
Sunset Yellow FCF (Yellow 6), 220, 233

Supermarkets, 26, 118–19
Surimi paste, 180
Sweden, 59, 232, 249
Sweeteners
　corn syrup, 272
　glycyrrhizin as, 216
　mannitol, 295–96
　sorbitol, 329–30
　See also Artificial sweeteners; Sugars
Synergism between chemicals, 192, 197, 207, 271, 309
Synthetic sugar, 198

Tabouli, 120–21
Tang, 135
Tannin (tannic acid), 190–91, 218, 340–42
Tartaric acid, 342–43
Tartrazine (Yellow 5), 220, 232–33
Taste specialists, 237
TBHQ (tertiary butylhydroquinone), 343
Tea, 132–33
　tannin in, 190–91, 340–42
Teeth, 6
　See also Tooth decay
Tepper, Lloyd, 146
Teratogens, 192–94
　See also Birth defects
Textured vegetable protein (TVP), 343–44
Thalidomide, 191, 196
Thiamin (vitamin B_1), 344
Thickeners, 180
　alginates, 213
　guar gum, 283
　karaya gum, 188, 288
　larch gum, 218–19
　starch, 331
Tiger Milk Nutrition, 154
Tin: biological effects of, 330–31
Titanium dioxide, 345
Tooth decay, 43, 145, 147, 330
　snacking and, 155
Total cereal, 145, 179, 288
Toward Healthful Diets (Food and Nutrition Board report), 16–17
Trace minerals, 105–7, 308–9
Tragacanth gum, 345
Trapnell, Susan, 337
Treasury, U.S., 354
Trichloroethylene, 205
Triethyl citrate, 271–72
Turner, James S., 242–43, 245
Type A personality, 110

UHT milk, 129
Ulland, B. M., 253

Universities Associated for Research and Education in Pathology (UAREP), 243
Unnecessary diseases, 5–6
Upton, Arthur, 59–60
Urethan, 355–56

Valone, Jo, 337
Vanderveen, John, 229
Vanik, Charles, 354
Vanilla, 345–46
Vanillin (ethyl vanillin), 345–46
Vegetable oils, 21, 185, 347–48
  See also Oils
Vegetables, 136–42
  consumption of, 137
  cooking of, 137–40
  fat content of, 65
  preserving Vitamin C in, 95
  sodium content of, 80, 84, 85
  sugar content of, 51
Vegetarianism, 127, 130
Verrett, Jacqueline, 354
Vinegar, 211
Violet 1, 357–59
Vitamin A (retinol), 89–92, 248, 348
  score in Nutrition Scoreboard, 165
  storage of, 90
  supplements, 28
  in vegetables, 138, 140
Vitamin B$_1$ (thiamin), 344
Vitamin B$_2$ (riboflavin) 92–93, 165, 314
Vitamin B$_3$ (niacin), 93–94, 165, 301
Vitamin B$_6$ (pyridoxine), 28, 311–12
Vitamin C (ascorbic acid), 94–97, 239–40, 327
  in fruit and fruit juice, 143
  score in Nutrition Scoreboard, 166
  sodium erythorbate compared to, 322
Vitamin D, 144, 278, 349
  calcium absorption and, 99
Vitamin D$_2$, 349
Vitamin E (alpha tocopherol), 214
Vitamins, 88–97
  definition of, 94
  as food additives, 178, 179
  in fruit, 143
  in refined foods, 119
Vitamin supplements, 27–28
  See also Megavitamin therapy
Voorhees, Charles, 249

Waffelos, 148
Warner-Lambert company, 293
Washington *Post,* 242
Washington University, 285
Wax, carnauba, 266
Waxman, Henry, 206
Weight control, 102–3
  See also Diets
Weisburger, J. H., 253
Weiss, Bernard, 222
Weiss, Ted, 228
Wendy's hamburgers, 124
Western Electric company: cancer study of, 90–91
Wheatena, 148
Wheat germ, 121, 145
Wheaties, 145, 179
Whelan, Elizabeth, 16
White House Office of Science and Technology Policy, 190
WIC (women/infants/children) program, 4
Wiley, Harvey, 315
Willett, Walter, 106
Wilson, J. G., 192–93
Winick, Myron, 287
Wolf, Isabel D., 88
World Health Organization, 210, 265, 267, 270, 339
Wurtman, Judith, 103
Wurtman, Richard, 103, 244
Wyden, Ron, 340
Wynder, Ernst, 40

Xanthan gum, 249–50
Xerophthalmia ("dry eye"), 89
Xylitol, 350–51

Yellow 5 (tartrazine), 21, 22, 220, 232–33
Yellow 6 (Sunset Yellow FCF), 220, 233
Yellow prussiate of soda, 351
Yogurt
  as condiment, 157
  fat content of, 63
  lactose intolerance and, 130
  nutritional rating of, 130
Young, Frank, 204, 221–22, 228, 340
Yudkin, John, 44

Zinc deficiency, 106, 120
Zinc gluconate, 282

About the Author

MICHAEL F. JACOBSON was born and raised in Chicago and graduated from the University of Chicago in 1965 with an AB in chemistry. Further studies in biology led him to the University of California at San Diego and finally to MIT, where he received his doctorate in microbiology in 1969. Dr. Jacobson was a research associate of the Salk Institute and served as a consultant to Ralph Nader's Center for the Study of Responsive Law in Washington, D.C. In 1971 he joined with several colleagues in the formation of the Center for Science in the Public Interest (CSPI), of which he is presently executive director.

CSPI seeks to represent the consumer's viewpoint in the development of national health and environmental policies. The Center sponsored National Food Day, which was celebrated in 1975–77; sought an end to junk food ads on children's television shows; promotes accurate food labeling and honest advertising; and in the past decade has been the citizens' group most active in promoting good nutrition. The Center's work has contributed in no small part to improved national nutrition policies. Other ongoing concerns of the Center are alcohol abuse and alcoholism, chemicals that affect human behavior, and the social responsibility of scientists.